Tumor Immunology and
Immunotherapy Resistance

Tumor Immunology and Immunotherapy Resistance

Editors

Subbaya Subramanian
Timothy K. Starr
Xianda Zhao

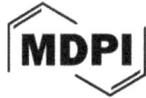

Basel • Beijing • Wuhan • Barcelona • Belgrade • Novi Sad • Cluj • Manchester

Editors

Subbaya Subramanian
University of Minnesota
Minneapolis, MN, USA

Timothy K. Starr
University of Minnesota
Minneapolis, MN, USA

Xianda Zhao
University of Minnesota
Minneapolis, MN, USA

Editorial Office
MDPI
St. Alban-Anlage 66
4052 Basel, Switzerland

This is a reprint of articles from the Special Issue published online in the open access journal *Cancers* (ISSN 2072-6694) (available at: https://www.mdpi.com/journal/cancers/special_issues/ Tumor_Immunology_Immunotherapy_Resistance).

For citation purposes, cite each article independently as indicated on the article page online and as indicated below:

Lastname, A.A.; Lastname, B.B. Article Title. *Journal Name* **Year**, *Volume Number*, Page Range.

ISBN 978-3-0365-8702-8 (Hbk)
ISBN 978-3-0365-8703-5 (PDF)
doi.org/10.3390/books978-3-0365-8703-5

Cover image courtesy of Subbaya Subramanian

© 2023 by the authors. Articles in this book are Open Access and distributed under the Creative Commons Attribution (CC BY) license. The book as a whole is distributed by MDPI under the terms and conditions of the Creative Commons Attribution-NonCommercial-NoDerivs (CC BY-NC-ND) license.

Contents

About the Editors vii

Xianda Zhao, Timothy Starr and Subbaya Subramanian
Advancing Cancer Immunotherapy: From Molecular Mechanisms to Clinical Applications
Reprinted from: *Cancers* 2023, 15, 4197, doi:10.3390/cancers15164197 1

Nikita Choudhary, Robert C. Osorio, Jun Y. Oh and Manish K. Aghi
Metabolic Barriers to Glioblastoma Immunotherapy
Reprinted from: *Cancers* 2023, 15, 1519, doi:10.3390/cancers15051519 5

Giovanni Monteleone, Eleonora Franzè, Claudia Maresca, Marco Colella, Teresa Pacifico and Carmine Stolfi
Targeted Therapy of Interleukin-34 as a Promising Approach to Overcome Cancer Therapy Resistance
Reprinted from: *Cancers* 2023, 15, 971, doi:10.3390/cancers15030971 23

Małgorzata Frak, Anna Grenda, Paweł Krawczyk, Janusz Milanowski and Ewa Kalinka
Interactions between Dietary Micronutrients, Composition of the Microbiome and Efficacy of Immunotherapy in Cancer Patients
Reprinted from: *Cancers* 2022, 14, 5577, doi:10.3390/cancers14225577 35

Xianyuan Wei, Meng Du, Zhiyi Chen and Zhen Yuan
Recent Advances in Bacteria-Based Cancer Treatment
Reprinted from: *Cancers* 2022, 14, 4945, doi:10.3390/cancers14194945 61

Giuseppe Fanciulli, Roberta Modica, Anna La Salvia, Federica Campolo, Tullio Florio, Nevena Mikovic, et al.
Immunotherapy of Neuroendocrine Neoplasms: Any Role for the Chimeric Antigen Receptor T Cells?
Reprinted from: *Cancers* 2022, 14, 3991, doi:10.3390/cancers14163991 91

Walter Hanel, Polina Shindiapina, David A. Bond, Yazeed Sawalha, Narendranath Epperla, Timothy Voorhees, et al.
A Phase 2 Trial of Ibrutinib and Nivolumab in Patients with Relapsed or Refractory Classical Hodgkin's Lymphoma
Reprinted from: *Cancers* 2023, 15, 1437, doi:10.3390/cancers15051437 105

Julius Drachneris, Allan Rasmusson, Mindaugas Morkunas, Mantas Fabijonavicius, Albertas Cekauskas, Feliksas Jankevicius and Arvydas Laurinavicius
CD8+ Cell Density Gradient across the Tumor Epithelium–Stromal Interface of Non-Muscle Invasive Papillary Urothelial Carcinoma Predicts Recurrence-Free Survival after BCG Immunotherapy
Reprinted from: *Cancers* 2023, 15, 1205, doi:10.3390/cancers15041205 119

Jiyong Liang, Dexing Fang, Joy Gumin, Hinda Najem, Moloud Sooreshjani, Renduo Song, et al.
A Case Study of Chimeric Antigen Receptor T Cell Function: Donor Therapeutic Differences in Activity and Modulation with Verteporfin
Reprinted from: *Cancers* 2023, 15, 1085, doi:10.3390/cancers15041085 131

Sascha Troschke-Meurer, Maxi Zumpe, Lena Meißner, Nikolai Siebert, Piotr Grabarczyk, Hannes Forkel, et al.
Chemotherapeutics Used for High-Risk Neuroblastoma Therapy Improve the Efficacy of Anti-GD2 Antibody Dinutuximab Beta in Preclinical Spheroid Models
Reprinted from: *Cancers* **2023**, *15*, 904, doi:10.3390/cancers15030904 . . . . **145**

Xuan Zou, Yu Liu, Xuan Lin, Ruijie Wang, Zhengjie Dai, Yusheng Chen, et al.
Characterization of Estrogen Receptors in Pancreatic Adenocarcinoma with Tertiary Lymphoid Structures
Reprinted from: *Cancers* **2023**, *15*, 828, doi:10.3390/cancers15030828 . . . . **165**

Nikolai Siebert, Justus Leopold, Maxi Zumpe, Sascha Troschke-Meurer, Simon Biskupski, Alexander Zikoridse and Holger N. Lode
The Immunocytokine FAP-IL-2v Enhances Anti-Neuroblastoma Efficacy of the Anti-GD$_2$ Antibody Dinutuximab Beta
Reprinted from: *Cancers* **2022**, *14*, 4842, doi:10.3390/cancers14194842 . . . . **181**

Chenyu Pi, Ping Jing, Bingyu Li, Yan Feng, Lijun Xu, Kun Xie, et al.
Reversing PD-1 Resistance in B16F10 Cells and Recovering Tumour Immunity Using a COX2 Inhibitor
Reprinted from: *Cancers* **2022**, *14*, 4134, doi:10.3390/cancers14174134 . . . . **199**

Thomas J. Gerton, Allen Green, Marco Campisi, Minyue Chen, Iliana Gjeci, Navin Mahadevan, et al.
Development of a Patient-Derived 3D Immuno-Oncology Platform to Potentiate Immunotherapy Responses in Ascites-Derived Circulating Tumor Cells
Reprinted from: *Cancers* **2023**, *15*, 4128, doi:10.3390/cancers15164128 . . . . **215**

About the Editors

Subbaya Subramanian

Dr. Subbaya Subramanian completed his postdoctoral fellowship at Stanford University and joined the faculty at the University of Minnesota in 2007. Dr. Subramanian has established an internationally recognized cancer research program focused on deciphering the molecular mechanisms of immune evasion in cancer. His current research focuses on understanding how cancer cells and the gut microbiome manipulate the anti-tumor immune response in colorectal cancer. Specifically, Dr. Subramanian's research has shed light on how cancer cells and the gut microbiome collaborate to suppress the immune response in patients with colorectal cancer. Dr. Subramanian and his team have revealed a previously unknown mechanism affecting T cell costimulation in colorectal cancer by identifying the immune suppression mediated by cancer-secreted exosomes. These findings have immense clinical relevance, offering new insights into treating advanced-stage colorectal cancer.

Dr. Subramanian's extensive publication record, including over 120 peer-reviewed articles, attests to his high-quality research and impact. He serves as the section Editor-in-Chief of the journal Vaccines and the Associate section Editor-in-Chief of Cancers. Dr. Subramanian is at the forefront of developing clinical-grade engineered exosomes to treat advanced-stage colorectal cancer patients. Moreover, as a leader in his field, Dr. Subramanian is dedicated to training the next generation of scientists and making a difference in people's lives. Beyond his research and teaching, Dr. Subramanian is committed to giving back to his community, a testament to his dedication to scientific advancement and social responsibility.

Timothy K. Starr

Dr. Starr received his Bachelor's degree from Stanford University and his Ph.D. in Molecular, Cellular, Developmental Biology and Genetics at the University of Minnesota. He currently has Professor Emeritus status in the Department of Ob-Gyn and Women's Health at the University of Minnesota. Dr. Starr's initial research took place in the laboratory of Dr. Kristin Hogquist where he did seminal work in the field of immunology that increased our understanding of T cell development in the thymus, with important implications for cell-based and antibody-based cancer treatments. After receiving his doctorate, Dr. Starr transitioned into the field of cancer research and worked as a post-doctoral fellow in Dr. David Largaespada's laboratory, where he developed a novel system using transgenic mice capable of identifying cancer genes. Dr. Starr went on to head his own cancer research program at the University of Minnesota. The Starr lab focused on understanding the genetics of ovarian and colorectal cancer. In collaboration with others, he helped launch several clinical trials based on adoptive cell therapy that harnessed the power of the immune system. Dr. Starr retired in 2023, but continues to mentor graduate students and collaborate on several projects with colleagues at the University of Minnesota as a Professor Emeritus.

Xianda Zhao

Dr. Zhao earned his Bachelor of Medicine degree (equivalent to M.D.) from Wuhan University, China, and obtained his Ph.D. in Microbiology, Immunology, and Cancer Biology from the University of Minnesota, USA. Bridging the realms of medicine and science, he excels as a physician–scientist with a focus on translational research. Dr. Zhao's work encompasses the development of innovative methodologies for establishing clinically relevant colorectal cancer models and unveiling crucial immunoregulatory mechanisms in colorectal cancer. Following his extensive training, including postdoctoral work at the University of Minnesota, he is currently a physician–scientist resident at the Mayo Clinic's Department of Laboratory Medicine and Pathology. Dr. Zhao's current and future clinical and research interests include precise cancer diagnostics, molecular test development, gastrointestinal malignancies, and cancer immunology.

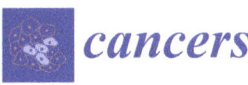

Editorial

Advancing Cancer Immunotherapy: From Molecular Mechanisms to Clinical Applications

Xianda Zhao [1], Timothy Starr [2] and Subbaya Subramanian [1,2,3,*]

[1] Department of Surgery, University of Minnesota Medical School, Minneapolis, MN 55455, USA; zhaox714@umn.edu
[2] Department of Obstetrics, Gynecology and Women's Health, Masonic Cancer Center, University of Minnesota, Minneapolis, MN 55455, USA; star0044@umn.edu
[3] Center for Immunology, University of Minnesota, Minneapolis, MN 55455, USA
* Correspondence: subree@umn.edu

In recent years, cancer immunotherapy research has made remarkable progress, completely transforming the cancer treatment landscape. In 2021, we proudly introduced the Special Issue "Cancer Immunology" in the journal *Cancers*, featuring a collection of 17 highly acclaimed research and review articles [1]. Building upon the success of this prior endeavor, we are excited to present this new Special Issue, which aims to delve deeper into the most recent advancements, state-of-the-art technologies, and prospects in fundamental cancer immunology, pre-clinical assessments, and clinical trials.

Increased understanding of the molecular mechanisms governing the anti-tumor immune response has led to a surge in the utilization of innovative cancer immunotherapies across various cancer types. However, it is important to acknowledge that the response to cancer immunotherapies remains limited to a small subset of patients with solid tumors and specific hematopoietic malignancies, with the underlying reasons for its failure in other patients largely unidentified [2,3]. In this Special Issue, we have collected seven meticulously conducted original studies and five expertly written review articles, highlighting the unmet challenges and needs of cancer immunotherapies.

Over the past decade, the blockade of programmed cell death protein 1 (PD-1), programmed death-ligand 1 (PD-L1), and cytotoxic T-lymphocyte–associated antigen 4 (CTLA-4) has emerged as a cornerstone of cancer immunotherapy. Our initial series of articles focuses on the latest advancements in immune checkpoint inhibitors. Classical Hodgkin lymphomas, particularly in cases of relapse or refractory diseases, pose a significant treatment challenge. In their phase 2 clinical trial, Hanel et al. [4] explored the combination of nivolumab with Bruton's tyrosine kinase inhibitor ibrutinib and observed durable responses, even among patients who had previously progressed on nivolumab therapy. In another study, Pi et al. [5] demonstrated a correlation between COX2 expression and resistance to anti-PD-1 therapy in a B16F10 animal model. Notably, inhibiting COX2 or knocking out the Ptgs2 gene in the B16F10 model reversed its resistance to anti-PD-1 treatment. These noteworthy findings provide valuable insights into potential strategies to overcome immune checkpoint inhibitor resistance.

Chimeric antigen receptor (CAR) T cell therapy represents another vital branch of tumor immunotherapy. Liang et al. [6] made an important discovery, demonstrating that the pharmacological facilitation of CAR-induced autophagy with verteporfin can effectively inhibit the trogocytic expression of tumor antigens on CARs. This breakthrough finding not only enhances CAR persistence and efficacy in mice, but also holds the potential to extend the duration of CAR T cell therapy in patients.

Conventional cancer treatments, such as chemotherapy, radiation therapy, and inhibitors targeting oncogenic pathways, have demonstrated remarkable immunoregulatory effects within tumor tissues [7]. Monoclonal antibodies designed to target oncogenic

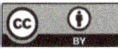

Citation: Zhao, X.; Starr, T.; Subramanian, S. Advancing Cancer Immunotherapy: From Molecular Mechanisms to Clinical Applications. *Cancers* 2023, *15*, 4197. https://doi.org/10.3390/cancers15164197

Received: 17 August 2023
Accepted: 18 August 2023
Published: 21 August 2023

Copyright: © 2023 by the authors. Licensee MDPI, Basel, Switzerland. This article is an open access article distributed under the terms and conditions of the Creative Commons Attribution (CC BY) license (https://creativecommons.org/licenses/by/4.0/).

pathways can activate antibody-dependent cell-mediated cytotoxicity (ADCC), thereby eliminating cancer cells through immunological mechanisms. Troschke-Meurer et al. [8] revealed that combining chemotherapeutics with Dinutuximab beta in the presence of immune cells significantly enhanced their cytotoxic efficacy against neuroblastoma, with the effect specific to the GD2 antigen. Additionally, the same group reported that the immunocytokine, FAP-IL-2v, in combination with the anti-GD2 antibody Dinutuximab beta, substantially increased ADCC against neuroblastoma cells. This synergistic approach involving Dinutuximab beta and FAP-IL-2v resulted in a significant reduction in tumor growth and improved survival in experimental mice [9].

Two insightful studies conducted by Zou et al. [10] and Drachneris et al. [11] have delved into potential biomarkers associated with the response to cancer immunotherapy. In their research, Drachneris et al. [11] examined a cohort of 157 high-risk, non-muscle invasive papillary urothelial carcinoma patients who underwent Bacille Calmette–Guerin immunotherapy following a transurethral resection. They discovered that gradient indicators of $CD8^+$ cell densities at the tumor epithelium-stroma interface, in conjunction with routine clinical and pathology data, significantly enhanced the prediction of recurrence-free survival. On the other hand, in the context of pancreatic adenocarcinoma, Zou et al. [10] established a correlation between estrogen receptor expression and the development of tertiary lymphoid structures, indicating that estrogen receptors may potentially contribute to anti-tumor immune responses.

In addition to the original articles presented, this Special Issue includes a selection of timely review articles that provide comprehensive insights into the latest advancements. Fanciulli et al. [12] conducted a meticulous analysis of pre-clinical and clinical data concerning CAR T cell therapy in neuroendocrine neoplasms, highlighting its promising potential in clinical practice. Choudhary et al. [13] discussed the metabolic alterations observed in glioblastoma tumor cells, which have been investigated as contributing factors to immunosuppression and resistance against immunotherapies. Monteleone et al. [14] reviewed the current body of evidence supporting the role of IL-34 in the differentiation and function of immune suppressive cells. Frak et al. [15] and Wei et al. [16] summarized recent progress in understanding how bacteria can influence the immune response against cancer, and their potential as a novel avenue for cancer immunotherapy. In addition, Gerton et al., showed epigenetic reprogramming and patient-derived 3D platforms could also be used to enhance immunotherapeutic responses in high-grade serous ovarian cancer [17].

In recent years, cancer immunotherapy has made remarkable progress, transforming cancer treatment. The Special Issue "Tumor Immunology and Immunotherapy Resistance" highlighted breakthroughs, technologies, and prospects in cancer immunology. While immune checkpoint inhibitors have been revolutionary, addressing limited responses is crucial. Studies in this Special Issue suggest strategies to overcome resistance, including combination therapies and specific pathway targeting.

Chimeric antigen receptor (CAR) T cell therapy is an important branch of immunotherapy. Facilitating CAR-induced autophagy has shown promise in enhancing CAR T cell therapy's effectiveness. Conventional treatments and monoclonal antibodies can also activate immunological mechanisms, offering synergistic approaches to enhance cytotoxic efficacy against specific cancers. Moreover, identifying biomarkers associated with treatment response is essential for personalized cancer immunotherapy. Studies in this Special Issue discuss potential biomarkers, such as immune cell densities and estrogen receptor expression, enabling more effective interventions. Notably, the review articles cover advancements in CAR T cell therapy, metabolic alterations in tumors, the role of immune suppressive cells, and the influence of bacteria on the immune response against cancer.

As we embark on the next generation of cancer immunotherapy, an increasing body of work has demonstrated that tumor-derived extracellular vesicles are key immune modulators in tumor signaling and the determinants of the antitumor immune response [18]. This Special Issue is an invaluable resource for researchers, clinicians, and industry professionals. The knowledge and discoveries presented within these articles will guide future developments, bringing us closer to realizing more effective and personalized cancer immunotherapies.

Conflicts of Interest: The authors declare no conflict of interest.

References

1. Zhao, X.; Subramanian, S. Cancer Immunology and Immunotherapies: Mechanisms That Affect Antitumor Immune Response and Treatment Resistance. *Cancers* **2021**, *13*, 5655. [CrossRef] [PubMed]
2. Zhao, X.; Subramanian, S. Intrinsic Resistance of Solid Tumors to Immune Checkpoint Blockade Therapy. *Cancer Res.* **2017**, *77*, 817–822. [CrossRef] [PubMed]
3. Zhao, X.; Wangmo, D.; Robertson, M.; Subramanian, S. Acquired Resistance to Immune Checkpoint Blockade Therapies. *Cancers* **2020**, *12*, 1161. [CrossRef] [PubMed]
4. Hanel, W.; Shindiapina, P.; Bond, D.A.; Sawalha, Y.; Epperla, N.; Voorhees, T.; Welkie, R.L.; Huang, Y.; Behbehani, G.K.; Zhang, X.; et al. A Phase 2 Trial of Ibrutinib and Nivolumab in Patients with Relapsed or Refractory Classical Hodgkin's Lymphoma. *Cancers* **2023**, *15*, 1437. [CrossRef] [PubMed]
5. Pi, C.; Jing, P.; Li, B.; Feng, Y.; Xu, L.; Xie, K.; Huang, T.; Xu, X.; Gu, H.; Fang, J. Reversing PD-1 Resistance in B16F10 Cells and Recovering Tumour Immunity Using a COX2 Inhibitor. *Cancers* **2022**, *14*, 4134. [CrossRef] [PubMed]
6. Liang, J.; Fang, D.; Gumin, J.; Najem, H.; Sooreshjani, M.; Song, R.; Sabbagh, A.; Kong, L.Y.; Duffy, J.; Balyasnikova, I.V.; et al. A Case Study of Chimeric Antigen Receptor T Cell Function: Donor Therapeutic Differences in Activity and Modulation with Verteporfin. *Cancers* **2023**, *15*, 1085. [CrossRef] [PubMed]
7. Zhao, X.; Subramanian, S. Oncogenic pathways that affect antitumor immune response and immune checkpoint blockade therapy. *Pharmacol. Ther.* **2018**, *181*, 76–84. [CrossRef] [PubMed]
8. Troschke-Meurer, S.; Zumpe, M.; Meissner, L.; Siebert, N.; Grabarczyk, P.; Forkel, H.; Maletzki, C.; Bekeschus, S.; Lode, H.N. Chemotherapeutics Used for High-Risk Neuroblastoma Therapy Improve the Efficacy of Anti-GD2 Antibody Dinutuximab Beta in Preclinical Spheroid Models. *Cancers* **2023**, *15*, 904. [CrossRef] [PubMed]
9. Siebert, N.; Leopold, J.; Zumpe, M.; Troschke-Meurer, S.; Biskupski, S.; Zikoridse, A.; Lode, H.N. The Immunocytokine FAP-IL-2v Enhances Anti-Neuroblastoma Efficacy of the Anti-GD(2) Antibody Dinutuximab Beta. *Cancers* **2022**, *14*, 4842. [CrossRef] [PubMed]
10. Zou, X.; Liu, Y.; Lin, X.; Wang, R.; Dai, Z.; Chen, Y.; Ma, M.; Tasiheng, Y.; Yan, Y.; Wang, X.; et al. Characterization of Estrogen Receptors in Pancreatic Adenocarcinoma with Tertiary Lymphoid Structures. *Cancers* **2023**, *15*, 828. [CrossRef] [PubMed]
11. Drachneris, J.; Rasmusson, A.; Morkunas, M.; Fabijonavicius, M.; Cekauskas, A.; Jankevicius, F.; Laurinavicius, A. CD8+ Cell Density Gradient across the Tumor Epithelium-Stromal Interface of Non-Muscle Invasive Papillary Urothelial Carcinoma Predicts Recurrence-Free Survival after BCG Immunotherapy. *Cancers* **2023**, *15*, 1205. [CrossRef] [PubMed]
12. Fanciulli, G.; Modica, R.; La Salvia, A.; Campolo, F.; Florio, T.; Mikovic, N.; Plebani, A.; Di Vito, V.; Colao, A.; Faggiano, A.; et al. Immunotherapy of Neuroendocrine Neoplasms: Any Role for the Chimeric Antigen Receptor T Cells? *Cancers* **2022**, *14*, 3991. [CrossRef] [PubMed]
13. Choudhary, N.; Osorio, R.C.; Oh, J.Y.; Aghi, M.K. Metabolic Barriers to Glioblastoma Immunotherapy. *Cancers* **2023**, *15*, 1519. [CrossRef] [PubMed]
14. Monteleone, G.; Franze, E.; Maresca, C.; Colella, M.; Pacifico, T.; Stolfi, C. Targeted Therapy of Interleukin-34 as a Promising Approach to Overcome Cancer Therapy Resistance. *Cancers* **2023**, *15*, 971. [CrossRef] [PubMed]
15. Frak, M.; Grenda, A.; Krawczyk, P.; Milanowski, J.; Kalinka, E. Interactions between Dietary Micronutrients, Composition of the Microbiome and Efficacy of Immunotherapy in Cancer Patients. *Cancers* **2022**, *14*, 5577. [CrossRef]
16. Wei, X.; Du, M.; Chen, Z.; Yuan, Z. Recent Advances in Bacteria-Based Cancer Treatment. *Cancers* **2022**, *14*, 4945. [CrossRef] [PubMed]
17. Gerton, T.J.; Green, A.; Campisi, M.; Chen, M.; Gjeci, I.; Mahadevan, N.; Lee, C.A.; Mishra, R.; Vo, H.V.; Haratani, K.; et al. Development of a Patient-Derived 3D Immuno-Oncology Platform to Potentiate Immunotherapy Responses in Ascites-Derived Circulating Tumor Cells. *Cancers* **2023**, *15*, 4128. [CrossRef]
18. Prakash, A.; Gates, T.; Zhao, X.; Wangmo, D.; Subramanian, S. Tumor-derived extracellular vesicles in the colorectal cancer immune environment and immunotherapy. *Pharmacol. Ther.* **2023**, *241*, 108332. [CrossRef] [PubMed]

Disclaimer/Publisher's Note: The statements, opinions and data contained in all publications are solely those of the individual author(s) and contributor(s) and not of MDPI and/or the editor(s). MDPI and/or the editor(s) disclaim responsibility for any injury to people or property resulting from any ideas, methods, instructions or products referred to in the content.

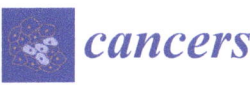

Review

Metabolic Barriers to Glioblastoma Immunotherapy

Nikita Choudhary, Robert C. Osorio, Jun Y. Oh and Manish K. Aghi *

Department of Neurosurgery, University of California San Francisco, San Francisco, CA 94143, USA
* Correspondence: manish.aghi@ucsf.edu

Simple Summary: Glioblastoma (GBM) is an aggressive brain tumor with limited prognosis despite multimodal treatment approaches. Various immunotherapies have been investigated to address the need for novel therapeutic options in GBM with limited success. Recently, alterations in the metabolism of cancer cells which allow for tumor proliferation, but simultaneously alter immune populations leading to an immunosuppressive tumor microenvironment, have been investigated as contributory to therapeutic resistance. This review discusses metabolic alterations in GBM tumor cells which have been investigated as contributory to immunosuppression and resistance to immunotherapies.

Abstract: Glioblastoma (GBM) is the most common primary brain tumor with a poor prognosis with the current standard of care treatment. To address the need for novel therapeutic options in GBM, immunotherapies which target cancer cells through stimulating an anti-tumoral immune response have been investigated in GBM. However, immunotherapies in GBM have not met with anywhere near the level of success they have encountered in other cancers. The immunosuppressive tumor microenvironment in GBM is thought to contribute significantly to resistance to immunotherapy. Metabolic alterations employed by cancer cells to promote their own growth and proliferation have been shown to impact the distribution and function of immune cells in the tumor microenvironment. More recently, the diminished function of anti-tumoral effector immune cells and promotion of immunosuppressive populations resulting from metabolic alterations have been investigated as contributory to therapeutic resistance. The GBM tumor cell metabolism of four nutrients (glucose, glutamine, tryptophan, and lipids) has recently been described as contributory to an immunosuppressive tumor microenvironment and immunotherapy resistance. Understanding metabolic mechanisms of resistance to immunotherapy in GBM can provide insight into future directions targeting the anti-tumor immune response in combination with tumor metabolism.

Keywords: glioblastoma; immunotherapy; metabolism; tumor microenvironment; glycolysis; glutamine metabolism; lipid metabolism; tryptophan metabolism

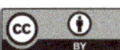

1. Introduction

Glioblastoma (GBM) is the most common primary brain tumor with a limited prognosis and a median survival of 15 months despite an aggressive standard of care treatment consisting of maximal safe surgical resection followed by radiation and chemotherapy with temozolomide [1]. Since the addition of temozolomide to the standard of care treatment in 2005, subsequent efforts to develop new therapeutic candidates have failed to outperform standard of care treatment in clinical trials [2]. Developing effective novel therapies for GBM therefore remains an unmet need.

One novel emerging area of cancer therapeutics is immunotherapies, which target one of the hallmarks of cancer—the ability to evade cellular immunity that would otherwise result in immunological targeting of tumor cells [3]. While in recent years immunotherapies have become standard treatment options for several cancer types, a variety of immune-based therapies including checkpoint inhibitors, vaccines, CAR-T cells, oncolytic viruses, and myeloid-targeted therapies have failed to benefit patients with GBM in trials [4]. The uniquely immunosuppressive tumor microenvironment in GBM is thought to contribute significantly to immunotherapy resistance [4,5].

The tumor microenvironment is affected by unique cancer cell metabolism that not only promotes tumor cell growth but also alters the pH, oxygen, and metabolite contents that affect the survival and function of immune cells in the tumor microenvironment [6]. Metabolic reprogramming within tumor cells diminishes the function of effector immune cells through depletion of essential metabolites and promotes enrichment of suppressive immune populations [7]. More recently, therapies targeting metabolic factors in the tumor microenvironment that adversely impact the antitumor immune response such as low glucose, low pH, hypoxia, and the generation of suppressive metabolites have been explored as immunotherapeutic anticancer strategies [7]. Similar findings have also been reported in GBM, where metabolic reprogramming in tumor cells plays a significant role in driving survival, proliferation, and invasion. However these metabolic adaptations additionally alter the GBM tumor immune microenvironment [8]. In this review, we discuss how GBM tumor cell metabolism of four nutrients (glucose, glutamine, tryptophan, and lipids) leads to an immunosuppressive tumor microenvironment and the implications of these metabolic changes on immune based treatment strategies for GBM.

2. Effects of Increased Tumor Cell Reliance on Glycolysis on the Immune Microenvironment of Glioblastoma

Glycolysis is the most prominent metabolic pathway implicated in cancer metabolism as contributory to sustaining the energetic cost of growth and proliferation. During glycolysis, glucose is catabolized to pyruvate which is then converted to lactate to either be secreted or enter the TCA cycle generating ATP and NADH in the process. Glucose metabolism plays a significant role in the brain microenvironment given the high metabolic demand of the brain and lack of glycogen storage within the brain. High blood glucose levels and increased neuronal expression of glucose transporters have been linked to decreased survival in glioblastoma patients [9].

Altered glucose metabolism in tumor cells results in preferential aerobic glycolysis—increased glycolytic activity despite the presence of oxygen enabling alternate metabolic pathways, a phenomenon known as the Warburg effect. Though glycolysis is an inefficient pathway for energy production relative to mitochondrial oxidation, increased glycolysis in proliferating tumor cells generates metabolic precursors such as lactate which are thought to be the rate-limiting factors during cellular proliferation. In tumor cells, glucose transporters and glycolytic enzymes essential for the conversion of pyruvate to lactate are upregulated. In glioblastoma, the significantly increased rate of glycolysis drives energy production [10]. Tumor cells develop alterations to allow for this increased glycolysis and tumor growth [10]. Genome-wide transcriptomic analysis of patient-derived GBM cells demonstrate strong upregulation of glycolysis-related genes [11]. Hexokinase 2 (HK2), an isoform of the enzyme which catalyzes the conversion of glucose to glucose-6-phosphate in the first step of glycolysis is strongly expressed in GBM [12]. Knockdown or silencing of glycolytic genes such as *HK2, PKFP, ALDOA, PGAM1, ENO1, ENO2*, or *PDK1* inhibits GBM tumor growth and prolongs survival in a mouse xenograft model [11]. These differentially regulated genes were involved in glycolysis and downstream hypoxia response signaling pathways, suggesting that the glycolytic enzymes encoded by these genes are essential for GBM growth [11].

More recently, attention has been given to the impact of alterations in glycolytic pathways on not only proliferating tumor cells but also the tumor microenvironment and resulting changes in immune cell metabolism and function (Figure 1) [13]. Glycolysis alters the immune response in cancer as shown by glycolysis-related genes with prognostic value found to be linked to varying immune cell infiltration and differential immune-related gene expression [14].

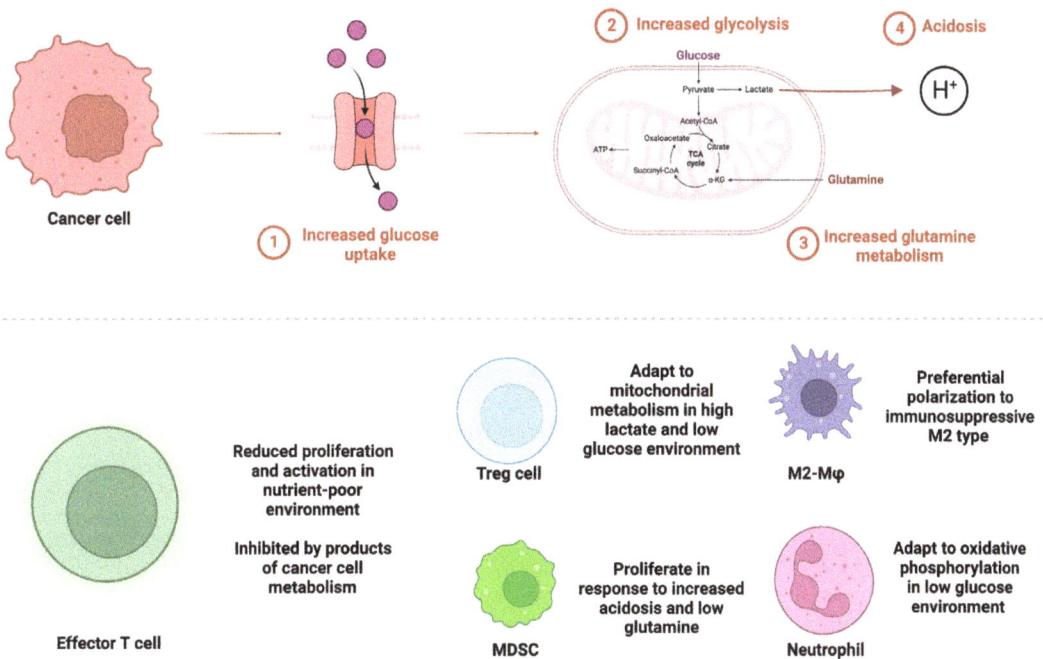

Figure 1. Glucose and glutamine metabolism in cancer cells alters immune cell populations in the glioblastoma tumor microenvironment. (**Top**) Cancer cells up regulate glucose transport into the cell (**1**) and increase glycolytic (**2**) and glutamine metabolism (**3**) leading to low levels of glucose and glutamine in the tumor microenvironment. Increased glycolysis results in acidosis from increased lactic acid production (**4**). (**Bottom**) Immune cell populations respond differentially to metabolic alterations in the tumor microenvironment. Anti-tumoral effector T cells have reduced function and proliferation. Pro-tumoral immunosuppressive populations of Tregs, MDSCs, M2 polarized macrophages, and neutrophils are enriched.

Glycolysis requires export of lactate from cells by transporters which co-transport lactate and protons (H+), leading to their accumulation in the tumor microenvironment and resulting in tumor acidosis which impacts the function of immune cells in the tumor microenvironment. Acidosis has been described in other cancers as contributory to immunosuppression [15]. Lactic acid produced by tumor cells inhibits the differentiation and activation of monocytes and T cells and regulates the expression and secretion of tumor-promoting cytokine interleukin 23 [16,17]. Lactate accumulation additionally inhibits type 1 interferon signaling and granzyme B expression which normally promotes cancer immunosurveillance through the activity of natural killer (NK) cells [18,19]. In melanoma, lactic acid production by tumor cells reduces the quantity and the cytotoxic activity of CD8 T cells and NK cells in culture and in vivo [20]. Activated T cells require the ability to co-transport lactate and protons as part of their own glycolytic metabolism. Increased lactic acid production by tumor cells has been shown to inhibit T cell glycolysis and function by altering the concentration gradient for lactate and proton export by the T cells [21]. In effect, increased glycolysis in tumor cells inhibits the ability of T cells to engage in glycolytic metabolism [20].

Strategies that free T cell glycolytic metabolism from the restrictions imposed on these cells by the tumor microenvironment have been evaluated in preclinical models. For example, genetic modification of tumor specific CD4 and CD8 T cells to overexpress phosphoenolpyruvate carboxykinase 1 (PCK1) increased the production of the glycolytic metabolite phosphoenolpyruvate, resulted in increased T cell glycolysis, increased T cell effector function, and restricted tumor growth and prolonged survival in a melanoma mouse model [22]. Further supporting the idea that increased tumor glycolysis results in a glucose-poor tumor microenvironment that diminishes T cell function, increased glycolytic metabolism in melanoma cells has been associated with resistance to adoptive T cell therapy and checkpoint blockade [23]. Another study in a mouse sarcoma model demonstrated that glucose consumption by tumors leads to metabolic restriction of T cells and reduced T cell glycolytic capacity allowing for tumor progression [24]. In this study, an antigenic model that enhanced glycolysis of T cells led to slower tumor growth [24]. Calcinotto et al. demonstrated that increased acidosis resulted in mouse and human CD8 T cell anergy [25]. Combining proton pump inhibitors lowering pH with adoptive transfer of antigen specific T cells or vaccines to melanoma specific antigens resulted in increased therapeutic efficacy in a mouse model of melanoma [25]. In a separate study of mouse models of multiple cancer types, neutralizing tumor acidity increased T cell infiltration and impaired tumor growth [26]. Furthermore, combining bicarbonate therapy for neutralization of tumor acidosis with checkpoint inhibitors or adoptive T cell transfer improved antitumor responses [26].

Lactic acid production has also been suggested to not only reduce anti-tumoral immune cell populations but also promote immunosuppressive populations. Notably, myeloid cells are resistant to lactic acid-induced apoptosis [20]. In fact, in some studies, these cells have not only been resistant to the effects of lactic acid, but the most aggressive pro-tumoral myeloid cells often thrive in response to lactic acid. For example, accumulation of lactic acid in pancreatic tumor cells was shown to increase the number of myeloid derived suppressor cells (MDSCs) in mice [27]. Colegio et al. showed that lactic acid promotes polarization of macrophages towards the tolerogenic M2 type [28]. Suppressive Treg cells are not impaired by the low lactate levels that impair the function of effector T cells. In fact, Treg cells are able to generate NAD+ through mitochondrial metabolism in high lactate environments [29].

Glycolytic alterations may also specifically impact neutrophils. While less is understood about the metabolic utilization of neutrophils in the tumor microenvironment than leukocytes, neutrophils are generally regarded as highly glycolytic. Neutrophil function has been described to highly depend on glucose availability with lack of glucose abrogating function [30]. suggesting that increased glucose metabolism by tumor cells may limit the availability of glucose to neutrophils limiting their function. However, counterintuitively to a perhaps reduced function in a tumor microenvironment with low levels of glucose, neutrophil recruitment to the tumor site has been regularly described as immunosuppressive and inhibitory of the activity of T cells [31]. An elevated circulating neutrophil to lymphocyte ratio (NLR) has been found to be a negative prognostic factor in glioblastoma patients [32]. Rice et al. suggest a potential mechanism in which neutrophils maintain local immune suppression in the glucose-limited tumor microenvironment through the adaptation of a neutrophil subpopulation to an oxidative mitochondrial metabolism [33].

Interestingly, the interplay between glycolytic tumor metabolism and immune cell function may be bidirectional with immune cells able to regulate metabolic pathways as well. Zhang et al. show that macrophages produce interleukin-6 which leads to downstream phosphorylation of the glycolytic enzyme phosphoglycerate kinase 1 (PGK1) and facilitates a PGK1-catalyzed reaction towards glycolysis rather than gluconeogenesis through altered substate affinity [34]. PGK1 phosphorylation correlated with increased macrophage infiltration, higher grade, and worse prognosis in human GBM samples [34]. Further work will be necessary to elucidate this metabolic crosstalk and metabolic competition between tumor cells and immune cells and to understand whether immune cells can themselves alter the metabolic environment to support tumor growth, including through mechanisms, such as post-translational modifications, which regulate the functions of many glycolytic enzymes.

Studies of glycolysis in glioblastoma have paralleled the findings in other cancer types of the significance of increased glycolysis in creating an immunosuppressive tumor microenvironment. The shift to increased aerobic glycolysis from oxidative phosphorylation in glioblastoma is associated with immunosuppression and tumor progression [35]. In

GBM, hypoxia-inducible factor 1α (HIF-1α) directs the metabolic switch for Tregs from glycolysis in the glucose-poor tumor environment to oxidative phosphorylation which drives immunosuppression [36]. One recent study determined a glycolytic score for glioblastoma utilizing seven genes involved in expression of glycolytic enzymes and found that T cells, B cells, and NK cells were depressed while there was high infiltration of immunosuppressive cells in patients with high glycolytic scores [37]. One of the genes utilized in the glycolytic score, *ENO1*, promoted M2 microglia polarization promoting immunosuppression and glioblastoma cell malignancy. Another recent study utilizing differentially expressed genes between high and low glycolytic activity to assign risk scores to classify high and low risk GBM patients found differential infiltration of immune cells and immune checkpoints, suggesting a relationship between glycolytic activity and immunosuppression in patients with GBM [38].

3. Anti-Tumoral Immunologic Effects of Targeting Glutamine Metabolism in Cancer

Glutamine, an amino acid highly expressed in cancer cells, plays a critical role for cellular function and the generation of energy and metabolic precursors for macromolecule synthesis which help sustain anabolic growth. Glutamine is converted by glutaminase into glutamate which is then converted to α-ketoglutarate, a critical component of the TCA cycle and in the production of metabolic intermediates utilized in the production of lipids, nucleic acids, and proteins. Upregulated glutamine metabolism in cancer cells promotes tumor growth through supporting macromolecule biosynthesis, altered signaling pathways, and cancer cell proliferation and survival. The metabolism of glutamine provides carbons for the TCA cycle to sustain accelerated anabolism in cancer cells and promotes tumor growth [39–41].

Glutamine is amongst the most prevalent amino acids in the brain as a precursor to the excitatory neurotransmitter glutamate [9]. Glutamate transporters are upregulated in gliomas allowing for increased glutamine uptake [42]. The absence of glutamine in culture medium leads to loss of viability as determined by a trypan blue dye exclusion test in glioma cell lines [43]. Increased and rapid glutamine utilization has been described as characteristic of glioblastoma cell proliferation through promoting generation of NADPH for anabolic processes such as nucleotide biosynthesis and providing a source of carbon for fatty acid synthesis [44]. Glutamate secretion in glioma cells results in a growth advantage in vivo, and targeting glutamate secretion or antagonizing glutamate target receptors resulted in slowed tumor expansion in C6Glu+ tumors in rats [45].

Glutamine metabolic pathways are also upregulated in glioblastoma. Glutamate dehydrogenase (GDH), an enzyme which catalyzes the conversion of L-glutamate into α-ketoglutarate as part of glutaminolysis, is upregulated in many human cancers and shown to promote tumor growth [46]. An isoenzyme of GDH, GDH1, maintains glioma cell survival in glucose depleted conditions through activation of glutamine metabolism and the α-ketoglutarate generated drives glucose uptake and cell survival under low glucose [47]. Glutamine synthetase expression in glioblastoma is associated with poor prognosis, with absent or low intensity expression of glutamine synthetase in neoplastic cells associated with longer survival [48]. Glutamine is hypothesized to be provided by surrounding astrocytes to feed GBM cells negative for glutamine synthetase cells [49].

Glutamine metabolism in cancer cells impacts the tumor microenvironment and the immune populations within it in ways similar to glucose metabolism (Figure 1). Cancer cells relying on exogenous glutamine synthesis utilize glucose, further depleting it in the tumor microenvironment and contributing to the reduced function of immunostimulatory effector T cells and NK populations that require glucose for function [7]. Glutaminolysis also results in the downstream production of lactate, mirroring the effect of aerobic glycolysis in generating an acidic tumor microenvironment which contributes to immunosuppression as described earlier in this review.

Increased uptake of glutamine by tumor cells may result in its depletion in the tumor microenvironment and affect the function of immune cells which utilize glutamine for their own metabolic programs. Activated T cells upregulate glutamine metabolism to generate α-ketoglutarate to enter the TCA cycle and generate ATP to fulfill the energetic demands of T cell proliferation [50]. Glutamine depletion in the tumor microenvironment compromises activation-induced T cell growth and proliferation. Addition of the macromolecular products of glutamine synthesis (nucleotides and polyamines) does not rescue T cell growth in a glutamine depleted environment, implicating the specific role of glutamine in meeting the bioenergetic and biosynthetic precursor requirements of activated T cells [50].

Targeting glutamine metabolism in a mouse model of colon cancer through a glutamine antagonist 6-Diazo-5-oxo-L-norleucine, which broadly inhibits several glutamine-using enzymes, led to suppression of both oxidative phosphorylation and glycolytic metabolism in cancer cells and decreased tumor-related changes in the microenvironment with decreased hypoxia, acidosis, and nutrient depletion [51]. In contrast, glutamine blockade in effector T cells resulted in upregulated oxidative metabolism and increased survival and activation [51]. PD-1-targeted checkpoint blockade co-administered with glutamine antagonism resulted in a complete therapeutic response and a memory response with tumor rechallenge [51]. The efficacy of glutamine antagonism was entirely dependent on the activity of CD8 T cells, indicating that the mechanism through which glutamine antagonism promoted anti-tumoral activity was through enhancing cytotoxic T cell anti-tumor response [51]. These findings highlight a common theme for glutamine and glycolytic metabolism in which tumor cells and anti-tumor immune cells compete for metabolites to promote their individual function. It additionally offers insights for metabolic targeting in cancer that leverages the therapeutic window created by the differential metabolic plasticity of immune cells versus cancer cells in which cancer cells are highly metabolically interdependent (targeting glutamine metabolism leads to widespread metabolic inhibition), whereas T cells exhibit adaptive metabolic reprogramming (targeting glutamine metabolism activates upregulation of alternate pathways allowing survival).

Additionally, glutamine metabolism by cancer cells leads to the enrichment of various immunosuppressive populations in cancer. Notably, α-ketoglutarate generated through glutaminolysis restricts anti-tumoral macrophage M1 activation [52]. A separate study also supports the role of α-ketoglutarate in promoting an immunosuppressive macrophage phenotype by showing that higher production of α-ketoglutarate results in M2 activation of macrophages (an immunotolerant phenotype) [53].

Targeting glutamine metabolism in cancers with known resistance to checkpoint blockade (triple negative breast cancer and lung carcinoma) with a small molecule inhibitor led to the marked inhibition of the generation and recruitment of immunosuppressive myeloid-derived suppressor cells (MDSCs) through apoptosis of these MDSCs [54]. Additionally, glutamine antagonism promoted the generation of antitumor inflammatory tumor-associated macrophages [54]. Combining glutamine antagonism with checkpoint blockade in immunotherapy-resistant tumors was shown to enhance the efficacy of checkpoint blockade [54].

Targeting glutamine metabolism may enhance endogenous anti-tumor immunity through independent mechanisms promoting the metabolic programs of cytotoxic populations while inhibiting immunosuppressive populations. Given the success of combining targeting glutamine metabolism with checkpoint inhibitors in other immunotherapy resistant tumors, it may be worthwhile to explore this combination in GBM.

4. Inhibition of Tryptophan Degrading Enzymes as a Strategy to Promote an Anti-Tumoral Immune Response

Tryptophan is an essential amino acid utilized for protein biosynthesis and a biochemical precursor to physiologically important compounds such as serotonin and melatonin. The majority of tryptophan which is not incorporated into proteins is broken down into degradation products (kynurenines) via the kynurenine pathway [55]. Physiologically, tryptophan degradation into kynurenines enables the generation of the essential metabolic cofactor nicotinamide adenine dinucleotide (NAD+). In cancer, the production of kynurenine metabolites by tumor cells contributes to tumor growth by generating an immunosuppressive tumor microenvironment through the recruitment and differentiation of immunosuppressive Treg cells and MDSCs [56]. Tryptophan is degraded into kynurenine metabolites by the two enzymes indoleamine-2,3-dioxygenase-1 (IDO1) or tryptophan-2,3-dioxygenase (TDO2) which catalyze the rate limiting reactions in the kynurenine pathway.

Tryptophan catabolism and alterations in kynurenine pathway has been implicated in poor prognosis in several cancer types, including in GBM [57]. The correlation between overexpression of enzymes involved in tryptophan degradation and patient survival in primary and metastatic brain tumors has been well established [58,59]. Recurrent malignant gliomas are associated with increased levels of tryptophan metabolism compared to newly diagnosed patients in metabolic profiles obtained from CSF analysis [60]. IDO1 and TDO2 are highly expressed in glioma cells proportionally to glioma grade [55,61]. Additionally, amongst higher grade patients, those with strong IDO expression were noted to have significantly worse overall survival rates compared to patients with weak IDO expression [61]. IDO1 is expressed in the majority of malignant gliomas with mRNA and protein expression levels correlating with overall patient survival [59].

IDO1- and TDO2- mediated degradation of tryptophan by cancer cells is a driver of immune suppression in the tumor microenvironment through recruitment and activation of myeloid-derived suppressor cells (MDSCs) and induction of anergy of CD8+ T cells [62]. Degradation of tryptophan and reduced tryptophan availability within the tumor microenvironment resulting in arrest of T cell growth and activation has been well characterized [63]. Tryptophan-free media suppresses human T cell proliferation and activation [64]. Tryptophan catabolism by tumor cells allows for metabolic inhibition of T cells and promotes tumor evasion of immune destruction. Two mechanisms enable tumor cell tryptophan catabolism to inhibit anti-tumoral T cells: (1) tumor cell depletion of the essential metabolite tryptophan which is required for T cell metabolism (the competition for nutrients scenario between tumor cells and T cells described above for glucose and glutamine) and (2) generation of T cell inhibitory molecules from tryptophan metabolites such as kynurenine and its derivatives (Figure 2).

Tryptophan utilization by tumor cells leads to metabolic starvation of T cells which are unable to utilize tryptophan for their own functions and thus promotes immunosuppression in the tumor microenvironment. Inhibition of tryptophan degrading enzymes blocks enzymatic activity and restores cytotoxic T cell activity in vitro and in vivo [65]. T cells undergo rapid growth arrest in low tryptophan conditions due to a tryptophan-sensitive checkpoint inhibiting the cell cycle in the G1 phase [66]. High IDO expression in colorectal cancer cell lines was associated with significant reduction of CD3+ infiltrating T cells and increased frequency of liver metastases [67]. Additionally, intratumoral immunosuppressive cells—such as MDSCs, tumor associated macrophages (TAMs), and Treg cells—upregulate production of IDO and metabolize tryptophan into suppressive kynurenine which reduces the availability of tryptophan for cytotoxic T cells in the tumor microenvironment [68]. This mechanism is so crucial to MDSC immunosuppression that IDO has been shown to be required for MDSCs' immunosuppression of T cells with inhibition of IDO leading to decreased MDSC suppression of T cell proliferation in a murine melanoma model [68,69].

Given the role of IDO through kynurenine synthesis in generating the tumor microenvironment allowing for immune escape in cancer, IDO inhibition has been explored as an attractive therapeutic option in multiple cancers. Inhibition of IDO was found to effectively normalize plasma kynurenine levels in patients with various tumor types [70]. Interestingly, combinatorial inhibition of IDO1, IDO2, and TDO2 (together thought to be the predominant rate-limiting enzymes for the kynurenine pathway) did not impact tumor viability in patient derived GBM cells [55]. However, these findings are consistent with the mechanistic understanding that inhibition of the kynurenine pathway enzymes has anti-tumoral effects due to alterations in the survival and function of immune cells normally present in the tumor microenvironment that are not present in an in vitro model.

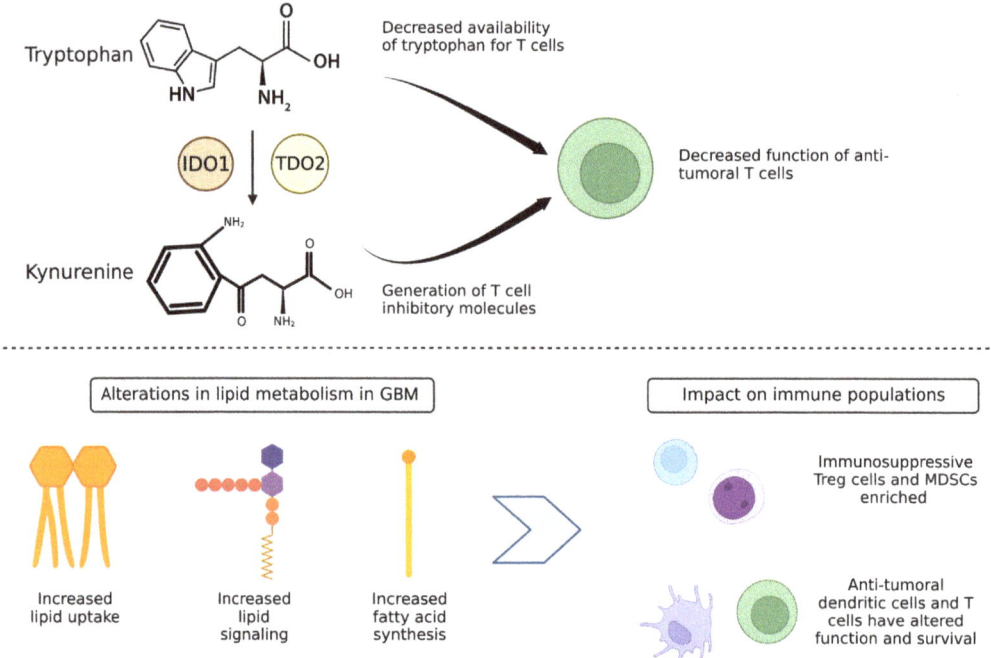

Figure 2. Altered tryptophan metabolism and lipid metabolism in GBM tumor cells contributes to an immunosuppressive population enriched tumor microenvironment. (**Top**) Tryptophan metabolism and generation of kynurenine degradation products by the enzymes IDO1 and TDO2 leads to decreased availability of tryptophan for T cells and generation of T cell inhibitory molecules, leading to decreased function of anti-tumoral T cells. (**Bottom**) Alterations in lipid metabolism lead to increased fatty acid oxidation and lipid signaling by immunosuppressive Treg and MDSC cells, leading to their enrichment over anti-tumor dendritic cells and cytotoxic T cells.

Kynurenine metabolites activate a ligand-activated transcription factor, aryl hydrocarbon receptor (AhR) which results in increased expression of IDO1 and IDO2 in a positive feedback loop. Targeting AhR in vitro led to decreased glioma cell viability [55]. Opitz et al. also showed that kynurenines generated by TDO act to suppress antitumor responses by T cell suppression and promotion of tumor cell survival through AhR mediated signaling in a murine glioma model [71]. Increased expression of AhR target genes involved in signaling pathways related to immune tolerance correlated with decreased survival in patients with glioma [71]. Additionally, AhR activity was found to drive T cell dysfunction through promotion of a Treg-macrophage suppressive axis [62]. This alternate pathway of AhR agonism may circumvent the anti-tumoral effects of tryptophan degradation inhibition through AhR agonism independent of immune function. This also suggests a potential limitation of previous clinical trials of IDO1 inhibitors, some of which have been AhR agonists themselves [72].

Tryptophan catabolism and its downstream metabolic pathways are known to contribute to the immunosuppressive tumor microenvironment and contribute to resistance to novel immunotherapies for malignant gliomas. Increased expression of IDO and TDO has been suggested as an acquired resistance mechanism to PD-1 and CTLA blockade in pre-clinical models of multiple cancers, including GBM [73,74]. The effect of CTLA-4 blockade synergized with IDO inhibitors in metastatic melanoma in both IDO-expressing and non-IDO-expressing poorly immunogenic tumors, and was shown to be effector T cell dependent [75].

The combination of targeting tryptophan metabolism with immune checkpoint blockade has been also explored in glioblastoma. Combining 1-methyltryptophan, which inhibits IDO, with dual immune checkpoint blockade significantly improved survival in an orthotropic mouse GBM model correlating with increased T-cell survival and synergistic decrease of Treg infiltration [76]. Likewise, immunotherapy simultaneously targeting IDO, CTLA-4, and PD-L1 in a mouse glioma model demonstrated a survival benefit [57]. However, combinatorial effects of IDO inhibition with checkpoint inhibitors have been observed in mouse models of other cancers but have not necessarily translated to success in clinical trials. Most prominently, a large phase 3 trial of an IDO1 enzyme inhibitor plus a PD-1 inhibitor in metastatic melanoma did not result in greater clinical benefit compared to PD-1 inhibition alone [77]. Subsequently, multiple phase 3 trials of various IDO1 inhibitors in combination with immune checkpoint inhibitors in other cancers were halted.

Potential limitations of IDO1 inhibition that led to failure in this phase 3 trial combining this approach with a PD-1 inhibitor include: insufficient inhibition of IDO1 at the doses being used; the ability of other enzymes involved in tryptophan metabolisms such as TDO2 or pathways downstream of IDO1 inhibition to compensate and still generate immunosuppressive tryptophan metabolites such as kynurenine and its derivatives when IDO1 is inhibited; and lack of patient selection based on IDO1 expression [65,78]. IDO1 may also suppress the antitumor immune response independent of its association with tryptophan metabolism [79]. Additionally, while overwhelming evidence suggests that IDO expression and tryptophan degradation results in immunosuppression and T cell dysfunction diminishing the efficacy of immunotherapy, the understanding of IDO interaction with immunotherapy remains incomplete. Counterintuitively, brain-tumor mice genetically deficient for IDO1 demonstrate decreased efficacy in dual and triple immunotherapy approaches [57]. Thus, IDO inhibition or deficiency may be evaded by alternate metabolic pathways that maintain continued immunosuppression. One study demonstrated that while IDO1 was identified as the top gene in determining low versus high tryptophan in GBM, another potential mediator of the high tryptophan metabolic phenotype in GBM, quinolinate phosphoribosyltransferase, was identified as well, suggesting alternate pathways that could be upregulated to evade IDO1 inhibition and maintain the high utilization of tryptophan in tumor cells [80]. Interestingly, targeting AhR in tumors with an active tryptophan catabolic pathway allows for the overcoming of immunosuppression and sensitization to anti-PD-1 therapy, suggesting a role for targeting alternate areas of tryptophan metabolism [62]. More work is needed to understand the role of compensatory pathways in targeting tryptophan metabolism.

Targeting tryptophan metabolism may also have implications for vaccine related cancer therapies which rely on T cell mediated antitumoral responses. IDO expression correlated with lack of specific T cell enrichment at the tumor site and prevented the rejection of tumor cells in mice who have been preimmunized against tumor antigens with a vaccine [58]. This effect was partially reversible with systemic administration of an IDO inhibitor, holding implications for combining cancer vaccines which utilize tumor specific antigenic peptides to generate a T cell antitumor response with IDO inhibitors to enhance the antitumoral effect of immunomodulatory vaccines.

5. Exogenous Induction of Lipid Peroxidation as a Strategy to Promote an Anti-Tumoral Immune Response

Lipid metabolism physiologically functions to allow for cellular energy storage, synthesis of cellular membranes, and cellular signaling. In cancer, alterations in lipid metabolism help meet high bioenergetic demands by generating energy through beta-oxidation. Utilization of fatty acid oxidation in addition to increased glycolysis allows for bioenergetic flexibility in promoting aggressive tumor growth and metastasis [81].

Glioma cells utilize lipid oxidation and upregulate transport of ketones generated from lipid metabolism to sustain growth [82]. Lipid metabolism is abnormally regulated in gliomas with altered expression of lipid-related genes, altered lipid composition, and lipogenesis [83]. Lipids provide energy to fuel GBM cellular proliferation and also play a role in mitigation of oxidative damage that is increased during proliferation [84]. Evidence supporting the role of lipid metabolism in GBM biology comes from studies in which targeting lipid homeostasis inhibits GBM cell proliferation [85]. Lipids are also utilized through lipolysis to maintain stem cell self-renewal in GBM and to allow for propagation of orthotopic tumor xenografts from GBM stem cells in mice [86]. Differential expression of nine genes related to lipid metabolism has been shown to allow the classification of GBM patients into high and low risk for poor outcome [87].

Altered lipid metabolism in GBM impacts immune cell function, particularly that of T cells [88]. T cells utilize lipids to promote their proliferation and differentiation by taking up exogenous lipids and oxidizing intracellular stores of lipids [89]. In GBM, T cells are sequestered in the bone marrow away from the tumor microenvironment via T cell internalization of the lipid sphingosine-1-phosphate receptor, which has been suggested to play a protumoral role through promotion of angiogenesis in GBM [90]. Notably, Treg cells also primarily utilize fatty acid oxidation for their metabolism [91].

While less is understood about the metabolic requirements of Treg cells, utilizing fatty acid oxidation over glycolysis may promote Treg survival over the survival of CD4 and CD8 T cells (Figure 2). Lipid signaling in intratumoral Treg cells additionally allows for cell survival and induces signaling pathways to promote oxidative phosphorylation in Treg cells [92]. Another class of suppressive immune cells, MDSCs, have also been found to demonstrate increased fatty acid uptake and activated fatty acid oxidation in multiple murine tumor models [93]. Pharmacological inhibition of fatty acid oxidation led to decreased production of inhibitory cytokines by MDSCs, blocking of immune inhibitory pathways, delayed tumor growth in a T-cell dependent manner, and enhanced efficacy of adoptive T-cell therapy [93].

GBM cells are also able to evade the anti-tumor immune response due to altered lipid metabolism impacting the function of antigen presenting cells. Exogenous induction of lipid peroxidation and ferroptosis resulted in release of damage-associated molecular patterns from glioma cells that stimulate dendritic cell activation and maturation and can lead to activation of cytotoxic T lymphocytes by dendritic cells [94,95]. Recurrent GBM reprogram metabolic processes to enrich fatty acid oxidation which allow for adaptive tumor resistance and anti-phagocytosis [96]. Fatty acid oxidation by GBM cells activates CD47 to mediate immune escape, representing a potential target for immunotherapy [96]. Notably, one class of fatty acids, arachidonic acids, also contributes to tumor progression in GBM [97]. However, targeting these molecules with steroids has been shown to also correlate with tumor progression and inhibits responses to oncolytic adenoviral therapy and checkpoint immunotherapy [98,99]. Further understanding of the specific role of individual classes of lipids in altering the immune response in the tumor microenvironment will be needed to develop specific anti-tumoral immune strategies targeting lipid utilization in GBM.

6. Implications of GBM Metabolic Alterations for Specific Immunotherapy Strategies

While initially the central nervous system was thought to be an immune-privileged site, current thought points to the presence of immune surveillance in the brain following findings revealing the presence of dedicated lymphatic channels running parallel to dural venous sinuses and allowing for lymphocyte priming from antigen presenting cells in the brain [96,100]. Despite this evidence supporting the possibility of immune responses in the central nervous system, immunotherapies have not met with anywhere near the level of success in GBM that they have encountered in other cancers. Indeed, GBMs have enriched immunosuppressive myeloid, microglia, and macrophage populations and depleted tumor infiltrating lymphocytes, and thus have been characterized as "cold" tumors due to their lack of response to immunotherapy [101]. Furthermore, each component of standard of care treatment (surgery, radiation, chemotherapy, steroids) for GBM elicits immunosuppressive effects as well [102].

The most studied immunotherapeutic approaches for GBM are vaccines, immune checkpoint inhibitors, and biologic therapies (Figure 3). The most advanced vaccine trial in GBM, a phase 3 trial of the peptide vaccine rindopepimut, which targets EGFR variant III (EGFRvIII), relied on adaptive immunity with the tumor based on a single immunogenic peptide and failed to demonstrate improvement in survival over standard of care in EGFRvIII positive patients [103]. Peptide vaccines such as rindopepimut have poor immunogenicity on their own and require an effective T cell response to have antitumoral effects, which may limit their efficacy in GBM due to metabolic alterations in the GBM microenvironment altering effector T cell proliferation and function (Figure 3). Another vaccine-based therapy in trials was based on utilizing dendritic cells with promising early phase 3 survival data. However, dendritic cells injected into the tumor may have altered function based on altered tumoral metabolism, such as changes in lipid metabolism [104]. Promisingly, there is much more limited evidence on metabolic alterations impacting dendritic cells as compared to T cells. However, these vaccines ultimately also depend on an effective T cell response.

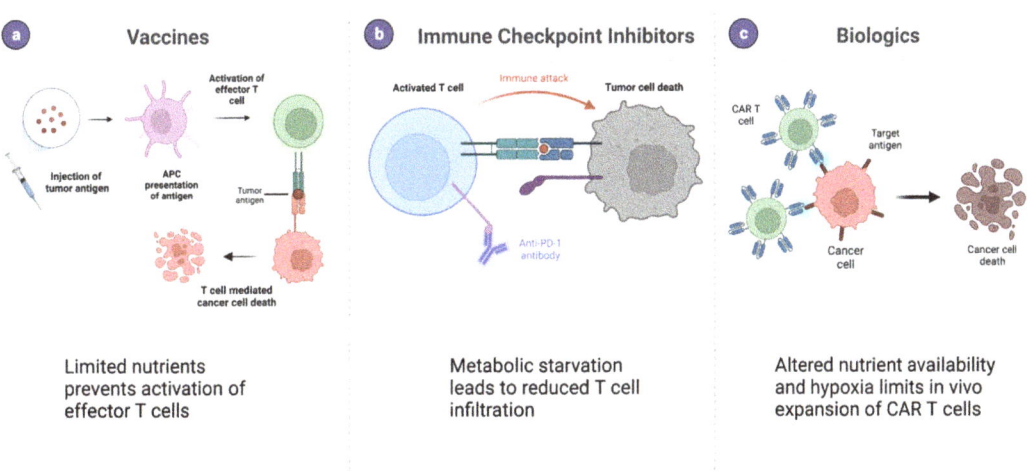

Figure 3. Immunosuppression and nutrient depletion in the tumor microenvironment limit efficacy of immunotherapies in glioblastoma. (**Top**) Cancer cell metabolism alters the pH, oxygen, and metabolite contents in the tumor microenvironment. (**Bottom**) Metabolic alterations result in resistance to different classes of immunotherapies such as vaccines (**a**), immune checkpoint inhibitors (**b**), and biologic therapies (**c**). Each of these mechanisms relies on an effective immune response which is diminished with metabolic alterations.

Immune checkpoint inhibitors targeting PD-1/PD-L1 and/or CTLA-4 are also being investigated in phase 3 trials in GBM, with initial results suggesting no clinical benefit [104,105]. While numerous factors may be responsible for the limited response observed thus far to immune checkpoint inhibitors, including the expression levels of the targets themselves, the reduced T cell infiltration in glioblastoma is a notable barrier (Figure 3). Both CTLA-4 and PD-1 mechanistically involve the T cell response—blocking CTLA-4 enhances T cell priming and blocking PD-1 enhances T cell differentiation. Addressing the metabolic restraints experienced by effector T cells within the tumor may have potential to enhance the respose to checkpoint inhibitors. Though combining metabolic targeting with immune checkpoint blockade has been investigated in other cancer types, this approach has not yet been explored in GBM. While enthusiasm for IDO inhibition combined with checkpoint inhibitors has diminished following failure in a metastatic melanoma phase 3 trial, alternate strategies could include targeting tryptophan metabolism, considering pathways that tumor cells may use to bypass IDO inhibition. Glycolytic targeting in combination with checkpoint inhibitors is another strategy that has been shown in preclinical studies as increasing T cell activation, viability, and effector function to improve the efficacy of checkpoint therapy [106].

Biologic therapies for GBM can be viral or cellular. Oncolytic viruses have overall met with limited success in GBM, and initial anti-tumor T cell immune responses generated by viral infiltration into tumor do not persist without serial treatment [107]. Metabolic alterations, particularly the limited glucose and acidosis in the tumor microenvironment, can inhibit viral replication as well as prevent the activation of CD8 T cells which are required for oncolytic viral stimulation of host anti-tumor immune responses [108]. Cellular therapies for GBM include chimeric antigen receptor (CAR) T cell therapy, in which T cells are engineered to express an activated phenotype and can be designed to recognize antigens not presented in the context of MHC molecules, potentially allowing this therapeutic approach to bypass some of the immunosuppressive metabolic limitations in the tumor microenvironment. However, in the first trial of CAR T cells directed at EGFRvIII in glioblastoma patients, tumor infiltration of CAR T cells was detected but overall survival was not affected [109]. Significantly, tumor samples from patients who underwent surgical resection after CAR T cell infusion revealed upregulation of IDO1 and increased T regulatory cells, implying the possibility of GBM escape mechanisms reinstating an immunosuppressive milieu. One potential strategy to enhance CAR T cell therapy involves culturing CAR T cells in metabolic conditions similar to the tumor microenvironment to allow for acclimation to low nutrient availability and potentially mititgate the metabolic immunosuppression in the tumor microenvironment (Figure 2). T cell expansion in media containing low levels of glutamine was shown to result in greater effective antitumor function compared to cells cultured in traditional media [110]. Ex vivo culturing of cells concurrent with glycolytic blockade demonstrated improved tumor clearance [111]. Targeting metabolic adaptations, such as increased fatty acid oxidation, in conjunction with adoptive T-cell therapy has also demonstrated success in preclinical models [93].

Metabolic pathways implicated in maintaining immunosuppression in the GBM microenvironment have been well elucidated. However, the potential for targeting these metabolic pathways to condition the tumor microenvironment to become more responsive to immunotherapies remains underexplored in GBM. Preclinical data targeting metabolic pathways in conjunction with immunotherapies largely come from models of more immunogenic cancers. This presents an attractive avenue for further study in GBM, in which modifying a largely immunosuppressive environment may meaningfully alter immunotherapeutic response.

While this review discusses the most studied metabolic pathways with respect to immunosuppression in GBM, several other metabolic pathway alterations occur to meet the energetic demands of GBM progression. Arginine metabolism reprogramming in GBM leads to increased intake and decreased degradation of arginine by tumor cells and has been linked to impaired T cell responses due to altered bioavailablity of arginine [112]. Targeting arginine metabolism has been explored preclinically in GBM and found to synergize with radiotherapy while promoting a protumor immune population, suggesting potential to explore targeting this pathway in combination with immunotherapies in GBM [112]. Another metabolite, 2-hydroxuglutarate (2-HG), has also been implicated in both tumor growth and modulation of anti-tumor immunity through inhibition of T cell activity, though 2-HG alterations in GBM are heterogenous and epigenetically regulated [113]. In IDH-1 mutant tumors which produce 2-HG, antitumor immunity induced by an IDH-1 specific vaccine or checkpoint inhibition is improved by simultaneously downregulating 2-HG production through inhibition of the enzymatic function of mutant IDH [113]. Several other metabolites have been described as altered in GBM such as aspartate, α-ketoglutarate, and methionine; however, less evidence exists regarding the contribution of these metabolic alterations to immunosuppression. Other molecular targets in GBM have also been noted to contrastingly impact tumor cell metabolism and immunosuppression in which tumor cell metabolism is slowed while T cell activatation promotes pro-tumoral effects on the immune microenvironment [114]. These suggest a range of alternative pathways that may be implicated in the limited response to immunotherapies and warrant further preclinical study.

7. Conclusions

While many immunotherapies are being investigated in GBM patients, none have resulted in major improvements in survival outcomes. Negative results from phase II and phase III clinical trials of vaccines and immune checkpoint inhibitors have challenged the potential of these approaches in GBM. Future directions for immune-based strategies for glioblastoma require treatment modalities that can convert a 'cold' tumor with significant local immunosuppression into a 'hot' tumor. The uniquely immunosuppressive environment generated by tumor cellular metabolism in GBM presents an opportunity for augmenting responses to immunotherapy. Combining immunotherapy with agents that target the metabolic alterations resulting in an immunosuppressive microenvironment may have greater success in generating an antitumor immune response. These combinations should be evaluated rigorously preclinically in order to ensure that the most biologically sound combination approaches addressing the antitumor immune response along with tumor metabolism are advanced to clinical trials.

Author Contributions: Conceptualization: N.C. and M.K.A. Drafting of the manuscript: N.C and M.K.A. Critical revision of the manuscript for important intellectual content: N.C., J.Y.O., R.C.O. and M.K.A. Supervision: M.K.A. All authors have read and agreed to the published version of the manuscript.

Funding: This research received no external funding.

Acknowledgments: We thank UCSF Helen Diller Family Comprehensive Cancer Center colleagues for their intellectual input. Figures in the manuscript were created with BioRender.

Conflicts of Interest: Authors declare no conflict of interest.

References

1. Tan, A.C.; Ashley, D.M.; López, G.Y.; Malinzak, M.; Friedman, H.S.; Khasraw, M. Management of glioblastoma: State of the art and future directions. *CA Cancer J. Clin.* **2020**, *70*, 299–312. [CrossRef]
2. Stupp, R.; Lukas, R.V.; Hegi, M.E. Improving survival in molecularly selected glioblastoma. *Lancet* **2019**, *393*, 615–617. [CrossRef]
3. Hanahan, D.; Weinberg, R.A. Hallmarks of Cancer: The Next Generation. *Cell* **2011**, *144*, 646–674. [CrossRef]
4. Yu, M.W.; Quail, D.F. Immunotherapy for Glioblastoma: Current Progress and Challenges. *Front. Immunol.* **2021**, *12*, 1637. [CrossRef]
5. Bausart, M.; Préat, V.; Malfanti, A. Immunotherapy for glioblastoma: The promise of combination strategies. *J. Exp. Clin. Cancer Res.* **2022**, *41*, 35. [CrossRef]
6. Leone, R.D.; Powell, J.D. Metabolism of immune cells in cancer. *Nat. Rev. Cancer* **2020**, *20*, 516–531. [CrossRef]
7. DePeaux, K.; Delgoffe, G.M. Metabolic barriers to cancer immunotherapy. *Nat. Rev. Immunol.* **2021**, *21*, 785–797. [CrossRef]
8. Zhou, W.; Wahl, D.R. Metabolic Abnormalities in Glioblastoma and Metabolic Strategies to Overcome Treatment Resistance. *Cancers* **2019**, *11*, 1231. [CrossRef]
9. Garcia, J.H.; Jain, S.; Aghi, M.K. Metabolic Drivers of Invasion in Glioblastoma. *Front. Cell Dev. Biol.* **2021**, *9*, 683276. [CrossRef]
10. Marin-Valencia, I.; Yang, C.; Mashimo, T.; Cho, S.; Baek, H.; Yang, X.-L.; Rajagopalan, K.N.; Maddie, M.; Vemireddy, V.; Zhao, Z.; et al. Analysis of tumor metabolism reveals mitochondrial glucose oxidation in genetically diverse human glioblastomas in the mouse brain in vivo. *Cell Metab.* **2012**, *15*, 827–837. [CrossRef]

11. Sanzey, M.; Rahim, S.A.A.; Oudin, A.; Dirkse, A.; Kaoma, T.; Vallar, L.; Herold-Mende, C.; Bjerkvig, R.; Golebiewska, A.; Niclou, S.P. Comprehensive analysis of glycolytic enzymes as therapeutic targets in the treatment of glioblastoma. *PLoS ONE* **2015**, *10*, e0123544. [CrossRef]
12. Wolf, A.; Agnihotri, S.; Munoz, D.; Guha, A. Developmental profile and regulation of the glycolytic enzyme hexokinase 2 in normal brain and glioblastoma multiforme. *Neurobiol. Dis.* **2011**, *44*, 84–91. [CrossRef]
13. Muir, A.; Vander Heiden, M.G. The nutrient environment affects therapy. *Science* **2018**, *360*, 962–963. [CrossRef]
14. Bi, J.; Bi, F.; Pan, X.; Yang, Q. Establishment of a novel glycolysis-related prognostic gene signature for ovarian cancer and its relationships with immune infiltration of the tumor microenvironment. *J. Transl. Med.* **2021**, *19*, 382. [CrossRef]
15. Li, F.; Simon, M.C. Cancer Cells Don't Live Alone: Metabolic Communication within Tumor Microenvironments. *Dev. Cell* **2020**, *54*, 183–195. [CrossRef]
16. Shime, H.; Yabu, M.; Akazawa, T.; Kodama, K.; Matsumoto, M.; Seya, T.; Inoue, N. Tumor-secreted lactic acid promotes IL-23/IL-17 proinflammatory pathway. *J. Immunol. Baltim. Md. 1950* **2008**, *180*, 7175–7183. [CrossRef]
17. Dietl, K.; Renner, K.; Dettmer, K.; Timischl, B.; Eberhart, K.; Dorn, C.; Hellerbrand, C.; Kastenberger, M.; Kunz-Schughart, L.A.; Oefner, P.J.; et al. Lactic acid and acidification inhibit TNF secretion and glycolysis of human monocytes. *J. Immunol. Baltim. Md. 1950* **2010**, *184*, 1200–1209. [CrossRef]
18. Zhang, W.; Wang, G.; Xu, Z.-G.; Tu, H.; Hu, F.; Dai, J.; Chang, Y.; Chen, Y.; Lu, Y.; Zeng, H.; et al. Lactate Is a Natural Suppressor of RLR Signaling by Targeting MAVS. *Cell* **2019**, *178*, 176–189.e15. [CrossRef]
19. Donnelly, R.P.; Loftus, R.M.; Keating, S.E.; Liou, K.T.; Biron, C.A.; Gardiner, C.M.; Finlay, D.K. mTORC1-dependent metabolic reprogramming is a prerequisite for NK cell effector function. *J. Immunol. Baltim. Md. 1950* **2014**, *193*, 4477–4484. [CrossRef]
20. Brand, A.; Singer, K.; Koehl, G.E.; Kolitzus, M.; Schoenhammer, G.; Thiel, A.; Matos, C.; Bruss, C.; Klobuch, S.; Peter, K.; et al. LDHA-Associated Lactic Acid Production Blunts Tumor Immunosurveillance by T and NK Cells. *Cell Metab.* **2016**, *24*, 657–671. [CrossRef]
21. Fischer, K.; Hoffmann, P.; Voelkl, S.; Meidenbauer, N.; Ammer, J.; Edinger, M.; Gottfried, E.; Schwarz, S.; Rothe, G.; Hoves, S.; et al. Inhibitory effect of tumor cell-derived lactic acid on human T cells. *Blood* **2007**, *109*, 3812–3819. [CrossRef]
22. Ho, P.-C.; Bihuniak, J.D.; Macintyre, A.N.; Staron, M.; Liu, X.; Amezquita, R.; Tsui, Y.-C.; Cui, G.; Micevic, G.; Perales, J.C.; et al. Phosphoenolpyruvate Is a Metabolic Checkpoint of Anti-tumor T Cell Responses. *Cell* **2015**, *162*, 1217–1228. [CrossRef]
23. Cascone, T.; McKenzie, J.A.; Mbofung, R.M.; Punt, S.; Wang, Z.; Xu, C.; Williams, L.J.; Wang, Z.; Bristow, C.A.; Carugo, A.; et al. Increased Tumor Glycolysis Characterizes Immune Resistance to Adoptive T Cell Therapy. *Cell Metab.* **2018**, *27*, 977–987.e4. [CrossRef]
24. Chang, C.-H.; Qiu, J.; O'Sullivan, D.; Buck, M.D.; Noguchi, T.; Curtis, J.D.; Chen, Q.; Gindin, M.; Gubin, M.M.; van der Windt, G.J.W.; et al. Metabolic Competition in the Tumor Microenvironment Is a Driver of Cancer Progression. *Cell* **2015**, *162*, 1229–1241. [CrossRef]
25. Calcinotto, A.; Filipazzi, P.; Grioni, M.; Iero, M.; De Milito, A.; Ricupito, A.; Cova, A.; Canese, R.; Jachetti, E.; Rossetti, M.; et al. Modulation of Microenvironment Acidity Reverses Anergy in Human and Murine Tumor-Infiltrating T Lymphocytes. *Cancer Res.* **2012**, *72*, 2746–2756. [CrossRef]
26. Pilon-Thomas, S.; Kodumudi, K.; El-Kenawi, A.; Russell, S.; Weber, A.; Luddy, K.; Damaghi, M.; Wojtkowiak, J.; Mulé, J.; Ibrahim-Hashim, A.; et al. Neutralization of tumor acidity improves anti-tumor responses to immunotherapies. *Cancer Res.* **2016**, *76*, 1381–1390. [CrossRef]
27. Husain, Z.; Huang, Y.; Seth, P.; Sukhatme, V.P. Tumor-derived lactate modifies antitumor immune response: Effect on myeloid-derived suppressor cells and NK cells. *J. Immunol. Baltim. Md. 1950* **2013**, *191*, 1486–1495. [CrossRef]
28. Colegio, O.R.; Chu, N.-Q.; Szabo, A.L.; Chu, T.; Rhebergen, A.M.; Jairam, V.; Cyrus, N.; Brokowski, C.E.; Eisenbarth, S.C.; Phillips, G.M.; et al. Functional polarization of tumour-associated macrophages by tumour-derived lactic acid. *Nature* **2014**, *513*, 559–563. [CrossRef]
29. Angelin, A.; Gil-De-Gómez, L.; Dahiya, S.; Jiao, J.; Guo, L.; Levine, M.H.; Wang, Z.; Quinn, W.J., III; Kopinski, P.K.; Wang, L.; et al. Foxp3 Reprograms T Cell Metabolism to Function in Low-Glucose, High-Lactate Environments. *Cell Metab.* **2017**, *25*, 1282–1293.e7. [CrossRef] [PubMed]
30. Rodríguez-Espinosa, O.; Rojas-Espinosa, O.; Moreno-Altamirano, M.M.B.; López-Villegas, E.O.; Sánchez-García, F.J. Metabolic requirements for neutrophil extracellular traps formation. *Immunology* **2015**, *145*, 213–224. [CrossRef]
31. Schmielau, J.; Finn, O.J. Activated granulocytes and granulocyte-derived hydrogen peroxide are the underlying mechanism of suppression of t-cell function in advanced cancer patients. *Cancer Res.* **2001**, *61*, 4756–4760.
32. Bambury, R.M.; Teo, M.Y.; Power, D.G.; Yusuf, A.; Murray, S.; Battley, J.E.; Drake, C.; O'Dea, P.; Bermingham, N.; Keohane, C.; et al. The association of pre-treatment neutrophil to lymphocyte ratio with overall survival in patients with glioblastoma multiforme. *J. Neurooncol.* **2013**, *114*, 149–154. [CrossRef]
33. Rice, C.M.; Davies, L.C.; Subleski, J.J.; Maio, N.; Gonzalez-Cotto, M.; Andrews, C.; Patel, N.L.; Palmieri, E.M.; Weiss, J.M.; Lee, J.-M.; et al. Tumour-elicited neutrophils engage mitochondrial metabolism to circumvent nutrient limitations and maintain immune suppression. *Nat. Commun.* **2018**, *9*, 5099. [CrossRef]
34. Zhang, Y.; Yu, G.; Chu, H.; Wang, X.; Xiong, L.; Cai, G.; Liu, R.; Gao, H.; Tao, B.; Li, W.; et al. Macrophage-Associated PGK1 Phosphorylation Promotes Aerobic Glycolysis and Tumorigenesis. *Mol. Cell* **2018**, *71*, 201–215.e7. [CrossRef] [PubMed]

35. Gong, L.; Ji, L.; Xu, D.; Wang, J.; Zou, J. TGF-β links glycolysis and immunosuppression in glioblastoma. *Histol. Histopathol.* **2021**, *36*, 1111–1124. [PubMed]
36. Miska, J.; Lee-Chang, C.; Rashidi, A.; Muroski, M.E.; Chang, A.L.; Lopez-Rosas, A.; Zhang, P.; Panek, W.K.; Cordero, A.; Han, Y.; et al. HIF-1α Is a Metabolic Switch between Glycolytic-Driven Migration and Oxidative Phosphorylation-Driven Immunosuppression of Tregs in Glioblastoma. *Cell Rep.* **2019**, *27*, 226–237.e4. [CrossRef]
37. Liang, X.; Wang, Z.; Dai, Z.; Zhang, H.; Zhang, J.; Luo, P.; Liu, Z.; Liu, Z.; Yang, K.; Cheng, Q.; et al. Glioblastoma glycolytic signature predicts unfavorable prognosis, immunological heterogeneity, and ENO1 promotes microglia M2 polarization and cancer cell malignancy. *Cancer Gene Ther.* **2022**, *22*, 1–16. [CrossRef] [PubMed]
38. Wang, F.; Liu, X.; Jiang, H.; Chen, B. A Promising Glycolysis- and Immune-Related Prognostic Signature for Glioblastoma. *World Neurosurg.* **2022**, *161*, e363–e375. [CrossRef]
39. Son, J.; Lyssiotis, C.A.; Ying, H.; Wang, X.; Hua, S.; Ligorio, M.; Perera, R.M.; Ferrone, C.R.; Mullarky, E.; Shyh-Chang, N.; et al. Glutamine supports pancreatic cancer growth through a KRAS-regulated metabolic pathway. *Nature* **2013**, *496*, 101–105. [CrossRef]
40. Willems, L.; Jacque, N.; Jacquel, A.; Neveux, N.; Maciel, T.T.; Lambert, M.; Schmitt, A.; Poulain, L.; Green, A.S.; Uzunov, M.; et al. Inhibiting glutamine uptake represents an attractive new strategy for treating acute myeloid leukemia. *Blood* **2013**, *122*, 3521–3532. [CrossRef]
41. Wang, J.-B.; Erickson, J.W.; Fuji, R.; Ramachandran, S.; Gao, P.; Dinavahi, R.; Wilson, K.F.; Ambrosio, A.L.; Dias, S.M.; Dang, C.V.; et al. Targeting mitochondrial glutaminase activity inhibits oncogenic transformation. *Cancer Cell* **2010**, *18*, 207–219. [CrossRef]
42. Gu, Y.; Albuquerque, C.P.; Braas, D.; Zhang, W.; Villa, G.R.; Bi, J.; Ikegami, S.; Masui, K.; Gini, B.; Yang, H.; et al. mTORC2 Regulates Amino Acid Metabolism in Cancer by Phosphorylation of the Cystine-Glutamate Antiporter xCT. *Mol. Cell* **2017**, *67*, 128–138.e7. [CrossRef] [PubMed]
43. Wise, D.R.; DeBerardinis, R.J.; Mancuso, A.; Sayed, N.; Zhang, X.-Y.; Pfeiffer, H.K.; Nissim, I.; Daikhin, E.; Yudkoff, M.; McMahon, S.B.; et al. Myc regulates a transcriptional program that stimulates mitochondrial glutaminolysis and leads to glutamine addiction. *Proc. Natl. Acad. Sci. USA* **2008**, *105*, 18782–18787. [CrossRef]
44. DeBerardinis, R.J.; Mancuso, A.; Daikhin, E.; Nissim, I.; Yudkoff, M.; Wehrli, S.; Thompson, C.B. Beyond aerobic glycolysis: Transformed cells can engage in glutamine metabolism that exceeds the requirement for protein and nucleotide synthesis. *Proc. Natl. Acad. Sci. USA* **2007**, *104*, 19345–19350. [CrossRef] [PubMed]
45. Takano, T.; Lin, J.H.-C.; Arcuino, G.; Gao, Q.; Yang, J.; Nedergaard, M. Glutamate release promotes growth of malignant gliomas. *Nat. Med.* **2001**, *7*, 1010–1015. [CrossRef]
46. Jin, L.; Li, D.; Alesi, G.N.; Fan, J.; Kang, H.-B.; Lu, Z.; Boggon, T.J.; Jin, P.; Yi, H.; Wright, E.R.; et al. Glutamate Dehydrogenase 1 Signals through Antioxidant Glutathione Peroxidase 1 to Regulate Redox Homeostasis and Tumor Growth. *Cancer Cell* **2015**, *27*, 257–270. [CrossRef] [PubMed]
47. Yang, C.; Sudderth, J.; Dang, T.; Bachoo, R.G.; McDonald, J.G.; DeBerardinis, R.J. Glioblastoma cells require glutamate dehydrogenase to survive impairments of glucose metabolism or Akt signaling. *Cancer Res.* **2009**, *69*, 7986–7993. [CrossRef]
48. Rosati, A.; Poliani, P.L.; Todeschini, A.; Cominelli, M.; Medicina, D.; Cenzato, M.; Simoncini, E.L.; Magrini, S.M.; Buglione, M.; Grisanti, S.; et al. Glutamine synthetase expression as a valuable marker of epilepsy and longer survival in newly diagnosed glioblastoma multiforme. *Neuro-Oncol.* **2013**, *15*, 618–625. [CrossRef]
49. Tardito, S.; Oudin, A.; Ahmed, S.U.; Fack, F.; Keunen, O.; Zheng, L.; Miletic, H.; Sakariassen, P.Ø.; Weinstock, A.; Wagner, A.; et al. Glutamine synthetase activity fuels nucleotide biosynthesis and supports growth of glutamine-restricted glioblastoma. *Nat. Cell Biol.* **2015**, *17*, 1556–1568. [CrossRef]
50. Wang, R.; Dillon, C.P.; Shi, L.Z.; Milasta, S.; Carter, R.; Finkelstein, D.; McCormick, L.L.; Fitzgerald, P.; Chi, H.; Munger, J.; et al. The transcription factor Myc controls metabolic reprogramming upon T lymphocyte activation. *Immunity* **2011**, *35*, 871–882. [CrossRef]
51. Leone, R.D.; Zhao, L.; Englert, J.M.; Sun, I.M.; Oh, M.H.; Sun, I.H.; Arwood, M.L.; Bettencourt, I.A.; Patel, C.H.; Wen, J.; et al. Glutamine blockade induces divergent metabolic programs to overcome tumor immune evasion. *Science* **2019**, *366*, 1013–1021. [CrossRef] [PubMed]
52. Wang, X.; Liu, R.; Qu, X.; Yu, H.; Chu, H.; Zhang, Y.; Zhu, W.; Wu, X.; Gao, H.; Tao, B.; et al. α-Ketoglutarate-Activated NF-κB Signaling Promotes Compensatory Glucose Uptake and Brain Tumor Development. *Mol. Cell* **2019**, *76*, 148–162.e7. [PubMed]
53. Liu, P.-S.; Wang, H.; Li, X.; Chao, T.; Teav, T.; Christen, S.; Di Conza, G.; Cheng, W.-C.; Chou, C.-H.; Vavakova, M.; et al. α-ketoglutarate orchestrates macrophage activation through metabolic and epigenetic reprogramming. *Nat. Immunol.* **2017**, *18*, 985–994. [CrossRef]
54. Oh, M.-H.; Sun, I.-H.; Zhao, L.; Leone, R.D.; Sun, I.M.; Xu, W.; Collins, S.L.; Tam, A.J.; Blosser, R.L.; Patel, C.H.; et al. Targeting glutamine metabolism enhances tumor-specific immunity by modulating suppressive myeloid cells. *J. Clin. Investig.* **2020**, *130*, 3865–3884. [CrossRef]
55. Guastella, A.R.; Michelhaugh, S.K.; Klinger, N.V.; Fadel, H.A.; Kiousis, S.; Ali-Fehmi, R.; Kupsky, W.J.; Juhász, C.; Mittal, S. Investigation of the aryl hydrocarbon receptor and the intrinsic tumoral component of the kynurenine pathway of tryptophan metabolism in primary brain tumors. *J. Neurooncol.* **2018**, *139*, 239–249. [CrossRef]
56. Kim, M.; Tomek, P. Tryptophan: A Rheostat of Cancer Immune Escape Mediated by Immunosuppressive Enzymes IDO1 and TDO. *Front. Immunol.* **2021**, *12*, 636081.

57. The Role of IDO in Brain Tumor Immunotherapy | SpringerLink. Available online: https://link.springer.com/article/10.1007/s1 1060-014-1687-8 (accessed on 15 December 2022).
58. Uyttenhove, C.; Pilotte, L.; Théate, I.; Stroobant, V.; Colau, D.; Parmentier, N.; Boon, T.; van den Eynde, B.J. Evidence for a tumoral immune resistance mechanism based on tryptophan degradation by indoleamine 2,3-dioxygenase. *Nat. Med.* **2003**, *9*, 1269–1274. [CrossRef] [PubMed]
59. Wainwright, D.A.; Balyasnikova, I.V.; Chang, A.L.; Ahmed, A.U.; Moon, K.-S.; Auffinger, B.; Tobias, A.L.; Han, Y.; Lesniak, M.S. IDO expression in brain tumors increases the recruitment of regulatory T cells and negatively impacts survival. *Clin. Cancer Res. Off. J. Am. Assoc. Cancer Res.* **2012**, *18*, 6110–6121. [CrossRef]
60. Locasale, J.W.; Melman, T.; Song, S.; Yang, X.; Swanson, K.D.; Cantley, L.C.; Wong, E.T.; Asara, J.M. Metabolomics of Human Cerebrospinal Fluid Identifies Signatures of Malignant Glioma*. *Mol. Cell. Proteom.* **2012**, *11*, M111.014688. [CrossRef]
61. Mitsuka, K.; Kawataki, T.; Satoh, E.; Asahara, T.; Horikoshi, T.; Kinouchi, H. Expression of indoleamine 2,3-dioxygenase and correlation with pathological malignancy in gliomas. *Neurosurgery* **2013**, *72*, 1031–1038; discussion 1038–1039. [CrossRef]
62. Campesato, L.F.; Budhu, S.; Tchaicha, J.; Weng, C.-H.; Gigoux, M.; Cohen, I.J.; Redmond, D.; Mangarin, L.; Pourpe, S.; Liu, C.; et al. Blockade of the AHR restricts a Treg-macrophage suppressive axis induced by L-Kynurenine. *Nat. Commun.* **2020**, *11*, 4011. [CrossRef] [PubMed]
63. Fallarino, F.; Grohmann, U.; Vacca, C.; Bianchi, R.; Orabona, C.; Spreca, A.; Fioretti, M.C.; Puccetti, P. T cell apoptosis by tryptophan catabolism. *Cell Death Differ.* **2002**, *9*, 1069–1077. [CrossRef] [PubMed]
64. Munn, D.H.; Sharma, M.D.; Baban, B.; Harding, H.P.; Zhang, Y.; Ron, D.; Mellor, A.L. GCN2 kinase in T cells mediates proliferative arrest and anergy induction in response to indoleamine 2,3-dioxygenase. *Immunity* **2005**, *22*, 633–642. [CrossRef]
65. van Baren, N.; Van den Eynde, B.J. Tumoral Immune Resistance Mediated by Enzymes That Degrade Tryptophan. *Cancer Immunol. Res.* **2015**, *3*, 978–985. [CrossRef] [PubMed]
66. Munn, D.H.; Shafizadeh, E.; Attwood, J.T.; Bondarev, I.; Pashine, A.; Mellor, A.L. Inhibition of T cell proliferation by macrophage tryptophan catabolism. *J. Exp. Med.* **1999**, *189*, 1363–1372. [CrossRef] [PubMed]
67. Brandacher, G.; Perathoner, A.; Ladurner, R.; Schneeberger, S.; Obrist, P.; Winkler, C.; Werner, E.R.; Werner-Felmayer, G.; Weiss, H.G.; G√∂Bel, G.; et al. Prognostic value of indoleamine 2,3-dioxygenase expression in colorectal cancer: Effect on tumor-infiltrating T cells. *Clin. Cancer Res. Off. J. Am. Assoc. Cancer Res.* **2006**, *12*, 1144–1151. [CrossRef]
68. Yu, J.; Du, W.; Yan, F.; Wang, Y.; Li, H.; Cao, S.; Yu, W.; Shen, C.; Liu, J.; Ren, X. Myeloid-derived suppressor cells suppress antitumor immune responses through IDO expression and correlate with lymph node metastasis in patients with breast cancer. *J. Immunol. Baltim. Md. 1950* **2013**, *190*, 3783–3797. [CrossRef]
69. Holmgaard, R.B.; Zamarin, D.; Li, Y.; Gasmi, B.; Munn, D.H.; Allison, J.P.; Merghoub, T.; Wolchok, J.D. Tumor-expressed IDO recruits and activates MDSCs in a Treg-dependent manner. *Cell Rep.* **2015**, *13*, 412–424. [CrossRef]
70. Beatty, G.L.; O'Dwyer, P.J.; Clark, J.; Shi, J.G.; Newton, R.C.; Schaub, R.; Maleski, J.; Leopold, L.; Gajewski, T. Phase I study of the safety, pharmacokinetics (PK), and pharmacodynamics (PD) of the oral inhibitor of indoleamine 2,3-dioxygenase (IDO1) INCB024360 in patients (pts) with advanced malignancies. *J. Clin. Oncol.* **2013**, *31*, 3025. [CrossRef]
71. Opitz, C.A.; Litzenburger, U.M.; Sahm, F.; Ott, M.; Tritschler, I.; Trump, S.; Schumacher, T.; Jestaedt, L.; Schrenk, D.; Weller, M.; et al. An endogenous tumour-promoting ligand of the human aryl hydrocarbon receptor. *Nature* **2011**, *478*, 197–203. [CrossRef]
72. Moyer, B.J.; Rojas, I.Y.; Murray, I.A.; Lee, S.; Hazlett, H.F.; Perdew, G.H.; Tomlinson, C.R. Indoleamine 2,3-dioxygenase 1 (IDO1) inhibitors activate the aryl hydrocarbon receptor. *Toxicol. Appl. Pharmacol.* **2017**, *323*, 74–80. [CrossRef] [PubMed]
73. Wirth, L.J.; Burtness, B.; Mehra, R.; Bauman, J.R.; Lee, J.; Smith, N.M.S.; Lefranc-Torres, A.; Westra, W.H.; Bishop, J.A.; Faquin, W.C.; et al. IDO1 as a mechanism of adaptive immune resistance to anti-PD1 monotherapy in HNSCC. *J. Clin. Oncol.* **2017**, *35*, 6053. [CrossRef]
74. Botticelli, A.; Cerbelli, B.; Lionetto, L.; Zizzari, I.; Salati, M.; Pisano, A.; Federica, M.; Simmaco, M.; Nuti, M.; Marchetti, P. Can IDO activity predict primary resistance to anti-PD-1 treatment in NSCLC? *J. Transl. Med.* **2018**, *16*, 219. [CrossRef] [PubMed]
75. Holmgaard, R.B.; Zamarin, D.; Munn, D.H.; Wolchok, J.D.; Allison, J.P. Indoleamine 2,3-dioxygenase is a critical resistance mechanism in antitumor T cell immunotherapy targeting CTLA-4. *J. Exp. Med.* **2013**, *210*, 1389–1402. [CrossRef]
76. Wainwright, D.A.; Chang, A.L.; Dey, M.; Balyasnikova, I.V.; Kim, C.K.; Tobias, A.; Cheng, Y.; Kim, J.W.; Qiao, J.; Zhang, L.; et al. Durable therapeutic efficacy utilizing combinatorial blockade against IDO, CTLA-4, and PD-L1 in mice with brain tumors. *Clin. Cancer Res. Off. J. Am. Assoc. Cancer Res.* **2014**, *20*, 5290–5301. [CrossRef] [PubMed]
77. Long, G.V.; Dummer, R.; Hamid, O.; Gajewski, T.; Caglevic, C.; Dalle, S.; Arance, A.; Carlino, M.; Grob, J.-J.; Kim, T.M.; et al. Epacadostat (E) plus pembrolizumab (P) versus pembrolizumab alone in patients (pts) with unresectable or metastatic melanoma: Results of the phase 3 ECHO-301/KEYNOTE-252 study. *J. Clin. Oncol.* **2018**, *36*, 108. [CrossRef]
78. Fujiwara, Y.; Kato, S.; Nesline, M.K.; Conroy, J.M.; DePietro, P.; Pabla, S.; Kurzrock, R. Indoleamine 2,3-dioxygenase (IDO) inhibitors and cancer immunotherapy. *Cancer Treat. Rev.* **2022**, *110*, 102461. [CrossRef]
79. Zhai, L.; Bell, A.; Ladomersky, E.; Lauing, K.L.; Bollu, L.; Nguyen, B.; Genet, M.; Kim, M.; Chen, P.; Mi, X.; et al. Tumor Cell IDO Enhances Immune Suppression and Decreases Survival Independent of Tryptophan Metabolism in Glioblastoma. *Clin. Cancer Res.* **2021**, *27*, 6514–6528. [CrossRef]
80. Kesarwani, P.; Prabhu, A.; Kant, S.; Chinnaiyan, P. Metabolic remodeling contributes towards an immune-suppressive phenotype in glioblastoma. *Cancer Immunol. Immunother.* **2019**, *68*, 1107–1120. [CrossRef]

81. Pascual, G.; Avgustinova, A.; Mejetta, S.; Martín, M.; Castellanos, A.; Attolini, C.S.-O.; Berenguer, A.; Prats, N.; Toll, A.; Hueto, J.A.; et al. Targeting metastasis-initiating cells through the fatty acid receptor CD36. *Nature* **2017**, *541*, 41–45. [CrossRef]
82. Hoang-Minh, L.B.; Siebzehnrubl, F.; Yang, C.; Suzuki-Hatano, S.; Dajac, K.; Loche, T.; Andrews, N.; Massari, M.S.; Patel, J.; Amin, K.; et al. Infiltrative and drug-resistant slow-cycling cells support metabolic heterogeneity in glioblastoma. *EMBO J.* **2018**, *37*, e98772. [CrossRef] [PubMed]
83. Shakya, S.; Gromovsky, A.D.; Hale, J.S.; Knudsen, A.M.; Prager, B.; Wallace, L.C.; Penalva, L.O.F.; Ivanova, P.; Brown, H.A.; Kristensen, B.W.; et al. Altered lipid metabolism marks glioblastoma stem and non-stem cells in separate tumor niches. *Acta Neuropathol. Commun.* **2021**, *9*, 101. [CrossRef] [PubMed]
84. Cheng, X.; Geng, F.; Pan, M.; Wu, X.; Zhong, Y.; Wang, C.; Tian, Z.; Cheng, C.; Zhang, R.; Puduvalli, V.; et al. Targeting DGAT1 Ameliorates Glioblastoma by Increasing Fat Catabolism and Oxidative Stress. *Cell Metab.* **2020**, *32*, 229–242.e8. [CrossRef] [PubMed]
85. Taïb, B.; Aboussalah, A.M.; Moniruzzaman, M.; Chen, S.; Haughey, N.J.; Kim, S.F.; Ahima, R.S. Lipid accumulation and oxidation in glioblastoma multiforme. *Sci. Rep.* **2019**, *9*, 19593. [CrossRef] [PubMed]
86. Sun, P.; Xia, S.; Lal, B.; Shi, X.; Yang, K.S.; A Watkins, P.; Laterra, J. Lipid metabolism enzyme ACSVL3 supports glioblastoma stem cell maintenance and tumorigenicity. *BMC Cancer* **2014**, *14*, 401. [CrossRef] [PubMed]
87. Wu, F.; Zhao, Z.; Chai, R.C.; Liu, Y.Q.; Li, G.Z.; Jiang, H.Y.; Jiang, T. Prognostic power of a lipid metabolism gene panel for diffuse gliomas. *J. Cell. Mol. Med.* **2019**, *23*, 7741–7748. [CrossRef]
88. Michalek, R.D.; Gerriets, V.A.; Jacobs, S.R.; Macintyre, A.N.; MacIver, N.J.; Mason, E.F.; Sullivan, S.A.; Nichols, A.G.; Rathmell, J.C. Cutting edge: Distinct glycolytic and lipid oxidative metabolic programs are essential for effector and regulatory CD4+ T cell subsets. *J. Immunol. Baltim. Md. 1950* **2011**, *186*, 3299–3303. [CrossRef]
89. Howie, D.; Ten Bokum, A.; Necula, A.S.; Cobbold, S.P.; Waldmann, H. The Role of Lipid Metabolism in T Lymphocyte Differentiation and Survival. *Front. Immunol.* **2017**, *8*, 1949. [CrossRef]
90. Abuhusain, H.J.; Matin, A.; Qiao, Q.; Shen, H.; Kain, N.; Day, B.W.; Stringer, B.; Daniels, B.; Laaksonen, M.A.; Teo, C.; et al. A Metabolic Shift Favoring Sphingosine 1-Phosphate at the Expense of Ceramide Controls Glioblastoma Angiogenesis. *J. Biol. Chem.* **2013**, *288*, 37355–37364. [CrossRef]
91. Kempkes, R.W.M.; Joosten, I.; Koenen, H.J.P.M.; He, X. Metabolic Pathways Involved in Regulatory T Cell Functionality. *Front. Immunol.* **2019**, *10*, 2839. [CrossRef]
92. Wang, H.; Franco, F.; Tsui, Y.-C.; Xie, X.; Trefny, M.P.; Zappasodi, R.; Mohmood, S.R.; Fernández-García, J.; Tsai, C.-H.; Schulze, I.; et al. CD36-mediated metabolic adaptation supports regulatory T cell survival and function in tumors. *Nat. Immunol.* **2020**, *21*, 298–308. [CrossRef] [PubMed]
93. Hossain, F.; Al-Khami, A.A.; Wyczechowska, D.; Hernandez, C.; Zheng, L.; Reiss, K.; Del Valle, L.; Trillo-Tinoco, J.; Maj, T.; Zou, W.; et al. Inhibition of Fatty Acid Oxidation Modulates Immunosuppressive Functions of Myeloid-Derived Suppressor Cells and Enhances Cancer Therapies. *Cancer Immunol. Res.* **2015**, *3*, 1236–1247. [CrossRef] [PubMed]
94. Turubanova, V.D.; Balalaeva, I.V.; Mishchenko, T.A.; Catanzaro, E.; Alzeibak, R.; Peskova, N.N.; Efimova, I.; Bachert, C.; Mitroshina, E.V.; Krysko, O.; et al. Immunogenic cell death induced by a new photodynamic therapy based on photosens and photodithazine. *J. Immunother. Cancer* **2019**, *7*, 350. [CrossRef]
95. Dastmalchi, F.; Karachi, A.; Yang, C.; Azari, H.; Sayour, E.J.; Dechkovskaia, A.; Vlasak, A.L.; Saia, M.E.; Lovaton, R.E.; Mitchell, D.A.; et al. Sarcosine promotes trafficking of dendritic cells and improves efficacy of anti-tumor dendritic cell vaccines via CXC chemokine family signaling. *J. Immunother. Cancer* **2019**, *7*, 321. [CrossRef]
96. Jiang, N.; Xie, B.; Xiao, W.; Fan, M.; Xu, S.; Duan, Y.; Hamsafar, Y.; Evans, A.C.; Huang, J.; Zhou, W.; et al. Fatty acid oxidation fuels glioblastoma radioresistance with CD47-mediated immune evasion. *Nat. Commun.* **2022**, *13*, 1511. [CrossRef]
97. Miska, J.; Chandel, N.S. Targeting fatty acid metabolism in glioblastoma. *J. Clin. Investig.* **2023**, *133*, e163448. [CrossRef] [PubMed]
98. Chiocca, E.A.; Yu, J.S.; Lukas, R.V.; Solomon, I.H.; Ligon, K.L.; Nakashima, H.; Triggs, D.A.; Reardon, D.A.; Wen, P.; Stopa, B.M.; et al. Regulatable interleukin-12 gene therapy in patients with recurrent high-grade glioma: Results of a phase 1 trial. *Sci. Transl. Med.* **2019**, *11*, eaaw5680. [CrossRef]
99. Iorgulescu, J.B.; Gokhale, P.C.; Speranza, M.C.; Eschle, B.K.; Poitras, M.J.; Wilkens, M.K.; Soroko, K.M.; Chhoeu, C.; Knott, A.; Gao, Y.; et al. Concurrent Dexamethasone Limits the Clinical Benefit of Immune Checkpoint Blockade in Glioblastoma. *Clin. Cancer Res. Off. J. Am. Assoc. Cancer Res.* **2021**, *27*, 276–287. [CrossRef]
100. Louveau, A.; Smirnov, I.; Keyes, T.J.; Eccles, J.D.; Rouhani, S.J.; Peske, J.D.; Derecki, N.C.; Castle, D.; Mandell, J.W.; Lee, K.S.; et al. Structural and functional features of central nervous system lymphatic vessels. *Nature* **2015**, *523*, 337–341. [CrossRef]
101. Nduom, E.K.; Weller, M.; Heimberger, A.B. Immunosuppressive mechanisms in glioblastoma. *Neuro-Oncol.* **2015**, *17* (Suppl. S7), vii9–vii14. [CrossRef]
102. Lim, M.; Xia, Y.; Bettegowda, C.; Weller, M. Current state of immunotherapy for glioblastoma. *Nat. Rev. Clin. Oncol.* **2018**, *15*, 422–442. [CrossRef] [PubMed]
103. Weller, M.; Butowski, N.; Tran, D.D.; Recht, L.D.; Lim, M.; Hirte, H.; Ashby, L.; Mechtler, L.; Goldlust, S.A.; Iwamoto, F.; et al. Rindopepimut with temozolomide for patients with newly diagnosed, EGFRvIII-expressing glioblastoma (ACT IV): A randomised, double-blind, international phase 3 trial. *Lancet Oncol.* **2017**, *18*, 1373–1385. [PubMed]

104. Liau, L.M.; Ashkan, K.; Tran, D.; Campian, J.; Trusheim, J.; Cobbs, C.; Heth, J.; Salacz, M.; Taylor, S.; D'Andre, S.D.; et al. First results on survival from a large Phase 3 clinical trial of an autologous dendritic cell vaccine in newly diagnosed glioblastoma. *J. Transl. Med.* **2018**, *16*, 142. [CrossRef] [PubMed]
105. Lukas, R.V.; Rodon, J.; Becker, K.; Wong, E.T.; Shih, K.; Touat, M.; Fassò, M.; Osborne, S.; Molinero, L.; O'Hear, C.; et al. Clinical activity and safety of atezolizumab in patients with recurrent glioblastoma. *J. Neurooncol.* **2018**, *140*, 317–328.
106. Renner, K.; Bruss, C.; Schnell, A.; Koehl, G.; Becker, H.M.; Fante, M.; Menevse, A.-N.; Kauer, N.; Blazquez, R.; Hacker, L.; et al. Restricting Glycolysis Preserves T Cell Effector Functions and Augments Checkpoint Therapy. *Cell Rep.* **2019**, *29*, 135–150.e9.
107. Todo, T.; Ito, H.; Ino, Y.; Ohtsu, H.; Ota, Y.; Shibahara, J.; Tanaka, M. Intratumoral oncolytic herpes virus G47Δ for residual or recurrent glioblastoma: A phase 2 trial. *Nat. Med.* **2022**, *28*, 1630–1639.
108. Woller, N.; Gürlevik, E.; Fleischmann-Mundt, B.; Schumacher, A.; Knocke, S.; Kloos, A.M.; Saborowski, M.; Geffers, R.; Manns, M.P.; Wirth, T.C.; et al. Viral Infection of Tumors Overcomes Resistance to PD-1-immunotherapy by Broadening Neoantigenome-directed T-cell Responses. *Mol. Ther. J. Am. Soc. Gene Ther.* **2015**, *23*, 1630–1640. [CrossRef]
109. O'Rourke, D.M.; Nasrallah, M.; Desai, A.; Melenhorst, J.; Mansfield, K.; Morrissette, J.; Martinez-Lage, M.; Brem, S.; Maloney, E.; Shen, A.; et al. A single dose of peripherally infused EGFRvIII-directed CAR T cells mediates antigen loss and induces adaptive resistance in patients with recurrent glioblastoma. *Sci. Transl. Med.* **2017**, *9*, eaaa0984. [CrossRef]
110. Nabe, S.; Yamada, T.; Suzuki, J.; Toriyama, K.; Yasuoka, T.; Kuwahara, M.; Shiraishi, A.; Takenaka, K.; Yasukawa, M.; Yamashita, M. Reinforce the antitumor activity of CD8+ T cells via glutamine restriction. *Cancer Sci.* **2018**, *109*, 3737–3750. [CrossRef]
111. Sukumar, M.; Liu, J.; Ji, Y.; Subramanian, M.; Crompton, J.G.; Yu, Z.; Roychoudhuri, R.; Palmer, D.C.; Muranski, P.; Karoly, E.D.; et al. Inhibiting glycolytic metabolism enhances CD8+ T cell memory and antitumor function. *J. Clin. Investig.* **2013**, *123*, 4479–4488.
112. Hajji, N.; Garcia-Revilla, J.; Soto, M.S.; Perryman, R.; Symington, J.; Quarles, C.C.; Healey, D.R.; Guo, Y.; Orta-Vázquez, M.L.; Mateos-Cordero, S.; et al. Arginine deprivation alters microglial polarity and synergizes with radiation to eradicate non-arginine-auxotrophic glioblastoma tumors. *J. Clin. Investig.* **2022**, *132*, e142137. [CrossRef]
113. Bunse, L.; Pusch, S.; Bunse, T.; Sahm, F.; Sanghvi, K.; Friedrich, M.; Alansary, D.; Sonner, J.K.; Green, E.; Deumelandt, K.; et al. Suppression of antitumor T cell immunity by the oncometabolite (R)-2-hydroxyglutarate. *Nat. Med.* **2018**, *24*, 1192–1203. [CrossRef]
114. Safaee, M.M.; Wang, E.J.; Jain, S.; Chen, J.-S.; Gill, S.; Zheng, A.C.; Garcia, J.H.; Beniwal, A.S.; Tran, Y.; Nguyen, A.T.; et al. CD97 is associated with mitogenic pathway activation, metabolic reprogramming, and immune microenvironment changes in glioblastoma. *Sci. Rep.* **2022**, *12*, 1464. [CrossRef]

Disclaimer/Publisher's Note: The statements, opinions and data contained in all publications are solely those of the individual author(s) and contributor(s) and not of MDPI and/or the editor(s). MDPI and/or the editor(s) disclaim responsibility for any injury to people or property resulting from any ideas, methods, instructions or products referred to in the content.

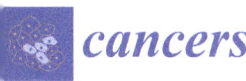

Review

Targeted Therapy of Interleukin-34 as a Promising Approach to Overcome Cancer Therapy Resistance

Giovanni Monteleone [1,2,*], Eleonora Franzè [1], Claudia Maresca [1], Marco Colella [1], Teresa Pacifico [1] and Carmine Stolfi [1]

[1] Department of Systems Medicine, University of Rome "Tor Vergata", 00133 Rome, Italy
[2] Gastroenterology Unit, Policlinico Universitario Tor Vergata, 00133 Rome, Italy
* Correspondence: gi.monteleone@med.uniroma2.it; Tel.: +39-06-20903702; Fax: +39-06-72596158

Simple Summary: In the last decades, identification of the factors/mechanisms leading to cancer development has advanced the way clinicians combat this pathology. Indeed, the use of adjuvant chemotherapies and targeted therapies has markedly contributed to prolonging the survival of cancer patients. Unfortunately, however, many cancer patients experience primary or acquired resistance to these therapies, and this has been linked to various factors, including the presence of a tumor microenvironment that restrains the anti-tumor immunity. In this article, we describe the ability of interleukin-34, a protein produced in excess in many cancers, to modulate the function of various immune cells, with the downstream effect of generating a tumor microenvironment that sustains cancer cell growth and, at the same time, enhances the resistance of cancers against chemotherapy and immunotherapy.

Abstract: Chemotherapy and immunotherapy have markedly improved the management of several malignancies. However, not all cancer patients respond primarily to such therapies, and others can become resistant during treatment. Thus, identification of the factors/mechanisms underlying cancer resistance to such treatments could help develop novel effective therapeutic compounds. Tumor-associated macrophages (TAMs), myeloid-derived suppressor cells (MDSCs), and regulatory T cells (Tregs) are major components of the suppressive tumor microenvironment and are critical drivers of immunosuppression, creating a tumor-promoting and drug-resistant niche. In this regard, therapeutic strategies to tackle immunosuppressive cells are an interesting option to increase anti-tumor immune responses and overcome the occurrence of drug resistance. Accumulating evidence indicates that interleukin-34 (IL-34), a cytokine produced by cancer cells, and/or TAMs act as a linker between induction of a tumor-associated immunosuppressive microenvironment and drug resistance. In this article, we review the current data supporting the role of IL-34 in the differentiation/function of immune suppressive cells and, hence, in the mechanisms leading to therapeutic resistance in various cancers.

Keywords: immunotherapy; chemotherapy; CSF1R; tumor-associated macrophages; myeloid-derived suppressor cells

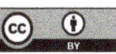

1. Introduction

Cancer is one of the major public health problems worldwide. It has been estimated that in 2022, nearly 2 million new cancer cases and more than half a million cancer deaths could occur in the United States [1]. However, it is noteworthy that the 5-year relative survival rate for all cancers combined has increased continuously in the last 3 decades, because of the better understanding of the factors/mechanisms driving cancer development. Hence, reduced exposure of the host to pro-carcinogenic insults (e.g., smoking), better surgical techniques, and accurate screening programs (e.g., mammography for women aged 45 to 74 for breast cancer; quantitative fecal immunochemical testing and colonoscopy for individuals between 50 and 74 years for colorectal cancer; prostate-specific antigen (PSA) testing for prostate cancer; esophagogastroduodenoscopy and the *Helicobacter pylori* test in regions with high gastric cancer incidence and mortality; the blood test for the CA 125 tumor marker in combination with ultrasound for women with a "high-risk" family history of ovarian cancer; and abdominal ultrasonography in combination with biomarkers, such as α-fetoprotein, in patients with a "high risk" of developing hepatocellular carcinoma (HCC), such as those with cirrhosis, including patients with hepatitis B virus (HBV) and hepatitis C virus (HCV) infections, as well as with nonalcoholic fatty liver disease) allow early detection of neoplastic lesions [1].

The decline in cancer death rate relies also on improvements in treatment protocols, including adjuvant chemotherapies and targeted therapies. For instance, the use of tyrosine-kinase inhibitors has markedly increased the 5-year relative survival rate of patients with chronic myeloid leukemia. Indeed, analysis of studies conducted between 2000 and 2012 showed that, for the whole population of patients with chronic myeloid leukemia in the chronic phase, the 5-year survival was only slightly lower than that of the matched general population [2]. More recently, immunotherapy (i.e., antibodies blocking programmed cell death protein 1 (PD-1) and/or cytotoxic T-lymphocyte-associated protein-4 (CTLA-4)) has changed the landscape of systemic therapy for metastatic solid tumors (e.g., metastatic melanoma, non-small-cell lung cancer, and genitourinary cancers), thereby improving the survival of cancer patients who were resistant to traditional therapies [3–6]. Concerning CTLA-4 immune checkpoint inhibitors, in addition to the fully human monoclonal IgG1 antibody ipilimumab (Yervoy), approved in March 2011 and currently used for the treatment of several cancers (e.g., melanoma, renal cell carcinoma (RCC), microsatellite instability-high (MSI-H) or mismatch repair deficient (dMMR) metastatic colorectal cancer (CRC), HCC, and non-small cell lung cancer (NSCLC)) [7], the Food and Drug Administration (FDA) has recently approved tremelimumab (Imjudo), a fully human monoclonal IgG2 antibody, as part of a first-line immunotherapy combination with the PD-L1 blocker durvalumab for non-resectable HCC [8].

To date, the FDA has approved three anti-PD-1 antibodies: pembrolizumab (Keytruda), nivolumab (Opdivo), and cemiplimab (Libtayo) [9]. Pembrolizumab, a humanized IgG4 antibody, was initially approved in September 2014, following the results of the KEYNOTE-001 clinical trial (clinicaltrials.gov/NCT01295827) studying patients with unresectable or metastatic melanoma and patients with NSCLC. Several additional indications without biomarker requirements have been approved since then, including indications for the treatment of patients with recurrent or metastatic cutaneous squamous cell carcinoma, adult and pediatric patients with refractory classical Hodgkin's lymphoma, individuals with advanced RCC, mediastinal large B cell lymphoma, and HCC, locally advanced or metastatic urothelial carcinoma for patients who are not eligible for chemotherapy containing cisplatin or who have had disease progression during or after platinum-containing chemotherapy [9].

Nivolumab, a fully human IgG4 monoclonal antibody, was approved following the pivotal trial CheckMate-037, in December 2014, for the treatment of patients with non-resectable metastatic melanoma who have experienced disease progression following ipilimumab and, if *BRAFV600* mutation positive, a BRAF inhibitor [10]. Since then, new indications have been approved, such as for treating patients with metastatic NSCLC with progression on or after platinum-based chemotherapy; for the treatment, either alone or in combination with ipilimumab, of patients with unresectable/metastatic melanoma; for treating individuals with advanced RCC, classical Hodgkin's lymphoma, recurrent or metastatic squamous cell carcinoma of the head and neck (HNSCC), locally advanced or metastatic urothelial carcinoma, HCC, or esophageal squamous cell carcinoma (ESCC); and for patients with unresectable malignant pleural mesothelioma [9].

Cemiplimab (Libtayo), a human IgG4 monoclonal antibody, was approved in 2018 for treating patients with metastatic cutaneous squamous cell carcinoma (CSCC) or locally advanced CSCC who are not candidates for curative surgery or radiation [11], and later for the treatment of NSCLC [9].

These approaches are based upon the demonstration that many cancers promote dysregulation of immune-checkpoint proteins (e.g., PD-1), which are physiologically crucial for limiting abnormal T-cell-driven immune responses [12]. Unlike many antibodies used for cancer therapy, immune checkpoint blockers do not target cancer cells directly; instead, they target lymphocyte receptors or their ligands, with the downstream effect of enhancing T cell-dependent antitumor activity [13,14].

Unfortunately, however, many cancer patients experience primary (existing before treatment) or acquired (generated after therapy) resistance to these drugs [15].

2. Mechanisms of Cancer Resistance to Standard Therapy and Immunotherapy

Drug resistance in cancer is a well-known phenomenon that occurs when cancer cells are, or become, tolerant to pharmaceutical treatment. Resistance to anticancer drugs is caused by a variety of factors, including genetic mutations and/or epigenetic changes, conserved but overregulated drug efflux, and various other cellular and molecular mechanisms.

Primary resistance can be caused by: (i) pre-existing (hereditary) mutations resulting in decreased responsiveness of cancer cells to both chemo- and immunotherapy (e.g., lack of the estrogen receptor (ER), progesterone receptor (PR), and amplification of HER-2/Neu in triple negative breast cancer cells [16] and HER2 overexpression resulting in a poorer outcome of cisplatin treatment in gastric cancer patients [17]); (ii) tumor heterogeneity in which pre-existing insensitive subpopulations, including cancer stem cells, will be selected after drug treatment, thus leading to relapse in later stages of the therapeutic regimen; and (iii) activation of intrinsic pathways used to defend the cell against environmental toxins (in this case, against anticancer drugs) (e.g., ATP binding cassette (ABC) transporter-mediated drug efflux [18] and glutathione (GSH)/glutathione S-transferase system [19] working to reduce cellular drug accumulation or detoxify drug treated cancer cells, respectively]

Acquired resistance can be identified by a gradual reduction in the anticancer efficacy of a given drug after treatment. Acquired resistance can be the result of: (i) activation of a second proto-oncogene that becomes the new driver gene; (ii) mutations or modified expression levels of the drug targets; and (iii) dynamic changes in the tumor microenvironment (TME)—that is, the surrounding space composed of immune cells, stroma, and vasculature—in the course of treatment [20].

With regard to the latter point, TME can mediate resistance to anticancer drugs through several mechanisms, including preventing immune clearance of tumor cells, inhibiting drug absorption, and stimulating paracrine growth factors to signal cancer cell growth [20]. For example, blockade of an immune-checkpoint protein can induce tumor regression only when there is a pre-existing antitumor immune response to be 'unlocked' when the pathway is blocked. In contrast, the presence of an immunosuppressive microenvironment, which inhibits intratumoral immune responses, can eventually hamper the efficacy of immunotherapy [21]. Recent studies have also shown that activation of the immune system is one of the mechanisms underlying the benefit of cytotoxic chemotherapy. Indeed, several chemotherapeutics trigger cancer cell death, thus promoting the release of a variety of factors that boost robust anti-tumor immune responses [22,23]. These discoveries have provided the rationale for many studies in cancer patients combining immune agents with chemotherapy. On the other hand, there is evidence that chemotherapy-treated cancer cells can release molecules, which in turn promote differentiation and activation of tumor-associated macrophages (TAMs) and myeloid-derived suppressor cells (MDSCs), thereby contributing to generating a tumor microenvironment that restrains the anti-tumor immunity [24].

One of such molecules is interleukin-34 (IL-34), a cytokine produced by cancer cells, TAMs, and stromal cells, which acts as a linker between induction of a tumor-associated immunosuppressive microenvironment and chemo/immunotherapy resistance.

In this article, we review the available evidence supporting the role of IL-34 in promoting cancer resistance to chemotherapy and immunotherapy.

3. Expression of IL-34 and IL-34 Receptors in Cancer

The functions of IL-34 are mediated by three distinct receptors or co-receptors, namely, CSF1R (CD115), CD138 (syndecan-1), and protein-tyrosine phosphatase zeta (PTP-ζ) [25–28]. Since its discovery, IL-34 has been indicated as a growth factor for monocytes, and it is now evident that IL-34 effects on monocyte viability occur through a mechanism independent of colony-stimulating factor 1 (CSF1), also known as the macrophage CSF (M-CSF), another ligand of CSF1R [25]. IL-34 and CSF1 bind to overlapping regions of CSF1R, but the two ligands can trigger distinct intracellular pathways, likely as a result of the different stability of the interaction of each cytokine with CSF1R [26,29–31]. This would explain the non-redundant functions of IL-34 and CSF1 on the survival, proliferation, and differentiation of monocytes/macrophages [29]. The differences between the two cytokines in modulating monocyte/macrophage functions could also be linked to the fact that, unlike IL-34, CSF1 does not interact with CD138 and PTP-ζ [27,28].

In physiological conditions, IL-34 RNA is expressed by many organs and tissues, but its protein levels are more pronounced in lymphoid tissues (i.e., spleen), the brain, and the skin [32–34]. In addition to monocytes/macrophages, many other cells produce IL-34 (e.g., neurons, peritubular cells, suprabasal keratinocytes, theca cells, Leydig cells, and fibroblasts) [35–38]. Recent studies have shown that IL-34 production is deregulated in many infectious, inflammatory, and neoplastic disorders, and they unveiled the contribution of the cytokine to several pathological states [39–41]. One of the first studies documenting the over-expression of IL-34 in neoplastic diseases was provided by Baud'huin and colleagues, who reported elevated levels of the cytokine in giant cell tumor (a benign bone tumor) and documented the ability of IL-34 to stimulate osteoclastogenesis via a CSF1-independent CSF1R activation [42]. Afterward, many authors have contributed to delineating the role of IL-34 in the control of the function of several cell types that sustain cancer initiation and progression (Figure 1).

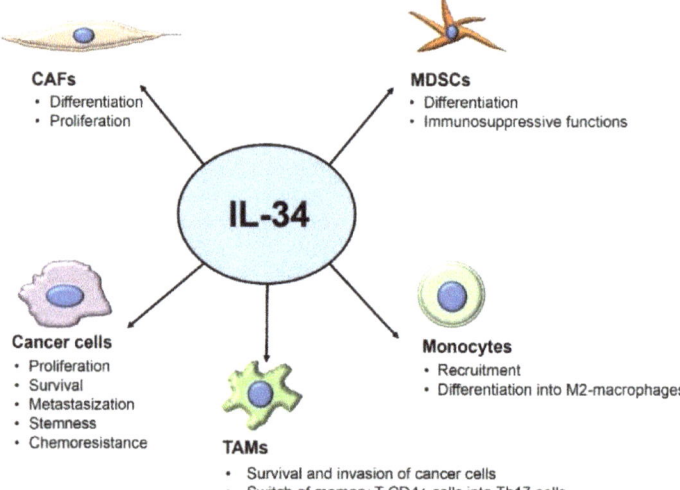

Figure 1. Overview of the tumor-promoting effects of IL-34 on its target cells. Arrows indicate the targets of IL-34 and the IL-34-driven tumor effects. Abbreviations: CAFs: cancer-associated fibroblasts; MDSCs: myeloid-derived suppressor cells; TAMs: tumor-associated macrophages.

IL-34 is overexpressed by cancers developing in the alimentary tract, such as esophageal squamous, gastric cancer, and CRC, as well as by ovarian, lung, hepatocellular, and pancreatic cancers, and metastatic melanoma (Table 1).

Table 1. Expression and function of IL-34 in various human cancers.

Cancer	System	IL-34 Functions	References
Colorectal	Cancer cell line	-Increases cell proliferation and invasion -Enhances resistance to oxaliplatin-induced death	[43]
	TAMs	-Induces type 2 macrophage markers -Enhances IL-6 production	[44]
	CAFs	-Promotes CAFs differentiation and proliferation	[45]
Breast	TAMs	-Enhances proliferation, Chemotaxis, and tumor infiltration	[46]
	Cancer cells	-Enhances metastatic properties	[47]
Ovarian	Macrophages and TAMs	-Promotes the switch of non-Th17 committed memory T cells into conventional Th17 cells	[48]
	Cancer cells	-Promotes survival of chemoresistant cancer cells	[49]
	TAMs	-Enhances the tumorigenic and immunosuppressive functions	[50]
Hepatocellular carcinoma	Cancer cell line	-Increases growth and metastatic properties	[51]
	TAMs	-Increases TGF-β production	[51]
Hepatoblastoma	Cancer cell line	-Increases cell growth and chemoresistance	[52]
	TAMs	-Promotes M2 polarization -Stimulates production of IL-6 -Enhances chemotaxis and tumor infiltration	[52]
Cholangiocarcinoma	TAMs	-Induces differentiation and activation and promotes tumor infiltration	[53]
	Cancer stem cells	-Promotes stemness features	[53]
Osteosarcoma	Cancer cells	-Induces cell proliferation and metastasis	[54]
	TAMs	-Increases recruitment into tumor tissue	[54]
	Endothelial cells	-Stimulates proliferation and vascular cord formation	[54]
Multiple myeloma	CD141$^+$Monocytes	-Accelerates multiple myeloma-induced osteoclast formation	[55]
Castration-resistant prostate cancer	TAMs	-Induces differentiation and chemotaxis and tumor infiltration	[56]
Adult T-cell leukemia/lymphoma	Cancer cell line	-Increases proliferation	[57]
Gastric cancer	Cancer cells line	-Increases proliferation, clone formation, migration, and invasion	[58]
Acute monocytic leukemia	Cancer cell line	-Increases proliferation and colony formation	[59]
Pancreatic ductal adenocarcinoma	Portal blood MDSCs	-Promotes differentiation and immune suppressive functions	[60]

Abbreviations: TAMs: tumor-associated macrophages; CAFs: cancer-associated fibroblasts; MDSCs: myeloid-derived suppressor cells.

IL-34 is also highly expressed in triple-negative breast cancer (TNBC), which is characterized by the lack of therapeutic receptors, epidermal growth factor-related 2, progesterone receptor, and estrogen receptor on the cell surface [61]. Although further work is needed to clarify the exact contribution of IL-34 in the initiation and progression of each of these malignancies, the overall evidence indicates that the expression of IL-34 in such tumors correlates with their metastatic behavior and poor survival of the patients [61]. This is in line with experimentation in mouse models of tumorigenesis showing a key role of IL-34 in promoting cancer metastasis [62].

4. IL-34 Contributes to Generating a Tumor Microenvironment That Restrains the Anti-Tumor Immunity

TAMs constitute the dominant immune cell population in various tumors. TAMs can be functionally divided into two main subtypes (M1-like and M2-like macrophages, respectively), depending on the profile of the molecules synthesized and, hence, their ability to either restrain or promote neoplastic growth and progression [63]. M1-like macrophages are pro-inflammatory and trigger robust T cell- and natural killer cell-mediated anti-tumoral responses, whereas alternatively activated, anti-inflammatory M2-like macrophages contribute to tissue remodeling and stimulate cancer cell growth, invasion, angiogenesis, and tumor metastasis [64]. Moreover, M2-type TAMs play a critical role in the therapeutic resistance of cancers, and increased infiltration of these cells into tumors following chemotherapy represents a hallmark of developing chemoresistance and correlates with poor clinical outcomes [65,66]. Therefore, in recent years, enormous efforts have been made to ascertain factors/mechanisms that promote the differentiation and function of M2-type TAMs, with the ultimate goal to identify new therapeutic targets to overcome chemoresistance. Accumulating evidence suggests that IL-34 could be one of such targets. Support for this hypothesis comes from studies in lung cancer showing that lung cancer cells exposed to chemotherapeutic agents exhibit enhanced NF-kB activation, which in turn sustains elevated production of IL-34 in chemoresistant cells [67]. These findings are in line with the demonstration that chemotherapy-driven NF-kB activation promotes cancer chemoresistance, mainly via the induction of anti-apoptotic genes [68]. Chemoresistant lung cancer cell-derived IL-34 activates an autocrine pathway, which enhances the survival of neoplastic cells, but at the same time, promotes the in vitro differentiation of monocyte-derived M2-polarized macrophages and enhances the immunosuppressive function of TAMs through a C/EBPβ-mediated mechanism [67]. Consistently, studies in a humanized mouse model of lung cancer showed that IL-34-producing chemoresistant tumors exhibit increased numbers of M2-type TAMs and reduced frequencies of tumor-infiltrating cytotoxic CD8+ T cells [67]. Along the same line are the results published by Nakajima and colleagues, who showed that neoadjuvant chemotherapy upregulates the induction of IL-34, but not CSF1, on esophageal squamous cell carcinoma cells. It was also shown that expression of IL-34 was more pronounced in patients not responsive to neoadjuvant chemotherapy than in those who were responsive, and patients with cancers expressing high levels of IL-34 had worse prognoses as compared with patients with IL34-low carcinoma [69]. Furthermore, human esophageal squamous cell carcinoma cell lines treated with 5-fluorouracil/cisplatin expressed high IL-34 and promoted induction of CD163, a marker of M2-type TAMs, in human peripheral blood monocytes [69]. Studies in ovarian cancer confirmed the induction of IL-34 in cancer cells by cytotoxic chemotherapy and the reduced overall survival of patients with high IL-34 expression. Moreover, in a mouse model of ovarian cancer, lack of IL-34 attenuated tumor progression, and this finding was associated with reduced increased infiltration of the tumors with T lymphocytes [49]. In CRC tissues, there is a positive correlation between IL-34 and CD163, and CRC-infiltrating immune cells respond to IL-34 by up-regulating M2-type macrophage-related markers [44]. In the MC38 CRC murine model, selective inhibition of CSF1R reduces the number of CD163+ macrophages [70] and increases the number of cytotoxic CD8+ T-cells within the tumor, thereby delaying tumor growth [71]. MDSCs, a heterogeneous population of immature myeloid cells, are generated in the bone marrow and can terminally differentiate into mature granulocytes, dendritic cells, or macrophages. In pathological conditions, such as cancer, the differentiation of precursor cells is partially blocked, thereby causing the accumulation of immature myeloid cells, defined as MDSCs [72]. Like TAMs, MDSCs constitute an important component of the immunosuppressive tumor microenvironment, and their infiltration into tumors is frequently associated with drug resistance and correlates with poor prognosis. MDSCs promote tumor immune escape via multiple mechanisms, including the production of immunosuppressive cytokines, expression of regulatory factors (e.g., arginase and indoleamine 2,3-dioxygenase), and interaction with and stimulation of other regulatory cells (e.g., Tregs) [73]. In cancer, MDSCs are relevant not only for promoting immunosuppression, but also for enhancing angiogenesis and tumor progression [73,74]. The mechanism of MDSCs-mediated chemoresistance acquisition in cancer is not well known, but recent studies support the contribution of IL-34 in the modulation of MDSCs differentiation and function. Kajihara and colleagues showed that TNBC-derived IL-34 induced differentiation of myeloid stem cells into monocytic MDSCs (M-MDSCs), which recruited Tregs and contributed to the creation of an immunosuppressive microenvironment [75]. At the same time, IL-34 decreased the differentiation of myeloid stem cells into polymorphonuclear MDSCs, thus leading to an acquisition of resistance to chemotherapy. The latter finding seems to rely on the suppression of angiogenesis as a blockade of IL-34 in mice with established tumor induced by the TNBC cell line 4T1, leading to a dramatic increase in vasculature, thereby restoring the penetration of chemotherapeutic agents and tumor sensitivity to paclitaxel (PTX), one of the standard treatments of TNBC. Importantly, analysis of the immune cells infiltrating the tumor showed that combination therapy with PTX and IL-34 blocker was superior to PTX monotherapy in reducing the fraction of M-MDSCs and increasing the number of T cells [75].

Although there is little evidence about the role of IL-34 in the differentiation and action of Tregs in cancer, studies in other systems demonstrated the involvement of IL-34 in human and rat Treg-mediated suppressive functions, as well as the ability of IL-34 to induce in vivo and in vitro $CD4^+$ and $CD8^+$ Tregs through monocytes polarization toward M2-type macrophages [76,77].

Altogether, these data suggest that the pro-tumorigenic action of IL-34 is, at least in part, mediated by the induction of immunosuppressive TAMs.

5. IL-34 and Cancer Immunotherapy

As pointed out above, the blockade of PD-1 and/or CTLA-4 enhances anti-tumor T cell-dependent immune response. However, such a therapeutic strategy does not always associate with benefits in cancer patients due to tumor-intrinsic or -extrinsic mechanisms for escaping immune surveillance [78]. In this regard, an abundance of M2-type TAMs, MDSCs, and Tregs in the tumor tissue contributes to immunotherapy resistance [79–81]. Preliminary evidence suggests that IL-34 signaling could make a contribution to cancer resistance to immunotherapy. Han and colleagues described a clinical case of a patient with metastatic refractory melanoma that acquired resistance to anti-PD-1 immunotherapy and exhibited enhanced expression of IL-34 in refractory melanoma tissues [82]. Studies conducted by Hama and colleagues showed that BALB/c mice inoculated with IL-34-expressing CT26 cells developed tumors resistant to anti-PD-1 antibody treatment. In the same model, combination therapy with anti-PD-1 and anti-CTLA-4 induced substantial tumor growth inhibition, which was further enhanced by anti-IL-34 treatment. Consistently, tumors generated by inoculation of mice with IL-34-deficient CT26 cells exhibited a good response to treatment with anti-PD-1 antibody [83]. The same group transplanted human lung cancer tissue expressing both IL-34 and PD-L1 in immunologically humanized mice to determine the effect of IL-34 neutralization, along with the immune checkpoint blockade, in human tumors. Combination therapy was superior to monotherapy in reducing tumor growth [84]. Indirect evidence comes from studies by Shi and colleagues, who treated mice bearing the CT26 and MC38 colon tumors with a combination of PLX3397 (an oral inhibitor of MCSF1R), anti-PD-1 antibody, and oncolytic viruses (OVs), which promote tumor T-cell infiltration due to their ability to selectively infect and kill tumor cells [85]. Combined treatment enhanced the number of T cells in the tumor and augmented anti-tumor $CD8^+$ T-cell function, thereby conferring tumor control and prolonged survival of mice. In particular, mice treated with PLX3397 exhibited reduced numbers of M2-type TAMs and enhanced response to anti-PD-1 therapy [85]. These observations are in line with findings of other studies showing that the limited efficacy of PD-1 and CTLA-4 antagonists, when used as single agents to restrain cancer growth, can be enhanced by MCSF1R blockers [86] Although these latter findings do not exclude the possibility that some of the benefit seen in animals receiving MCSF1R blockers are due to the inhibition of CSF1 function, the overall data would seem to indicate that IL-34 can target several regulatory cell types within the tumor and favors an anti-inflammatory environment, with the downstream effect of interfering with immunotherapy.

6. Conclusions

Accumulating evidence indicates that IL-34 is produced in many cancers and supports the hypothesis that this cytokine triggers multiple signals that enhance cancer cell growth and diffusion. Nonetheless, it is worth noting that some studies suggest a beneficial role for IL-34 in particular tumor contexts [87–89], thus raising the question of whether the role of IL-34 in cancer is dependent on tumor type, location, or even treatment regimens.

In some cancers, IL-34 production can be further increased by chemotherapies, and this is particularly evident in those patients who are, or become, resistant to chemotherapy and/or immunotherapy. The findings described here also indicate that IL-34 facilitates the differentiation of immunosuppressive cells within the tumor microenvironment, leading to therapeutic resistance and poor outcomes in various cancers. Therefore, the possibility to use inhibitors of IL-34 signaling to overcome cancer resistance could open up a promising opportunity for the treatment of such patients. However, before moving into the clinic, further pre-clinical work is needed to better clarify if IL-34-mediated cancer resistance to therapies is either a general phenomenon occurring in all the patients who do not respond to such treatments or restricted to specific subsets of cancers/patients. Experimentation will be also needed to understand if the circulating levels of IL-34 may contribute to the early identification of non-responders and whether the positive effect of IL-34 on the induction of the immunosuppressive cells is shared with and/or enhanced by CSF1. If this is the case, blockade of CSF1R, rather than IL-34 alone, could be more appropriate to overcome resistance to chemotherapy/immunotherapy.

Author Contributions: G.M. searched the literature for relevant articles and wrote the article; E.F., C.M., M.C., T.P. and C.S. searched the literature for relevant articles and revised the manuscript. All authors have read and agreed to the published version of the manuscript.

Funding: The study was supported by the Associazione Italiana per la Ricerca sul Cancro (IG2016-19223).

Conflicts of Interest: G.M. has served as an advisory board member for ABBVIE and First Wave BioPharma. The remaining authors declare that the research was conducted in the absence of any commercial or financial relationships that could be construed as a potential conflict of interest.

References

1. Siegel, R.L.; Miller, K.D.; Fuchs, H.E.; Jemal, A. Cancer statistics, 2022. *CA Cancer J. Clin.* **2022**, *72*, 7–33. [CrossRef]
2. Sasaki, K.; Strom, S.S.; O'Brien, S.; Jabbour, E.; Ravandi, F.; Konopleva, M.; Borthakur, G.; Pemmaraju, N.; Daver, N.; Jain, P.; et al. Relative survival in patients with chronic-phase chronic myeloid leukaemia in the tyrosine-kinase inhibitor era: Analysis of patient data from six prospective clinical trials. *Lancet Haematol.* **2015**, *2*, e186–e193. [CrossRef] [PubMed]
3. Cheng, W.; Fu, D.; Xu, F.; Zhang, Z. Unwrapping the genomic characteristics of urothelial bladder cancer and successes with immune checkpoint blockade therapy. *Oncogenesis* **2018**, *7*, 2. [CrossRef] [PubMed]
4. Garon, E.B.; Rizvi, N.A.; Hui, R.; Leighl, N.; Balmanoukian, A.S.; Eder, J.P.; Patnaik, A.; Aggarwal, C.; Gubens, M.; Horn, L.; et al. Pembrolizumab for the treatment of non-small-cell lung cancer. *N. Engl. J. Med.* **2015**, *372*, 2018–2028. [CrossRef]
5. Hodi, F.S.; O'Day, S.J.; McDermott, D.F.; Weber, R.W.; Sosman, J.A.; Haanen, J.B.; Gonzalez, R.; Robert, C.; Schadendorf, D.; Hassel, J.C.; et al. Improved survival with ipilimumab in patients with metastatic melanoma. *N. Engl. J. Med.* **2010**, *363*, 711–723. [CrossRef] [PubMed]
6. He, X.; Xu, C. Immune checkpoint signaling and cancer immunotherapy. *Cell Res.* **2020**, *30*, 660–669. [CrossRef]
7. Rotte, A. Combination of CTLA-4 and PD-1 blockers for treatment of cancer. *J. Exp. Clin. Cancer Res.* **2019**, *38*, 255. [CrossRef]
8. Mullard, A. Second CTLA4-targeted checkpoint inhibitor secures FDA approval. *Nat. Rev. Drug Discov.* **2022**, *21*, 868. [CrossRef]

9. Twomey, J.D.; Zhang, B. Cancer Immunotherapy Update: FDA-Approved Checkpoint Inhibitors and Companion Diagnostics. *AAPS J.* **2021**, *23*, 39. [CrossRef]
10. Weber, J.S.; D'Angelo, S.P.; Minor, D.; Hodi, F.S.; Gutzmer, R.; Neyns, B.; Hoeller, C.; Khushalani, N.I.; Miller, W.H., Jr.; Lao, C.D.; et al. Nivolumab versus chemotherapy in patients with advanced melanoma who progressed after anti-CTLA-4 treatment (CheckMate 037): A randomised, controlled, open-label, phase 3 trial. *Lancet Oncol.* **2015**, *16*, 375–384. [CrossRef] [PubMed]
11. Migden, M.R.; Rischin, D.; Schmults, C.D.; Guminski, A.; Hauschild, A.; Lewis, K.D.; Chung, C.H.; Hernandez-Aya, L.; Lim, A.M.; Chang, A.L.S.; et al. PD-1 Blockade with Cemiplimab in Advanced Cutaneous Squamous-Cell Carcinoma. *N. Engl. J. Med.* **2018**, *379*, 341–351. [CrossRef] [PubMed]
12. Pardoll, D.M. The blockade of immune checkpoints in cancer immunotherapy. *Nat. Rev. Cancer* **2012**, *12*, 252–264. [CrossRef]
13. Shiravand, Y.; Khodadadi, F.; Kashani, S.M.A.; Hosseini-Fard, S.R.; Hosseini, S.; Sadeghirad, H.; Ladwa, R.; O'Byrne, K.; Kulasinghe, A. Immune Checkpoint Inhibitors in Cancer Therapy. *Curr. Oncol.* **2022**, *29*, 3044–3060. [CrossRef] [PubMed]
14. Robert, C. A decade of immune-checkpoint inhibitors in cancer therapy. *Nat. Commun.* **2020**, *11*, 3801. [CrossRef] [PubMed]
15. Barrueto, L.; Caminero, F.; Cash, L.; Makris, C.; Lamichhane, P.; Deshmukh, R.R. Resistance to Checkpoint Inhibition in Cancer Immunotherapy. *Transl. Oncol.* **2020**, *13*, 100738. [CrossRef]
16. Nedeljkovic, M.; Damjanovic, A. Mechanisms of Chemotherapy Resistance in Triple-Negative Breast Cancer-How We Can Rise to the Challenge. *Cells* **2019**, *8*, 957. [CrossRef] [PubMed]
17. Huang, D.; Duan, H.; Huang, H.; Tong, X.; Han, Y.; Ru, G.; Qu, L.; Shou, C.; Zhao, Z. Cisplatin resistance in gastric cancer cells is associated with HER2 upregulation-induced epithelial-mesenchymal transition. *Sci. Rep.* **2016**, *6*, 20502. [CrossRef]
18. Chen, Z.; Shi, T.; Zhang, L.; Zhu, P.; Deng, M.; Huang, C.; Hu, T.; Jiang, L.; Li, J. Mammalian drug efflux transporters of the ATP binding cassette (ABC) family in multidrug resistance: A review of the past decade. *Cancer Lett.* **2016**, *370*, 153–164. [CrossRef]
19. Townsend, D.M.; Tew, K.D. The role of glutathione-S-transferase in anti-cancer drug resistance. *Oncogene* **2003**, *22*, 7369–7375. [CrossRef]
20. Sharma, P.; Hu-Lieskovan, S.; Wargo, J.A.; Ribas, A. Primary, Adaptive, and Acquired Resistance to Cancer Immunotherapy. *Cell* **2017**, *168*, 707–723. [CrossRef]
21. Binnewies, M.; Roberts, E.W.; Kersten, K.; Chan, V.; Fearon, D.F.; Merad, M.; Coussens, L.M.; Gabrilovich, D.I.; Ostrand-Rosenberg, S.; Hedrick, C.C.; et al. Understanding the tumor immune microenvironment (TIME) for effective therapy. *Nat. Med.* **2018**, *24*, 541–550. [CrossRef]
22. Bracci, L.; Schiavoni, G.; Sistigu, A.; Belardelli, F. Immune-based mechanisms of cytotoxic chemotherapy: Implications for the design of novel and rationale-based combined treatments against cancer. *Cell Death Differ.* **2014**, *21*, 15–25. [CrossRef] [PubMed]
23. Opzoomer, J.W.; Sosnowska, D.; Anstee, J.E.; Spicer, J.F.; Arnold, J.N. Cytotoxic Chemotherapy as an Immune Stimulus: A Molecular Perspective on Turning Up the Immunological Heat on Cancer. *Front. Immunol.* **2019**, *10*, 1654. [CrossRef]
24. Neophytou, C.M.; Pierides, C.; Christodoulou, M.I.; Costeas, P.; Kyriakou, T.C.; Papageorgis, P. The Role of Tumor-Associated Myeloid Cells in Modulating Cancer Therapy. *Front. Oncol.* **2020**, *10*, 899. [CrossRef] [PubMed]
25. Lin, H.; Lee, E.; Hestir, K.; Leo, C.; Huang, M.; Bosch, E.; Halenbeck, R.; Wu, G.; Zhou, A.; Behrens, D.; et al. Discovery of a cytokine and its receptor by functional screening of the extracellular proteome. *Science* **2008**, *320*, 807–811. [CrossRef] [PubMed]
26. Ma, X.; Lin, W.Y.; Chen, Y.; Stawicki, S.; Mukhyala, K.; Wu, Y.; Martin, F.; Bazan, J.F.; Starovasnik, M.A. Structural basis for the dual recognition of helical cytokines IL-34 and CSF-1 by CSF-1R. *Structure* **2012**, *20*, 676–687. [CrossRef]
27. Nandi, S.; Cioce, M.; Yeung, Y.G.; Nieves, E.; Tesfa, L.; Lin, H.; Hsu, A.W.; Halenbeck, R.; Cheng, H.Y.; Gokhan, S.; et al. Receptor-type protein-tyrosine phosphatase zeta is a functional receptor for interleukin-34. *J. Biol. Chem.* **2013**, *288*, 21972–21986. [CrossRef] [PubMed]
28. Segaliny, A.I.; Brion, R.; Mortier, E.; Maillasson, M.; Cherel, M.; Jacques, Y.; Le Goff, B.; Heymann, D. Syndecan-1 regulates the biological activities of interleukin-34. *Biochim. Biophys. Acta* **2015**, *1853*, 1010–1021. [CrossRef]
29. Chihara, T.; Suzu, S.; Hassan, R.; Chutiwitoonchai, N.; Hiyoshi, M.; Motoyoshi, K.; Kimura, F.; Okada, S. IL-34 and M-CSF share the receptor Fms but are not identical in biological activity and signal activation. *Cell Death Differ.* **2010**, *17*, 1917–1927. [CrossRef]
30. Droin, N.; Solary, E. Editorial: CSF1R, CSF-1, and IL-34, a "menage a trois" conserved across vertebrates. *J. Leukoc. Biol.* **2010**, *87*, 745–747. [CrossRef] [PubMed]
31. Felix, J.; Elegheert, J.; Gutsche, I.; Shkumatov, A.V.; Wen, Y.; Bracke, N.; Pannecoucke, E.; Vandenberghe, I.; Devreese, B.; Svergun, D.I.; et al. Human IL-34 and CSF-1 establish structurally similar extracellular assemblies with their common hematopoietic receptor. *Structure* **2013**, *21*, 528–539. [CrossRef]
32. Greter, M.; Lelios, I.; Pelczar, P.; Hoeffel, G.; Price, J.; Leboeuf, M.; Kundig, T.M.; Frei, K.; Ginhoux, F.; Merad, M.; et al. Stroma-derived interleukin-34 controls the development and maintenance of langerhans cells and the maintenance of microglia. *Immunity* **2012**, *37*, 1050–1060. [CrossRef] [PubMed]
33. Wang, Y.; Szretter, K.J.; Vermi, W.; Gilfillan, S.; Rossini, C.; Cella, M.; Barrow, A.D.; Diamond, M.S.; Colonna, M. IL-34 is a tissue-restricted ligand of CSF1R required for the development of Langerhans cells and microglia. *Nat. Immunol.* **2012**, *13*, 753–760. [CrossRef] [PubMed]
34. Lelios, I.; Cansever, D.; Utz, S.G.; Mildenberger, W.; Stifter, S.A.; Greter, M. Emerging roles of IL-34 in health and disease. *J. Exp. Med.* **2020**, *217*, e20190290. [CrossRef] [PubMed]

35. Franze, E.; Dinallo, V.; Laudisi, F.; Di Grazia, A.; Di Fusco, D.; Colantoni, A.; Ortenzi, A.; Giuffrida, P.; Di Carlo, S.; Sica, G.S.; et al. Interleukin-34 Stimulates Gut Fibroblasts to Produce Collagen Synthesis. *J. Crohn's Colitis* **2020**, *14*, 1436–1445. [CrossRef]
36. Franze, E.; Marafini, I.; De Simone, V.; Monteleone, I.; Caprioli, F.; Colantoni, A.; Ortenzi, A.; Crescenzi, F.; Izzo, R.; Sica, G.; et al. Interleukin-34 Induces Cc-chemokine Ligand 20 in Gut Epithelial Cells. *J. Crohn's Colitis* **2016**, *10*, 87–94. [CrossRef]
37. Franze, E.; Monteleone, I.; Cupi, M.L.; Mancia, P.; Caprioli, F.; Marafini, I.; Colantoni, A.; Ortenzi, A.; Laudisi, F.; Sica, G.; et al. Interleukin-34 sustains inflammatory pathways in the gut. *Clin. Sci.* **2015**, *129*, 271–280. [CrossRef]
38. Preisser, L.; Miot, C.; Le Guillou-Guillemette, H.; Beaumont, E.; Foucher, E.D.; Garo, E.; Blanchard, S.; Fremaux, I.; Croue, A.; Fouchard, I.; et al. IL-34 and macrophage colony-stimulating factor are overexpressed in hepatitis C virus fibrosis and induce profibrotic macrophages that promote collagen synthesis by hepatic stellate cells. *Hepatology* **2014**, *60*, 1879–1890. [CrossRef]
39. Franze, E.; Stolfi, C.; Troncone, E.; Scarozza, P.; Monteleone, G. Role of Interleukin-34 in Cancer. *Cancers* **2020**, *12*, 252. [CrossRef]
40. Baghdadi, M.; Endo, H.; Tanaka, Y.; Wada, H.; Seino, K.I. Interleukin 34, from pathogenesis to clinical applications. *Cytokine* **2017**, *99*, 139–147. [CrossRef]
41. Otsuka, R.; Wada, H.; Seino, K.I. IL-34, the rationale for its expression in physiological and pathological conditions. *Semin. Immunol.* **2021**, *54*, 101517. [CrossRef]
42. Baud'huin, M.; Renault, R.; Charrier, C.; Riet, A.; Moreau, A.; Brion, R.; Gouin, F.; Duplomb, L.; Heymann, D. Interleukin-34 is expressed by giant cell tumours of bone and plays a key role in RANKL-induced osteoclastogenesis. *J. Pathol.* **2010**, *221*, 77–86. [CrossRef]
43. Franze, E.; Dinallo, V.; Rizzo, A.; Di Giovangiulio, M.; Bevivino, G.; Stolfi, C.; Caprioli, F.; Colantoni, A.; Ortenzi, A.; Grazia, A.D.; et al. Interleukin-34 sustains pro-tumorigenic signals in colon cancer tissue. *Oncotarget* **2018**, *9*, 3432–3445. [CrossRef]
44. Franze, E.; Laudisi, F.; Di Grazia, A.; Maronek, M.; Bellato, V.; Sica, G.; Monteleone, G. Macrophages produce and functionally respond to interleukin-34 in colon cancer. *Cell Death Discov.* **2020**, *6*, 117. [CrossRef]
45. Franze, E.; Di Grazia, A.; Sica, G.S.; Biancone, L.; Laudisi, F.; Monteleone, G. Interleukin-34 Enhances the Tumor Promoting Function of Colorectal Cancer-Associated Fibroblasts. *Cancers* **2020**, *12*, 3537. [CrossRef]
46. Wang, Z.; Wang, F.; Ding, X.Y.; Li, T.E.; Wang, H.Y.; Gao, Y.H.; Wang, W.J.; Liu, Y.F.; Chen, X.S.; Shen, K.W. Hippo/YAP signaling choreographs the tumor immune microenvironment to promote triple negative breast cancer progression via TAZ/IL-34 axis. *Cancer Lett.* **2022**, *527*, 174–190. [CrossRef]
47. DeNardo, D.G.; Brennan, D.J.; Rexhepaj, E.; Ruffell, B.; Shiao, S.L.; Madden, S.F.; Gallagher, W.M.; Wadhwani, N.; Keil, S.D.; Junaid, S.A.; et al. Leukocyte complexity predicts breast cancer survival and functionally regulates response to chemotherapy. *Cancer Discov.* **2011**, *1*, 54–67. [CrossRef]
48. Foucher, E.D.; Blanchard, S.; Preisser, L.; Descamps, P.; Ifrah, N.; Delneste, Y.; Jeannin, P. IL-34- and M-CSF-induced macrophages switch memory T cells into Th17 cells via membrane IL-1alpha. *Eur. J. Immunol.* **2015**, *45*, 1092–1102. [CrossRef]
49. Endo, H.; Hama, N.; Baghdadi, M.; Ishikawa, K.; Otsuka, R.; Wada, H.; Asano, H.; Endo, D.; Konno, Y.; Kato, T.; et al. Interleukin-34 expression in ovarian cancer: A possible correlation with disease progression. *Int. Immunol.* **2020**, *32*, 175–186. [CrossRef]
50. Foucher, E.D.; Blanchard, S.; Preisser, L.; Garo, E.; Ifrah, N.; Guardiola, P.; Delneste, Y.; Jeannin, P. IL-34 induces the differentiation of human monocytes into immunosuppressive macrophages. antagonistic effects of GM-CSF and IFNgamma. *PloS ONE* **2013**, *8*, e56045. [CrossRef]
51. Zhou, S.L.; Hu, Z.Q.; Zhou, Z.J.; Dai, Z.; Wang, Z.; Cao, Y.; Fan, J.; Huang, X.W.; Zhou, J. miR-28-5p-IL-34-macrophage feedback loop modulates hepatocellular carcinoma metastasis. *Hepatology* **2016**, *63*, 1560–1575. [CrossRef] [PubMed]
52. Irie, T.; Yoshii, D.; Komohara, Y.; Fujiwara, Y.; Kadohisa, M.; Honda, M.; Suzu, S.; Matsuura, T.; Kohashi, K.; Oda, Y.; et al. IL-34 in hepatoblastoma cells potentially promote tumor progression via autocrine and paracrine mechanisms. *Cancer Med.* **2022**, *11*, 1441–1453. [CrossRef] [PubMed]
53. Raggi, C.; Correnti, M.; Sica, A.; Andersen, J.B.; Cardinale, V.; Alvaro, D.; Chiorino, G.; Forti, E.; Glaser, S.; Alpini, G.; et al. Cholangiocarcinoma stem-like subset shapes tumor-initiating niche by educating associated macrophages. *J. Hepatol.* **2017**, *66*, 102–115. [CrossRef]
54. Segaliny, A.I.; Mohamadi, A.; Dizier, B.; Lokajczyk, A.; Brion, R.; Lanel, R.; Amiaud, J.; Charrier, C.; Boisson-Vidal, C.; Heymann, D. Interleukin-34 promotes tumor progression and metastatic process in osteosarcoma through induction of angiogenesis and macrophage recruitment. *Int. J. Cancer* **2015**, *137*, 73–85. [CrossRef] [PubMed]
55. Baghdadi, M.; Ishikawa, K.; Nakanishi, S.; Murata, T.; Umeyama, Y.; Kobayashi, T.; Kameda, Y.; Endo, H.; Wada, H.; Bogen, B.; et al. A role for IL-34 in osteolytic disease of multiple myeloma. *Blood Adv.* **2019**, *3*, 541–551. [CrossRef]
56. Arora, H.; Panara, K.; Kuchakulla, M.; Kulandavelu, S.; Burnstein, K.L.; Schally, A.V.; Hare, J.M.; Ramasamy, R. Alterations of tumor microenvironment by nitric oxide impedes castration-resistant prostate cancer growth. *Proc. Natl. Acad. Sci. USA* **2018**, *115*, 11298–11303. [CrossRef]
57. Komohara, Y.; Noyori, O.; Saito, Y.; Takeya, H.; Baghdadi, M.; Kitagawa, F.; Hama, N.; Ishikawa, K.; Okuno, Y.; Nosaka, K.; et al. Potential anti-lymphoma effect of M-CSFR inhibitor in adult T-cell leukemia/lymphoma. *J. Clin. Exp. Hematop.* **2018**, *58*, 152–160. [CrossRef]
58. Li, C.H.; Chen, Z.M.; Chen, P.F.; Meng, L.; Sui, W.N.; Ying, S.C.; Xu, A.M.; Han, W.X. Interleukin-34 promotes the proliferation and epithelial-mesenchymal transition of gastric cancer cells. *World J. Gastrointest. Oncol.* **2022**, *14*, 1968–1980. [CrossRef]

59. Lv, X.; Hu, Y.; Wang, L.; Zhang, D.; Wang, H.; Dai, Y.; Cui, X.; Zheng, G. DDIT4 mediates the proliferation-promotive effect of IL-34 in human monocytic leukemia cells. *Blood Sci.* **2021**, *3*, 48–56. [CrossRef]
60. Arnoletti, J.P.; Reza, J.; Rosales, A.; Monreal, A.; Fanaian, N.; Whisner, S.; Srivastava, M.; Rivera-Otero, J.; Yu, G.; Phanstiel Iv, O.; et al. Pancreatic Ductal Adenocarcinoma (PDAC) circulating tumor cells influence myeloid cell differentiation to support their survival and immunoresistance in portal vein circulation. *PloS ONE* **2022**, *17*, e0265725. [CrossRef]
61. Kajihara, N.; Kitagawa, F.; Kobayashi, T.; Wada, H.; Otsuka, R.; Seino, K.I. Interleukin-34 contributes to poor prognosis in triple-negative breast cancer. *Breast Cancer* **2020**, *27*, 1198–1204. [CrossRef]
62. Poudel, M.; Kim, G.; Bhattarai, P.Y.; Kim, J.Y.; Choi, H.S. Interleukin-34-CSF1R Signaling Axis Promotes Epithelial Cell Transformation and Breast Tumorigenesis. *Int. J. Mol. Sci.* **2021**, *22*, 2711. [CrossRef] [PubMed]
63. Pan, Y.; Yu, Y.; Wang, X.; Zhang, T. Tumor-Associated Macrophages in Tumor Immunity. *Front. Immunol.* **2020**, *11*, 583084. [CrossRef] [PubMed]
64. Cendrowicz, E.; Sas, Z.; Bremer, E.; Rygiel, T.P. The Role of Macrophages in Cancer Development and Therapy. *Cancers* **2021**, *13*, 1946. [CrossRef]
65. Ruffell, B.; Coussens, L.M. Macrophages and therapeutic resistance in cancer. *Cancer Cell* **2015**, *27*, 462–472. [CrossRef] [PubMed]
66. Anestakis, D.; Petanidis, S.; Domvri, K.; Tsavlis, D.; Zarogoulidis, P.; Katopodi, T. Carboplatin chemoresistance is associated with CD11b(+)/Ly6C(+) myeloid release and upregulation of TIGIT and LAG3/CD160 exhausted T cells. *Mol. Immunol.* **2020**, *118*, 99–109. [CrossRef]
67. Baghdadi, M.; Wada, H.; Nakanishi, S.; Abe, H.; Han, N.; Putra, W.E.; Endo, D.; Watari, H.; Sakuragi, N.; Hida, Y.; et al. Chemotherapy-Induced IL34 Enhances Immunosuppression by Tumor-Associated Macrophages and Mediates Survival of Chemoresistant Lung Cancer Cells. *Cancer Res.* **2016**, *76*, 6030–6042. [CrossRef]
68. Karin, M.; Cao, Y.; Greten, F.R.; Li, Z.W. NF-kappaB in cancer: From innocent bystander to major culprit. *Nat. Rev. Cancer* **2002**, *2*, 301–310. [CrossRef]
69. Nakajima, S.; Mimura, K.; Saito, K.; Thar Min, A.K.; Endo, E.; Yamada, L.; Kase, K.; Yamauchi, N.; Matsumoto, T.; Nakano, H.; et al. Neoadjuvant Chemotherapy Induces IL34 Signaling and Promotes Chemoresistance via Tumor-Associated Macrophage Polarization in Esophageal Squamous Cell Carcinoma. *Mol. Cancer Res.* **2021**, *19*, 1085–1095. [CrossRef]
70. Ries, C.H.; Cannarile, M.A.; Hoves, S.; Benz, J.; Wartha, K.; Runza, V.; Rey-Giraud, F.; Pradel, L.P.; Feuerhake, F.; Klaman, I.; et al. Targeting tumor-associated macrophages with anti-CSF-1R antibody reveals a strategy for cancer therapy. *Cancer Cell* **2014**, *25*, 846–859. [CrossRef]
71. Lee, K.H.; Yen, W.C.; Lin, W.H.; Wang, P.C.; Lai, Y.L.; Su, Y.C.; Chang, C.Y.; Wu, C.S.; Huang, Y.C.; Yang, C.M.; et al. Discovery of BPR1R024, an Orally Active and Selective CSF1R Inhibitor that Exhibits Antitumor and Immunomodulatory Activity in a Murine Colon Tumor Model. *J. Med. Chem.* **2021**, *64*, 14477–14497. [CrossRef] [PubMed]
72. Yang, Y.; Li, C.; Liu, T.; Dai, X.; Bazhin, A.V. Myeloid-Derived Suppressor Cells in Tumors: From Mechanisms to Antigen Specificity and Microenvironmental Regulation. *Front. Immunol.* **2020**, *11*, 1371. [CrossRef] [PubMed]
73. Li, K.; Shi, H.; Zhang, B.; Ou, X.; Ma, Q.; Chen, Y.; Shu, P.; Li, D.; Wang, Y. Myeloid-derived suppressor cells as immunosuppressive regulators and therapeutic targets in cancer. *Signal Transduct. Target. Ther.* **2021**, *6*, 362. [CrossRef] [PubMed]
74. Groth, C.; Hu, X.; Weber, R.; Fleming, V.; Altevogt, P.; Utikal, J.; Umansky, V. Immunosuppression mediated by myeloid-derived suppressor cells (MDSCs) during tumour progression. *Br. J. Cancer* **2019**, *120*, 16–25. [CrossRef] [PubMed]
75. Kajihara, N.; Kobayashi, T.; Otsuka, R.; Nio-Kobayashi, J.; Oshino, T.; Takahashi, M.; Imanishi, S.; Hashimoto, A.; Wada, H.; Seino, K.I. Tumor-derived interleukin-34 creates an immunosuppressive and chemoresistant tumor microenvironment by modulating myeloid-derived suppressor cells in triple-negative breast cancer. *Cancer Immunol. Immunother.* **2022**, 1–14. [CrossRef]
76. Bezie, S.; Picarda, E.; Ossart, J.; Tesson, L.; Usal, C.; Renaudin, K.; Anegon, I.; Guillonneau, C. IL-34 is a Treg-specific cytokine and mediates transplant tolerance. *J. Clin. Investig.* **2015**, *125*, 3952–3964. [CrossRef]
77. Kim, J.I.; Turka, L.A. Transplant tolerance: A new role for IL-34. *J. Clin. Investig.* **2015**, *125*, 3751–3753. [CrossRef]
78. Gorzo, A.; Galos, D.; Volovat, S.R.; Lungulescu, C.V.; Burz, C.; Sur, D. Landscape of Immunotherapy Options for Colorectal Cancer: Current Knowledge and Future Perspectives beyond Immune Checkpoint Blockade. *Life* **2022**, *12*, 229. [CrossRef]
79. Kumar, V.; Patel, S.; Tcyganov, E.; Gabrilovich, D.I. The Nature of Myeloid-Derived Suppressor Cells in the Tumor Microenvironment. *Trends Immunol.* **2016**, *37*, 208–220. [CrossRef]
80. Prima, V.; Kaliberova, L.N.; Kaliberov, S.; Curiel, D.T.; Kusmartsev, S. COX2/mPGES1/PGE2 pathway regulates PD-L1 expression in tumor-associated macrophages and myeloid-derived suppressor cells. *Proc. Natl. Acad. Sci. USA* **2017**, *114*, 1117–1122. [CrossRef]
81. Ugel, S.; De Sanctis, F.; Mandruzzato, S.; Bronte, V. Tumor-induced myeloid deviation: When myeloid-derived suppressor cells meet tumor-associated macrophages. *J. Clin. Investig.* **2015**, *125*, 3365–3376. [CrossRef] [PubMed]
82. Han, N.; Baghdadi, M.; Ishikawa, K.; Endo, H.; Kobayashi, T.; Wada, H.; Imafuku, K.; Hata, H.; Seino, K.I. Enhanced IL-34 expression in Nivolumab-resistant metastatic melanoma. *Inflamm. Regen.* **2018**, *38*, 3. [CrossRef] [PubMed]
83. Hama, N.; Kobayashi, T.; Han, N.; Kitagawa, F.; Kajihara, N.; Otsuka, R.; Wada, H.; Lee, H.K.; Rhee, H.; Hasegawa, Y.; et al. Interleukin-34 Limits the Therapeutic Effects of Immune Checkpoint Blockade. *iScience* **2020**, *23*, 101584. [CrossRef] [PubMed]
84. Han, N.; Jang, H.Y.; Hama, N.; Kobayashi, T.; Otsuka, R.; Wada, H.; Seino, K.I. An optimized protocol for patient-derived xenograft in humanized mice to evaluate the role of IL-34 in immunotherapeutic resistance. *STAR Protoc.* **2021**, *2*, 100460. [CrossRef] [PubMed]

85. Shi, G.; Yang, Q.; Zhang, Y.; Jiang, Q.; Lin, Y.; Yang, S.; Wang, H.; Cheng, L.; Zhang, X.; Li, Y.; et al. Modulating the Tumor Microenvironment via Oncolytic Viruses and CSF-1R Inhibition Synergistically Enhances Anti-PD-1 Immunotherapy. *Mol. Ther. J. Am. Soc. Gene Ther.* **2019**, *27*, 244–260. [CrossRef]
86. Zhu, Y.; Knolhoff, B.L.; Meyer, M.A.; Nywening, T.M.; West, B.L.; Luo, J.; Wang-Gillam, A.; Goedegebuure, S.P.; Linehan, D.C.; DeNardo, D.G. CSF1/CSF1R blockade reprograms tumor-infiltrating macrophages and improves response to T-cell checkpoint immunotherapy in pancreatic cancer models. *Cancer Res.* **2014**, *74*, 5057–5069. [CrossRef]
87. Booker, B.E.; Clark, R.S.; Pellom, S.T.; Adunyah, S.E. Interleukin-34 induces monocytic-like differentiation in leukemia cell lines. *Int. J. Biochem. Mol. Biol.* **2015**, *6*, 1–16.
88. Wang, Z.; Zhu, J.; Wang, T.; Zhou, H.; Wang, J.; Huang, Z.; Zhang, H.; Shi, J. Loss of IL-34 Expression Indicates Poor Prognosis in Patients with Lung Adenocarcinoma. *Front. Oncol.* **2021**, *11*, 639724. [CrossRef]
89. Zins, K.; Heller, G.; Mayerhofer, M.; Schreiber, M.; Abraham, D. Differential prognostic impact of interleukin-34 mRNA expression and infiltrating immune cell composition in intrinsic breast cancer subtypes. *Oncotarget* **2018**, *9*, 23126–23148. [CrossRef]

Disclaimer/Publisher's Note: The statements, opinions and data contained in all publications are solely those of the individual author(s) and contributor(s) and not of MDPI and/or the editor(s). MDPI and/or the editor(s) disclaim responsibility for any injury to people or property resulting from any ideas, methods, instructions or products referred to in the content.

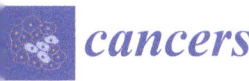

Review

Interactions between Dietary Micronutrients, Composition of the Microbiome and Efficacy of Immunotherapy in Cancer Patients

Małgorzata Frąk [1,*], Anna Grenda [1], Paweł Krawczyk [1], Janusz Milanowski [1] and Ewa Kalinka [2]

[1] Chair and Department of Pneumonology, Oncology and Allergology, Medical University of Lublin, 20-059 Lublin, Poland
[2] Department of Oncology, Polish Mother's Memorial Hospital—Research Institute, 93-338 Lodz, Poland
* Correspondence: malgorzata.frak@gmail.com

Simple Summary: Immunotherapy is a systemic therapy significant for numerous types of cancer. The search for factors which may improve the effectiveness of the therapy is still ongoing. The correlation between host microbiome and the efficacy of immunotherapy has been confirmed. Nutrients modulate the composition of the microbiome, which can be used to improve treatment. The paper presents the impact of probiotics, prebiotics and micronutrients on particular species of bacteria associated with a significant increase in response to anti-PD1, anti-PD-L1 and anti-CTLA4 immunotherapy. We also present our own investigation on the relationship between the gut microbiome and the effectiveness of immunotherapy in non-small-cell lung cancer patients.

Abstract: The effectiveness of immunotherapy in cancer patients depends on the activity of the host's immune system. The intestinal microbiome is a proven immune system modulator, which plays an important role in the development of many cancers and may affect the effectiveness of anti-cancer therapy. The richness of certain bacteria in the gut microbiome (e.g., *Bifidobacterium* spp., *Akkermanisa muciniphila* and *Enterococcus hire*) improves anti-tumor specific immunity and the response to anti-PD-1 or anti-PD-L1 immunotherapy by activating antigen-presenting cells and cytotoxic T cells within the tumor. Moreover, micronutrients affect directly the activities of the immune system or regulate their function by influencing the composition of the microbiome. Therefore, micronutrients can significantly influence the effectiveness of immunotherapy and the development of immunorelated adverse events. In this review, we describe the relationship between the supply of microelements and the abundance of various bacteria in the intestinal microbiome and the effectiveness of immunotherapy in cancer patients. We also point to the function of the immune system in the case of shifts in the composition of the microbiome and disturbances in the supply of microelements. This may in the future become a therapeutic target supporting the effects of immunotherapy in cancer patients.

Keywords: microbiome; micronutrients; immunotherapy; cancer

Citation: Frąk, M.; Grenda, A.; Krawczyk, P.; Milanowski, J.; Kalinka, E. Interactions between Dietary Micronutrients, Composition of the Microbiome and Efficacy of Immunotherapy in Cancer Patients. *Cancers* 2022, *14*, 5577. https://doi.org/10.3390/cancers14225577

Academic Editor: David Wong

Received: 17 October 2022
Accepted: 11 November 2022
Published: 14 November 2022

Publisher's Note: MDPI stays neutral with regard to jurisdictional claims in published maps and institutional affiliations.

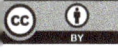

Copyright: © 2022 by the authors. Licensee MDPI, Basel, Switzerland. This article is an open access article distributed under the terms and conditions of the Creative Commons Attribution (CC BY) license (https://creativecommons.org/licenses/by/4.0/).

1. Introduction

The health of the human body consists of a series of processes and reactions occurring constantly in all its tissues. Perfect balance is the guarantee of a long and good quality life. Immunity is vital in protecting against various damaging factors from the external environment as well as from the inside of the body. The human microbiome is a well-known component of host immunity. It includes not only bacteria but also other microorganisms such as fungi, archaea and protozoa [1]. The microbiome influences numerous essential functions of the body. Human health and balance depend on its qualitative and quantitative composition. Its composition is unique to the individual and depends on the diet, lifestyle and medications taken. The microbiota is the body's first line of defense. It mediates the host's interactions with the external environment (including food, environmental toxins, bacteria, viruses, parasites and fungi) on the skin and mucous membranes in the intestines, lungs, vagina and even the cornea [2]. The digestive tract, especially the colon, has the largest concentration of microorganisms—the number of their cells is 10 times greater than the number of all host cells (1×10^{14}) weighing about 1.8 kg. The number of their genomes is a hundred times greater. In the human body, there are on average about 160 species of bacteria species [1,3]. The density of the microbiome (measured as colony-forming units (CFUs) per 1 mL) increases from the duodenum ($\simeq 10^{1-3}$ CFU/mL) to the ileocecal valve ($\simeq 10^{10}$ CFU/mL) and reaches the highest concentration in the colon ($\simeq 10^{11-12}$ CFU/mL) [4]. Most of the human bacteria are of the following types: *Firmicutes, Bacteroidetes, Actinobacteria* and *Proteobacteria*, and strictly anaerobic: *Bacteroides, Fusobacteria, Proteobacteria, Eubacteria, Bifidobacteria, Clostridia, Vermcomicrobia, Cyanobacteria, Spirochaeates, Peptostreocptocci,* and *Ruminococci*. The dominant types are *Firmicutes* and *Bacteroidetes* [4–6]. The consistency of the microbiome depends on the diet—for example, *Bacteroides* more often correlates with the high content of fats and animal proteins in the food, and the prevalence of *Prevotella* is associated with the high content of simple sugars [7].

The microbiome in the first place ensures the maintenance of the correct structure of the intestinal mucosa and protects against pathogens. It plays an active part in the fermentation of nutrients that human enzymes cannot digest. Furthermore, it processes endogenous compounds produced by microorganisms and the host itself, providing unique metabolites necessary for proper functioning, such as lipopolysaccharides (LPS), short-chain fatty acids (SCFAs) and tryptophan. It takes part in the synthesis of vitamins, among others K and B vitamins, mainly riboflavin, niacin, biotin, folic acid, pyroxidine, and cobalamin [8]. It breaks down mutagenic carcinogens (heterocyclic amines and N-nitroso compounds) deriving from a diet rich in red meat. In addition, intestinal microorganisms are involved in the synthesis of amino acids, including lysine and threonine. Fermentation by the intestinal microbiome provides up to 10% of energy from food [9]. Therefore, it may be involved in the regulation of body weight and the amount of adipose tissue present in the system [10]. It is believed that a rich, varied microbiome is most desirable, and a depleted microbiome promotes disease. A relationship between disturbances in the microbiome and the occurrence of at least 25 diseases has been shown [11].

Microbiome disorders are common in gastrointestinal diseases—inflammatory bowel disease (IBD), Crohn's disease, ulcerative colitis, food intolerance, digestive disorders, irritable bowel syndrome (IBS) and colorectal cancer [12,13]. Interestingly, the influence of microbiome extends well beyond the intestinal boundaries and affects not only intestinal homeostasis but also the entire organism. Its validity is observed in metabolic diseases such as non-alcoholic steatohepatitis (NASH), diabetes, dyslipidemia, glucose intolerance, insulin resistance, obesity, hypertension, bone density disorders, allergic diseases and autoimmune diseases such as rheumatoid arthritis and multiple sclerosis [11,14,15]. Also, the correlation with disorders of the nervous system such as Alzheimer's disease, autism spectrum disorders, depression, chronic fatigue syndrome and Parkinson's disease has also been shown [9,16]. The subject of this paper, dysbiosis of the intestinal microbiome, mediates the development of numerous neoplastic diseases and influences the effects of oncological treatment [17,18].

By correlating the above information with the scientific reports of the last decade, it should be understood that humans and their microbiota do not exist in isolation, independently of each other, but form a complex meta-organism called "holobiont". The microbiome regulates itself as well. The huge number of microorganisms requires the implementation of control mechanisms by which the host assesses the state of colonization and reacts to deviations from homeostasis [19,20]. Identifying the mechanisms of interaction between the organism and the gut microbiome is a major challenge for public health in developing new preventive or therapeutic strategies. Owing to achievements in the fields of genetics, molecular biology and bioinformatics, it has become possible to study the microbiome in more detail.

2. The Immunomodulatory Activity of the Intestinal Microbiome

Microorganisms participate in the host's immune system maturation process. They contribute to the formation of innate and adaptive immunity on many levels. In experiments with mice, it was shown that germ-free (GF) individuals devoid of gut microbiota had severe immunodeficiencies. Inter alia, absence of mucosa, altered IgA secretion, reduced size and functionality of Peyer's patches and mesenteric lymph nodes were observed [21]. Studies at the molecular matter have shown that the differentiation of T cells into T regulatory cells (Tregs) and their functional maturation do not take place in the thymus but in the intestine, with the participation of the commensal microbiome [22].

From the immunological point of view, microbes are acknowledged as pathogens by the host's immune system which recognizes and eliminates them. The relationship with the microbiome is different—the immune system has evolved to coexist with microbes in symbiosis. These bilateral interactions enable tolerance of commensal bacteria and food antigens, and, at the same time, intestinal bacteria enable the recognition and destruction of opportunistic bacteria, thus preventing bacterial invasion and infection [23]. The intestines contain gut-associated lymphoid tissue (GALT) organized into lymphoid follicles (Peyer's patches) and containing antigen-presenting cells (APCs), innate lymphoid cells (ILCs), CD4+ and CD8+ T cells and B cells, and many other immune cells. Communication between the GALT system and the intestinal lumen is provided by the intestinal epithelium (IEC) rich in intraepithelial lymphocytes (IELs) and Paneth cells that secrete antimicrobial peptides. In the intestinal epithelium, there are microfold cells (M cells). M cells have the unique ability to take up antigens from the small intestine lumen via endocytosis, phagocytosis or transcytosis. These antigens are delivered to dendritic cells (DCs) and other APCs [23].

The pathogen-related molecular patterns (PAMPs), which are recognized by the pattern recognition receptors of immune cells, mainly Toll-like receptors (TLRs), are of great importance in immunological communication and distinguishing one's own cells from pathogens [24]. It has been proven that the activation of TLRs led to an increased synthesis of peptides against microorganisms: diptericins (against Gram-negative bacteria), defensins (against Gram-positive bacteria) and drosomycins (antifungal). So far, 10 types of TLR have been identified in humans. They are located in the intestinal epithelial wall: on dendritic cells, macrophages, mast cells, natural killer cells (NK), eosinophils, and on T (including Treg cells) and B cells, as well as in epithelial cells, vascular endothelium, fibroblasts, cardiomyocytes, keratinocytes and adipocytes. The immune response through Toll-like receptors is part of the non-specific (innate) response. PAMPs include mainly lipopolysaccharide, flagellin (a protein of cilia from Gram-negative bacteria) and peptidoglycan, as well as lipoproteins, bacterial polysaccharides, lipoteichoic acid, unmethylated CpG sequences and bacterial wall proteins derived from their breakdown (e.g., under the influence of an antibiotic). TLR2, TLR3, TLR4 and TLR5 are of the greatest importance in PAMP-mediated activation of the immune system [25]. TLR2 ligands are bacterial lipoproteins, peptidoglycan, lipoteichoic acid, zymosan, glycolipids, bacterial porins and lipoarabinomannan. The ligand for the TLR4 receptor is lipopolysaccharide, while the TLR5 receptor recognizes flagellin. The TLR3 receptor is involved in the recognition of microbial nucleic acids—double strand RNA (dsRNA) and synthetic polyinosinic polycytidylic acid (poly I:C). Activation of TLRs in antigen-presenting cells enhances the processes that result in the induction of a specific response [26–28].

Upon activation by an antigen, dendritic cells migrate to the mesentery lymph nodes of the small intestine and colon, where they stimulate the conversion of naïve T cells to CD4+ T lymphocytes. Newly formed regulatory CD4+ T and Th17 cells are particularly important due to their intestinal tropism [23]. Tregs return to the gut where they induce immune tolerance directly as well as through the production of immunosuppressive cytokines such as interleukin 10 (IL-10), TGF-β (tumor growth factor) and IL-35 to prevent autoimmunity [4]. Moreover, some bacteria have the ability to maturate Tregs and stimulate

TGF-β via an alternative pathway involving polysaccharide A (PSA) and TLR2 receptors on dendritic cells [23]. Live bacteria can also induce an IgA plasma cell response [29].

Th17 cells are located in the *lamina propria* of the mucosa of the small and large intestines and protect the body against bacterial and fungal infections. By producing cytokines, they stimulate the intestinal epithelium to produce tight junctions that seal the intestinal barrier and produce proteins against pathogens. Th17 cells secrete, inter alia, IL-17, which stimulates epithelial and endothelial cells, fibroblasts and macrophages to produce other cytokines, such as IL-6, IL-8 and TNF (tumor necrosis factor). Moreover, it increases secretion of granulocyte and macrophage colony stimulating factor (GM-CSF) and stimulates the maturation of DCs. When activated by dendritic cells, B and T cells (including Tregs and Th17) have the ability to migrate throughout the body wherever they are needed [30]. It is worth noting that migrating Th17 cells have significant plasticity of action, altering cytokine production depending on the presence or absence of inflammation. Thanks to the cascade of reactions taking place with the participation of the microbiome, the body is able to trigger a strong immune reaction even in distant places.

Therefore, the gut microbiome contributes to the establishment of a proper Th1/Th2 balance. Dysbiosis stimulates the prevalence of Th2, which may manifest in allergic disorders. In germ-free mice, administration of *Bacteroides fragilis* has been observed to correct T cells deficiency and PSA-mediated Th1/Th2 imbalance [30]. *Bernesiella intestinihominis* stimulates cytotoxic T cells (CTLs). *Bernesiella intestinihominis* and *Bilophila* increase the pro-inflammatory Th1 response. *Escherichia coli* and *Escherichia coli Nissle* (EcN) increase the production of cytokines such as IL-6, IL-8 and IL-1β via TLR [31]. *Enterococcus hirae* enhances the Th17 cells response and may increase the ratio of CTLs and Tregs [30]. Some intestinal bacteria have the ability to produce anti-inflammatory cytokines, including IL-10, IL-25, IL-33, TGF-β, and thymic stromal lymphopoietins. These include *Bacteroides*, *Lactobacillus acidophilus*, *Lactobacillus murinus*, *Lactobacillus reuteri*, *Helicobacter hepaticus*, *Faecalibacterium* and some strains of *Clostridia* [22,30]. Particularly noteworthy is *Bacteroides thetaiotaomicron*, which has a significant role in the production of defensins. These bacteria stimulate the intestinal epithelium to produce α- and β-defensins, antimicrobial peptides (AMP), type C lectins and hydrolytic enzymes. They also promote the expression of matrix metalloproteinases (MMPs), which are necessary for the activation of defensins. *B. thetaiotaomicron* has the ability to disrupt NFκB activation in the peroxisome proliferator-activated γ-receptor (PPARγ) pathway and thus reduce the inflammatory response of the immune system. In the absence of danger, it is possible to maintain a non-inflammatory state [7].

3. The Role of Dietary Fiber and Short-Chain Fatty Acids

Short-chain fatty acids (SCFAs) are products of intestinal bacterial metabolism, resulting from the fermentation of dietary fiber [32]. Dietary fiber (DF) are edible carbohydrate polymers with at least three monomeric units, either derived from natural sources such as cereals, legumes, fruits and vegetables or obtained from food raw materials by physical, enzymatic, chemical or synthetic methods [33]. These polymers are resistant to endogenous digestive enzymes in the human small intestine and fermented by bacteria in the large intestine. Soluble fiber is highly fermented, and it is the main source of energy for the microbiome and thus causes the formation of metabolites such as short-chain fatty acids [34]. Soluble fiber includes pectins, inulin, β-glucans, arabinoxylans, oligosaccharides and guar gum. Insoluble fiber (lignin, cellulose, hemicellulose) is poorly fermented by bacteria due to its inability to retain water. Fermentation is possible in the presence of species and strains with the enzymatic ability to metabolize fiber [33]. *Bifidobacterium*, *Bacteroides* and *Prevotella* have a major part in this process. DF fermentation is associated with a strong anti-inflammatory effect, lowering the pH of the colon, increasing the bacterial diversity of the large intestine, reducing pathogens, stimulating the production of antioxidant compounds and vitamins, as well as regulating the epithelial barrier.

SCFAs are organic compounds consisting mainly of acetate, propionate and butyrate. In addition to lowering intestinal pH, they increase the bioavailability of some metals, e.g., iron [35]. *Bacteroides thetaiotaomicron*, responsible for the production of acetate and propionate, promotes the differentiation of goblet cells in the intestine and the expression of mucin-related genes. *Faecalibacterium prausnitzii*, by consuming acetate reduces its influence on mucus and prevents its overproduction. *F. prausnitzii* is responsible for the production of butyrate, thanks to which it maintains the appropriate structure and composition of the intestinal epithelium [36].

SCFAs lead to GPR43-dependent stimulation of Tregs, and also by induction of histone H3 acetylation [37,38]. This ensures a balance between anti-inflammatory Tregs and pro-inflammatory Th17 cells [39]. They increase the concentration of IL-10 which is produced after the recognition of polysaccharide A by plasma dendritic cells and reduces inflammation [40]. Microbial SCFAs and dietary fiber fermentation products can stimulate the population of myeloid DCs in the bone marrow and stimulate the phagocytic capacity of these cells. SCFAs also show anti-inflammatory effects by inhibiting NF-κB, binding to G protein-coupled receptors 43 and 41 (GPR43 and GPR41) [31]. Higher amount of SCFAs inhibit the expression of proinflammatory tumor necrosis factor in mononuclear cells and neutrophils and may lead to inactivation of NF-κB. This interaction promotes signal transduction and alleviates the effects of hypoxia, increases intestinal integrity and prevents LPS translocation to combat inflammation. Additionally, SCFAs increase the activation of histone acetyltransferase and inhibit the histone deacetylase, which influence the development of anti-inflammatory phenotypes in the intestinal microbiome [41]. Moreover, they are involved in epigenetic regulation of inflammation through free fatty acid receptors (FFARs) [31,42]. The most important SCFA-producing bacteria are *Faecalibacterium prausnitzii, Eubacterium, Roseburia, Bifidobacterium longum, Ruminococcus, Alistipes* and *Lactobacillus*. Polysaccharide A is produced by *Bacteroidales, Erysipelotrichales, Clostridiales* and *Bacillales* [39].

Numerous studies reflecting the effects of fiber on the microbiota have been conducted. The use of β-glucan in the diet after 4 weeks resulted in an increase in the generalized diversity of the microbiome and an increase in the total amount of bacteria as well as the richness of *Bifidobacterium* spp.and *Akkermansia municiphila* compared to the control group without β-glucan in the diet [43]. The inclusion of 6.3 g of fiber per day and 2.9 g of β-glucan per day for 6 weeks resulted in an increase in the total amount of intestinal bacteria and a significant increase in *Bifidobacterium* spp.and *Lactobacillus* spp.compared to the control group. The use of a diet containing 3 g of fiber per day excluding β-glucan, however, resulted in a significant decrease in the amount of the above-mentioned bacteria [44]. A study evaluating the effect of β-glucan at a dose of 6 g per day showed a significant increase in microbiological diversity and richness after 4 weeks and an increase in the number of *Bifidobacterium* spp.and *Akkermansia municiphila* compared to the control group without β-glucan in the diet [43]. An increased amount of propionate and a decreased amount of acetate in the faeces has also been shown. The application of a diet with the content of 16 g of fiber/1000 kcal showed a reduction in the contents of *Enterobacteriaceae* after 6 weeks and the growth of *Lachnospira* and *Roseburia* compared to the application of a diet of 8 g of fiber/1000 kcal [45]. Immediate reaction in the composition of the intestinal microbiome after diet modification was proven in KovatchevDatchary's study. In only 3 days of a high-fiber diet (37.5 g/day), an increase in the amount of *Bacteroidetes* and in the *Prevotella/Bacteroides* ratio was observed [46]. A high-fiber diet leads to the growth of SCFA-producing bacteria, including *Lachnospira, Akkermansia, Bifidobacterium, Lactobacillus, Ruminococcus, Roseburia, Clostridium, Faecalibacterium* and *Dorea* [45,47,48].

4. The Effectiveness of Cancer Immunotherapy Depends on the Microbiome

Immunotherapy is widely used in systemic treatment of many types of cancers. In the late nineteenth century, American surgeon William Coley observed spontaneous remission of a malignant sarcoma in a patient with comorbid bacterial infection (erysipelas). Inspired by that experiment, Coley started to infect cancer patients with *Staphyloccocus aureus* which causes erysipelas, or by injecting bacterial culture supernatants. In his studies, he achieved remission of various types of cancers. This became the basis of nonspecific active immunotherapy, used, inter alia, in BCG vaccine (Bacillus Calmette-Guérin) for intravesical infusion in patients with surgically removed bladder cancer.

Immunotherapy is based on the immune potential of the host. Under regular conditions the human immune system destroys cancer cells that arise spontaneously in the body. To avoid this, cancer cells have developed mechanisms to escape from the surveillance of the immune system, thus ensuring their survival and further growth. This phenomenon was discovered in 1967 by Burnet and Thomas and ushered in a new era of cancer treatment. The avoiding process is various and multi-stage. First, cancer cells tend to be invisible by reducing or completely removing the expression of major histocompatibility complex class I molecules (MHC), their antigens and co-stimulatory molecules. The expression of proteins related to the recognition and transport of antigens across the cell membrane is inhibited. As a result, tumor cells are not recognized by cytotoxic T cells. The second mechanism of cancer cells' defense is the production of anti-inflammatory factors such as prostaglandins, histamine, epinephrine, arginase, TGF-β and IL-1 [6]. An "immune desert" is formed, poor in non-specific (NK cells, macrophages, neutrophils) and specific (effector cytotoxic T cells, Tregs, T helper cells) immune cells as well as pro-inflammatory cytokines (e.g., IL-2, IL-12, TNF-α). A non-immunogenic "cold tumor" is characterized by a low response to immunotherapy. The third mechanism by which a tumor escapes from immune surveillance is the most important in the context of immunotherapy. It consists in the direct neutralization of immune cells by interaction of immune checkpoints such as cytotoxic T cell antigen 4 (CTLA-4) and programmed death 1 (PD-1, CD279). PD-1 is located on the surface of macrophages, monocytes as well as T and B cells. It performs a major role in suppressing the immune system. Tumor cells develop ligands for PD-1 (PD-L1 and PD-L2) that bind the PD-1 receptor on T cells and inhibit their activity. CTLA-4 is located on lymphocytes, and its displacement of CD28 (costimulatory molecule) from binding to CD80 (B7-1) and CD86 (B7-2) on APCs causes T cells anergy [5]. To defeat these mechanisms is a challenge for immunotherapy research. Its action is based on the use of anti-CTLA-4, anti-PD-1 or anti-PD-L1 antibodies, which, after binding to immune checkpoints, lead to the activation of lymphocytes. Tumors become rich in immune cells and pro-inflammatory cytokines such as TNF-α, which is a prerequisite for the effectiveness of immunotherapy. This ensures the destruction of the tumor not by a cytotoxic drug but by the host's own immune cells, so it is potentially possible to cure the tumor even at a very advanced stage.

Immune cells' responses depend on many factors. One of them is the gut microbiome [30,31]. The first scientific reports indicated an increased incidence of colorectal cancer in patients with intestinal dysbiosis, which is beyond doubt. Chronic inflammation, IBD, food intolerance, infections, colonization with pathogenic strains, butyrate deficiency, a high-protein diet and products of its metabolism leading to a decrease in the pH in the colon, all create favorable conditions for the intensification of the inflammatory process and carcinogenesis.

However, in the development of clinical trials, a correlation was observed between the effectiveness of immunotherapy (but also chemotherapy and radiotherapy) for various types of cancer located outside the large intestine (e.g., in the lung) and the composition of the intestinal microbiome. Initial observations were made in mice with solid tumors receiving broad-spectrum antibiotic therapy. A significantly worse response to the immunotherapeutic PD-1 blockade has been demonstrated. A similar dependence took place in a group of mice grown in germ-free conditions. The reason was the significantly low level of TNF-α and T cells activation. Oral supplementation with intestinal bacteria strains restored the ability to respond to immunotherapy [49]. High levels of TNF-α correlated with a good response to immunotherapy and increased levels of *Alistipes shahii* in mice gut [50,51]. The enrichment of the microbiome of mice with bacteria of the *Bifidobacterium* species resulted in an increase in the level of T CD8+ cells in the tumor microenvironment and a delay in tumor growth. The combination of *Bifidobacterium* supplementation with anti-PD-L1 antibody resulted in almost complete tumor remission in mice [50]. An analogous response was observed for anti-CTLA-4 antibody in mice with melanoma, sarcoma and colorectal cancer. *Bacteroides thetaiotamicron* and *Bacteriodes fragilis* were necessary for the efficacy of the anti-CTLA4 antibody. These bacteria induced interleukin-12-dependent antitumor T-helper 1 lymphocyte responses [52].

In the group of patients not treated with antibiotics or with short-term exposure to antibiotics (<7 days), longer overall survival (OS) and progression-free survival (PFS) were reported, compared to patients with longer exposure [53]. The effect of antibiotic administration was strongest within 30 days prior to treatment with checkpoint blockade [54]. Of 60 patients with advanced cancer (including lung, kidney, melanoma, hepatocellular carcinoma, head and neck cancer and urothelial carcinoma) treated with anti-PD-1 antibodies, 17 patients were receiving antibiotics within 2 weeks before or after starting treatment for various bacterial infections. These patients had a worse response to immunotherapy. Treatment with broad-spectrum antibiotics (against Gram-positive and Gram-negative bacteria, both aerobic and anaerobic) resulted in shorter overall survival compared to patients treated with narrow-spectrum antibiotics (Gram-positive bacteria only) [55,56]. Heumer et al. conducted a study of 30 patients with non-small-cell lung cancer (NSCLC) of whom 11 received an antibiotic within a month before or after starting treatment with immune-checkpoint inhibitors (ICIs). Authors observed a significantly shorter PFS and OS in patients treated with antibiotics (2.9 and 7.5 months) versus patients without antibiotics (13.1 and 15.1 months) ($p = 0.028$ and $p = 0.026$) [57]. The above observations are justified by a decrease in the diversity and richness of the gut microbiome, which leads to a reduction in the production of pro-inflammatory cytokines and less pronounced tumor necrosis.

5. Gut Microbiota Species Associated with the Efficacy of Immunotherapy

The influence of the intestinal microbiota on the efficacy of ICIs has been noted through the remote modulation of lymphoid and myeloid cells. The microbiome triggers the activation mechanism of IL-12 dependent Th1 cells with cross-reactivity to tumor and bacterial antigens and stimulates DCs [7]. Mucin-eating bacteria (i.a. *Bifidobacterium longum* or *Akkermansia muciniphila*) have been linked to a better response to treatment [58]. It was confirmed that *Bacteroides* (*Bacteroides thetaiotaomicron* and *Bacteroides fragilis*) increases the effectiveness of anti-CTLA-4 therapy and restores its effects after administration of antibiotics [59,60]. Patients whose gut microbiome was rich in *Bacteroides* had increased Th1 cells and decreased Tregs cells and myeloid suppressor cells (MDSC). In mice with large numbers of *Bacteroides* (mainly *B. fragilis*) and *Burkholderia* in the intestines, slower growth of various tumors was observed [7]. In mice, a reduction in MCA205 sarcoma was observed during anti-CTLA-4 therapy when *Bacteroides fragilis*, *Bacteroides thetaiotamicron* and *Burkholderia* species were present in their organisms. These bacterial species may influence the IL-12 dependent Th1 immune response, which enables better disease control [52]. However, it is believed that other common species of *Bacteroides* do not have an impact on the efficacy of anti-CTLA-4 treatment [61].

Patients with melanoma treated with anti-CTLA-4, and with high *Faecalibacterium* abundance and low abundance of *Bacteroidales*, had significantly prolonged PFS compared to those with low and high abundance of these bacteria ($p = 0.03$ and $p = 0.05$) [62,63]. However, the presence of more *Bacteroidetes*, including *Bacteroidaceae*, *Rikenellaceae* and *Barnesiellaceae*, had a preventive effect against the onset of complications of immunotherapy in the form of autoimmune colitis after immunotherapy [63,64].

The presence of *Bifidobacterium* spp.in the gut microbiome has been associated with greater anti-PD-L1 treatment efficacy in melanoma patients. Oral administration of probiotics containing *Bifidobacterium* to mice increased the anti-tumor efficacy of PD-L1 blockade and led to an almost complete inhibition of tumor growth [50]. Gopalakrishnan et al. showed that in melanoma patients, a higher level of *Faecalibacterium prausnitzii*, *Ruminococcus bromii*, *Enterococcus faecium*, *Collinsella aerofaciens*, *Bifidobacterium adolescentis*, *Klebsiella pneumoniae*, *Veillonella parvula*, *Parabac-teroides merdae* and *Lactococcus formicus* correlated with a better response to anti-PD-1 immunotherapy [49,61,62,65]. In metastatic melanoma patients, the richness of *Bifidobacterium longum*, *Bifidobacterium adolescentis*, *Enterococcus faecium*, *Collinsella aerofaciens*, *Lactobacillus species*, *Klebsiella pneumoniae*, *Veillonella parvula* and *Parabacteroides merdae* was higher among responders to anti-PD-L1 treatment, whereas *Roseburia intestinalis* and *Ruminococcus obeum* were significantly higher among the non-responders [65].

More detailed studies were carried out in a group of patients treated with anti-PD-1 with various types of cancer (NSCLC, melanoma, renal cell carcinoma, etc.). Multiparameter immunohistochemistry (IHC) confirmed a higher density of CD8+ T cells in the tumor environment in patients with a better response than in patients with a worse response to immunotherapy ($p = 0.04$). A high level of T CD8+ in tumor tissue correlated with an increased abundance of the genus *Faecalibacterium* of the *Ruminococcaceae* family and of the order *Clostridiales*. Flow cytometric analysis showed that patients with high levels of *Clostridiales*, *Ruminococcaceae* or *Faecalibacterium* in the gut had higher levels of CD4+ and CD8+ effector T cells in the peripheral blood. These patients responded more frequently to anti-PD-1 therapy. However, the patients with high abundance of *Bacteroidales* in gut microbiome had higher levels of regulatory Tregs and MDSC in the peripheral blood and they were less responsive to ICIs treatment [66,67]. Higher content of *Faecalibacterium* in the gut microbiome was connected with a high density of immune cells and high concentration of pro-inflammatory and antigen-presenting cytokines compared to patients with a large amount of *Bacteroidales* [68].

In other research, Tanoue et al. indicate 11 commensal strains which induce CD8+ T cells and interferon-γ in the intestine of germ-free mice and cause significant increase of the response to anti-PD-1 or anti-CTLA-4 antibodies [69]. These strains are: *Ruthenibacterium lactatiformans*, *Bacteroides uniformis*, *Bacteroides dorei*, *Fusobacterium ulcerans*, *Eubacterium limosum*, *Phascolarctobacterium succinatutens*, *Paraprevotella xylaniphila*, *Parabacteroides distasonis* and *Parabacteroides johnsonii*. Bacteria may increase the efficacy of checkpoint inhibitors therapy by stimulating dendritic cells to secrete IL-12 and stimulate differentiation of cytotoxic T cells [56,61].

Song et al. analyzed the gut microbiome in NSCLC patients treated with ICIs. PFS ≥ 6 months was associated with significantly increased diversity in the gut microbiome compared to the PFS < 6 months. In the PFS ≥ 6 months group, a richness of *Methanobrevibacter* and *Parabacteroides* was observed, while in the PFS group < 6 months an enrichment in *Selenomonadales*, *Negativicutes* and *Veillonella* was noted [70]. Jin et al. showed a relationship between high abundance of *Alistipes putredinis*, *Prevotella copri* and *Bifidobacterium longum* and greater efficacy of anti-PD-1 treatment in NSCLC patients. Multicolor flow cytometry showed that patients with a greater variety of gut microbes had a higher percentage of peripheral blood NK cells and memory CD8+ T cells [71]. Valuable research was also presented by Lee et al., who demonstrated the richness of the microbiome in *Bifidobacterium bifidum* in a group of NSCLC patients with a better response to anti-PD-L1 treatment [72]. The presence of *Bifidobacterium spp.* is associated with a response due to an increase in CD8+ T cells and DCs in the tumor microenvironment. Consequently, a higher level of IFN-γ is produced [62]. *Bifidobacterium spp.* improves tumor-specific immunity and the response to anti-PD-L1 immunotherapy by activating antigen-presenting cells inside the tumor [50].

Akkermansia muciniphila and *Alistipes indistinctus* have a marked effect on the anti-PD-1 response in NSCLC and renal cell carcinoma (RCC). Their disproportionate number was recorded in the stool of people with a better response to treatment (partial response or stable disease) compared to those without response (progression). High abundance of *Akkermanasia muciniphila* was significantly associated with response to ICIs therapy in NSCLC and RCC patients ($p = 0.004$). *A. muciniphila* was also more frequent in the stool of patients with PFS longer than 3 months ($p = 0.028$) [49]. Oral supplementation with specific *Akkermansia muciniphila* may restore the responsive phenotype in non-responders [49,73]. A high proportion of the following species among microbiota increases the effectiveness of anti-PD-1 immunotherapy in NSCLC patients: *Akkermansia muciniphila*, *Alistipes indistinctus*, *Bifidobacterium breve*, *Propionibacterium acnes*, *Prevotella copri*, *Rikenellaceae*, *Staphylococcus* aureus, *Streptocptoccus prausnitzi*, *Bacteroides plebeius*, *Enterococcus hirae* and *Enterobacteriaceae* [Table 1]. In contrast, in patients with a good response to anti-PD-1 therapy, *Ruminococcus bromii*, *Dialister* and *Sutterella* occurred less [7,71,73]. Moreover, abundance of *Ruminococcus* unclassified was detected in the gut microbiome of patients with a poor response [71].

Table 1. Gut microbiota species associated with efficacy of cancer immunotherapy.

Malignancy	Treatment	Bacteria Correlated with Positive Immunotherapy Response	Reference
Non-small-cell lung cancer	anti-PD-L1	*Akkermansia muciniphila, Alistipes, Enterococcus hirae*	[49,50,71]
		Bifidobacterium bifidum	[50,72]
		Alistipes putredinis, Prevotella copri, Bifidobacterium longum	[71]
		Methanobrevibacter and *Parabacteroides*	[70]
		Bifidobacterium breve, Propionibacterium acnes, Prevotella copri, Rikenellaceae, Staphylococcus aureus, Streptococcus, Peptostreptococcus, Oscillospira, Faecalibacterium prausnitzi, Bacteroides plebeius, Enterococcus hirae, Enterobacteriaceae	[7,71,73,74]
Melanoma	anti-PD-L1	*Bifidobacterium, Akkermansia muciniphila, Alistipes, Enterococcus hirae, Faecalibacterium prausnitzii, Bacteroides thetaiotamicron, Holdemania filiformis, Bacteroides caccae*	[62]
	anti-PD-L1, anti-CTLA-4	*Ruthenibacterium lactatiformans, Eubacterium limosum, Fusobacterium ulcerans, Phascolarctobacterium succinatutens, Bacteroides uniformis, Bacteroides dorei, Paraprevotella xylaniphila, Parabacteroides distasonis, Parabacteroides johnsonii*	[56,68]
		Enterococcus faecium, Collinsella aerofaciens, Bifidobacterium adolescentis, Klebsiella pneumoniae, Veillonella parvula, Parabacteroides merdae, Lactobacillus spp., Bifidobacterium longum	[69]
		Bifidobacterium longum, Collinsella aerofaciens, Enterococcus faecium	[49,61]
Sarcoma	anti-PD1 or anti-CTLA-4	*Bacteroides fragilis, Bacteroides thetaiotamicron, Burkholderia, Akkermansia muciniphila, Enterococcus hirae, Alistipes*	[49,52]
Colorectal cancer	anti-PD1 or anti-CTLA-4	*Ruthenibacterium lactatiformans, Eubacterium limosum, Fusobacterium ulcerans, Phascolarctobacterium succinatutens, Bacteroides uniformis, Bacteroides dorei, Paraprevotella xylaniphila, Parabacteroides johnsonii, Parabacteroides gordonii, Alistipes senegalensis*	[68]
Renal cell carcinoma	anti-PD-L1	*Akkermansia muciniphila, Lachnospiraceae, Erisypelotrichaceae lacteria, Enterocous faevium, Alistipes indistinctus, Bacteroidaceae, Bacteriodes xylanisolvens, Bacteroides nordii*	[49]
Carcinoma hepatocellulare	anti-PD-1	*Streptococcus thermophilus, Fusobacterium ulcerans, Candidatus Liberibacter, Lactobacillus mucosae, Ruminococcus obeum,* unclassified *Lachnospiracae, Ruminococcus bromii, Subdoligranulum, Bacteroides cellulosyticus, Lactobacillus gasseri, Anaerotruncus colihominis, Eubacterium hallii, Dorea formicigenerans, Lactobacillus vaginalis, Dalister invisus, Lactobacillus oris, Akkermansia muciniphila, Bifidobacterium dentium, Megasphera micronuciformis, Coproccus comes*	[75]

Abbreviations: PD-1—programmed death-1, PD-L1—programmed death-1 ligand, CTLA4—cytotoxic T cell antigen 4.

6. Our Own Observations on the Relationship between the Gut Microbiome and the Effectiveness of Anti-PD-1 or Anti-PD-L1 Immunotherapy in NSCLC Patients

The study of the microbiome is possible thanks to next-generation sequencing (NGS), which allows the identification of the composition of the broad range of microbiota without the need for culture. The bacterial hypervariable region of 16S RNA genes, which are characteristic of individual bacteria, is analyzed in this approach. In our preliminary study of the gut microbiome of patients with advanced non-small-cell lung cancer treated with anti-PD-1 or anti-PD-L1 antibodies, we found that high abundance of the *Akkermansiaceae* family (of which *Akkermansia muciniflla* is a major member) is a favorable predictor of immunotherapy efficacy (PFS prolongation), thus confirming the results in the literature [76]. Nevertheless, an excessively high percentage of *Akkermansiaceae* may be an indicator of dysbiosis and low diversity of the gut microbiome, occurring, for example, as a result of the use of antibiotics (especially broad-spectrum antibiotics). This is a very important factor, due to the fact that a high diversity in the composition of the microbiome is associated with stimulation of the immune system in oncological diseases, and with an increase in the efficacy of immunotherapy.

In 37 NSCLC patients not treated previously with antibiotics, the abundance of *Oscillospirales* (especially *Oscillospirales UCG-010*) was significantly positively correlated with PFS duration. Moreover, high content of *Staphylococcaceae* and *Leuconostocaeae* was associated with a significantly shorter PFS (data not published). In the whole group of patients treated and not treated with antibiotics (n = 47), we observed even more significant correlations between PFS and the abundance of the mentioned bacterial groups. In addition, we noticed that in the whole group of patients a high abundance of *Veillonellaceae* was correlated with shorter PFS, which seems to be in line with the results of Song et al. [70]. Moreover, Cekikij et al. indicated that patients with CRC non-resistant to ICIs therapy had an increased content of *Akkermansia, Clostridium sensu stricto 1* and *Oscillospiraceae* and decreased content of *Streptococcus* and *Leuconostoc* [77]. Due to the fact that PFS is not the best indicator of the effectiveness of immunotherapy, our 47 advanced NSCLC patients with microbiome genotyping are under surveillance in order to obtain prospective long-term observations in terms of overall survival.

7. Probiotics and Prebiotics

Knowing the influence of particular species of bacteria on the immune system and the effectiveness of cancer immunotherapy, it is worth considering how we can interfere with the quantitative and qualitative composition of the microbiome to a patient's benefit. The experiences to date confirm that even a few days' diet modification has a clear impact on the microbiome [46]. Modifying the microbiome through the diet can be directly through the supply of live bacteria (probiotics), which are a natural component of food. In this way, we provide the organism with fermenting bacteria, such as *Lactobacillus, Bifodobacterium, Enterococcus* or *Pediococcus* [7,78,79]. Dairy products, mainly yoghurts, kefirs and cheeses, are commonly enriched with *Bifidobacterium longum, B. lactis, Lactobacillus acidophilus, L. casei* and *L. paracasei* [80]. Buttermilk provides *L. lactis* and *L. bulgaricus*. Fermented vegetables such as pickled cucumbers or cabbage are rich in *Lactobacillus* species, especially *L. plantarum* and *L. brevis*, while kimchi provides *Lactococcus lactis*. Fermented soybean products such as tempeh and miso contain large amounts of *Enterococcus faecium* and *Lactobacillus* species. Live bacteria can also be supplied in the form of ready-made preparations, standardized in relation to the quantitative and qualitative composition [78]. It should be strongly emphasized that the safety and efficacy of large amounts of probiotics in cancer patients has not been demonstrated. There are also no data regarding whether such a procedure has an impact on the effectiveness of immunotherapy. Probiotics can disrupt the natural composition of the microbiome, which may be counterproductive.

Modification of the microbiome is also possible by supplying the body with ingredients that contribute to its enrichment. Prebiotics are commonly known substrates in the form of non-digestible food ingredients (carbohydrates) which are components of the dietary fiber fraction, primarily oligosaccharides, among which the most important are fructooligosaccharides, lactulose and soy oligosaccharides, and polysaccharides, among which the most important are inulin, β-glucans, and pectin [78]. Foods naturally rich in prebiotics include chicory, onions, asparagus, garlic, potatoes, bananas, soybeans (including soybean whey), artichokes, wheat, oats, barley, Jerusalem artichoke, tomatoes and honey. Fiber selectively stimulates growth and increases the activity of microorganisms that are beneficial to health in the intestinal microbiota, regulates the pH of the intestinal contents, and provides a breeding ground for bacteria, stimulating the production of SCFAs, butyric acid and vitamins. A diet rich in dietary fiber results in an increase in the total amount of intestinal bacteria, increasing the diversity of the microbiome with a significant increase in *Bifidobacterium spp.* and *Lactobacillus spp.* [43]. A high-fiber diet enriches the microbiome with bacteria, which has been associated with increased immunotherapy effectiveness in various cancers, which was widely described above.

8. Micronutrients, Gut Microbiome and Cancer

As opposed to the commonly known beneficial effects of fiber, knowledge about the influence of micronutrients on the development of intestinal microbiota beneficial for humans is less widespread. However, micronutrient deficiencies have been linked to changes of bacterial species in the human gut microbiota affecting the host regulation of immune responses. Moreover, malnutrition is one of the common symptoms of cancer [81]. The supply of selected elements and vitamins could promote the richness of the intestinal microbiome and increase the amount of bacteria that are vital to higher effectiveness of oncological treatment (Table 2).

8.1. Vitamin A

In a large study involving 306 children, vitamin A supplementation compared to the placebo resulted in a higher concentration of *Bifidobacterium* in the faeces. These observations were made in boys, but this difference was not present in girls [82]. In girls in late infancy, a positive correlation was found between the concentration of retinol in the plasma with *Bifidobacterium* and *Akkermansia* abundance. In a group of patients with retinol deficiency, a higher concentration of *Enterococcus faecalis* in the faeces was demonstrated [83]. Studies by Mandala et al. showed that an increase in retinol consumption was associated with the increase in *Proteobacteria* to *Actinobacteria* and *Proteobacteria* to *Firmicutes* ratios [84]. However, research results on the influence of vitamin A supplementation on the composition of the microbiome are inconsistent. Another study in a group of 64 children showed that after vitamin A intake, stool samples were dominated by *Bacteroidetes* (46%) as well as *Proteobacteria, Actinobacter, Enterobacter* and *Bifidobacterium* [85].

Consumption of carotenoids in the diet may reduce the risk of colon cancer, and conversely, dietary beta-carotene consumption was inversely related to the incidence of colorectal adenoma. A link has been shown between vitamin A deficiency and an increased incidence of different cancers, e.g., breast, cervix, lung, skin, mouth, prostate and leukemia [86,87]. Vitamin A has been used in clinical trials, alone or in combination with chemotherapy, to treat breast cancer, colorectal cancer, hepatocellular carcinoma, melanoma, neuroblastoma, glioblastoma, skin T-cell lymphoma, lung cancer, prostate cancer, gastric cancer and pancreatic cancer [88]. Interesting results were presented by Pastorino and co-authors. In a group of 307 patients with stage I NSCLC after surgery, the adjuvant effect of high-dose vitamin A was examined. One group of patients received retinol palmitate (orally 300,000 IU daily for 12 months) and the control group received a placebo [89]. After a median follow-up of 46 months, 131 relapses were observed. Recurrence of the disease occurred in 56 patients receiving vitamin A (37%) and in 75 patients in the control arm (48%) [89]. The development of the second primary tumor occurred with a similar frequency in patients receiving and not receiving vitamin A supplementation (29% vs. 33%). Carotenoids in human breast cancer cell lines inhibit cell proliferation and increase cancer cell apoptosis [90,91]. Vitamin A supplementation reduced the liver metastases of colon cancer [92] and reduced melanoma metastases in mice [93]. Despite numerous scientific studies and clinical trials, Vitamin A has not been widely used in the prevention and treatment of cancer. Only all-trans retinoic acid (ATRA) has been registered for the treatment of acute promyelocytic leukemia (APL).

In the context of cancer therapy, vitamin A has a wide range of effects on the immune system. Retinol is required for B cells stimulation, thymocytes growth, myeloid-derived suppressor cells (MDSC) maturation and NK cells activation [94]. Vitamin A is involved in regulating the function of mitochondria and microRNA and it influences tumor stem cells. Retinoids bind to selective proteins in the target cells, such as RAR (retionoic acid receptor),

RXR (retinoid X receptor), EGFR (epidermal growth factor receptor), JAK2 and caspase-3 [95]. On the other hand, receptor complexes bind to a selective region of nuclear DNA, which enables the regulation of gene expression and protein synthesis. A total of seventeen gene signaling pathways have been involved in the anti-tumor mechanisms of retinoids [88]. Modulating the appropriate signaling pathways of vitamin A results in inhibition of tumor cells proliferation and tumor growth arrest [88]. There are no scientific reports examining the effect of vitamin A on the effectiveness of cancer immunotherapy, either directly or through the influence of this vitamin on the immune system or microbiome, except for one phase II clinical trial. Five melanoma patients received ipilimumab alone and another five patients ipilimumab plus ATRA. ATRA significantly decreased the frequency of circulating MDSCs compared to ipilimumab treatment alone in advanced-stage melanoma patients. Additionally, ATRA reduced the expression of immunosuppressive genes, including PD-L1, IL-10 and indoleamine 2,3-dioxygenase (IDO), by MDSCs. Furthermore, ATRA did not increase the frequency of grade 3 or 4 adverse events [96].

8.2. B Vitamins

The effect of vitamin B1 (thiamine) was demonstrated on lymphoid tissue—lymph nodes and spleen were smaller in the group of mice that were not given vitamin B1. Upon commencement of supplementation, tissues increased in volume and returned to normal size in 14 days [97]. In studies in mice infected with *Mycobacterium tuberculosis* that were treated with vitamin B1, increased levels of TNF-α and IL-6 in the lungs and enhanced upregulation of CD86 and MHC-II expression on antigen-presenting cells were shown. Further observations indicate that vitamin B1 could regulate the functions of macrophages and regulate the NF-κB signal in macrophages to promote the protective immune response [98]. In a group of 257 patients, the influence of the supply of vitamin B1 in a dose of up to 0.6 mg/1000 kcal/day on the intestinal microbiota was examined. The study showed a significant increase in *Bacteroides*, *Faecalibacterium* and *Prevotella*. The greatest correlation was found between the *Ruminococcaceae* family and the vitamin B1 supplementation [99].

It has been observed that the microbial pathway of vitamin B2 (riboflavin) synthesis produces metabolites that stimulate the activation of mucosa-bound T cells in intestines and airways, promote a tissue repair response and help to maintain the integrity of the epithelial barrier [100]. Vitamin B2 supplementation resulted in an enrichment of the overall diversity of the microbiome, in particular in *Faecalibacterium* and *Roseburia*, as well as a reduction in the number of *Enterobacteriaceae* [101,102]. The use of high doses of vitamin B2 (100 mg daily) resulted in an increase in *Faecalibacterium prausnitzii* (one of the main producers of butyrate) within 2 weeks of supplementation. A reduction in the number of these bacteria was observed after the end of supplementation. An increase in the number of *Roseburia* species and a decrease in *Escherichia coli* were also shown. Randomized studies of vitamin B2 supplementation at a dose of 75 mg/day showed an increase in *Alistipes shahii* in the gut microbiome [103]. In a study of patients who received vitamin B2 for 2 weeks, there was an increase in *Faecalibacterium prausnitzii* in the faeces, which is a strong producer of SCFAs. Another study, in which supplementation lasted for 3 weeks, showed a reduction in the number of potentially pathogenic *Enterobacteriaceae* (including *Escherichia coli*) [101].

Studies conducted in a group of people supplementing orally with vitamin B3 (nicotinic acid) indicate the effect of this vitamin on the growth of *Bacteroidetes* [103]. To confirm this concept, 10 volunteers received vitamin B3: nicotinic acid (30–300 mg) and nicotinamide (900–3000 mg) to the ileo-colonic region to evaluate direct effects on the gut microbiome. After a period of 6 weeks, a significant increase in the amount of *Bacteroidetes* was observed in the group using nicotinic acid compared to the group using nicotinamide [104]. Vitamin B3 suppresses monocytes by inhibiting the release of inflammatory mediators such as TNF-α, IL-6 and monocyte chemotactic protein-1, and it also reduces the production of pro-inflammatory cytokines by macrophages [105].

Vitamin B12 in food is present in the form of a protein complex and it is released free via pepsin in the stomach. It is absorbed in the small intestine via the intrinsic factor (IF).

Vitamin B12 is also produced by intestinal bacteria, which include *Bifidobacterium animalis*, *B. infantis*, *B. longum*, *Lactobacillus plantarum*, *L. coryniformis*, *Bacteroides fragilis*, *Prevotella copri*, *Faecalibacterium prausnitzii* and *Ruminococcus lactaris* [106]. Vitamin B12 produced by *Eubacterium hallii* promotes *Akkermansia muciniphila* growth and propionate production [107]. Additionally, *A. muciniphila* stimulates the growth of *E. hallii* and *Anaerostipes caccae*, which are responsible for the participation in the vitamin B12 biosynthetic pathway. In murine models, vitamin B12 deficiency reduces the number of lymphocytes and CD8+ T cells, increases the ratio of CD4+ cells to CD8+ cells and inhibits the activity of NKT cells. This effect can be reversed with vitamin B12 supplementation. These observations confirm that vitamin B12 contributes to the immune response mediated by CD8+ T cells and NK T cells. Vitamin B12 supplements may reduce the direct toxic side effects of therapy as vitamin B12 is required for DNA synthesis, neural functions and reduction of the severity of drug-induced peripheral neuropathy in patients who receive chemotherapy (especially pemetrexed) [108].

8.3. Vitamin C

Vitamin C supplementation significantly increases the biodiversity of the gut microbiome, with a particular abundance of *Collinsella* and fecal SCFA levels, especially butyrate and propionate [103]. In vitro studies showed that high vitamin C concentration causes the growth of *Roseburia*, *Faecalibacterium*, *Akkermansia* and *Bifidobacterium*, but this trend has not yet been confirmed in humans. Vitamin C is essential for the survival of commensal anaerobes such as *Bacteroides* [109]. Vitamin C acts as an absorber for radicals (e.g., hydroxyl OH− or superoxide O_2-), thus generating ascorbyl free radical (AFR) and hydrogen peroxide (H_2O_2) or water [94]. Neoplastic cells coexist with increased expression of vitamin C transporters and intensified oxidative processes. In this way, the accumulation of free radicals occurs, which causes an imbalance in the activity of mitochondria and the production of reactive oxygen species. This in turn causes demethylation, damage to DNA strands and biological membranes. In the mechanism outlined above, vitamin C inhibits cancer proliferation and enhances cancer cell apoptosis.

Vitamin C deficiency has been correlated with a higher frequency of gastric cancer and prostate cancer occurrence [94]. Vitamin C stimulates and strengthens the function of leukocytes and neutrophils. Supplementation may enhance the proliferation of T cells and increase the production of cytokines. Numerous studies examine the usefulness of vitamin C as monotherapy or in combination with chemotherapy or immunotherapy in the treatment of many types of cancer [110]. Leukemia, colorectal cancer, melanoma, pancreatic cancer, prostate cancer, NSCLC, breast cancer, ovarian cancer, hepatocellular carcinoma, mesothelioma, thyroid cancer, oral squamous cell carcinoma, neuroblastoma and glioma were the most commonly studied. Studies conducted in animal models have shown inhibition of tumor growth (40–60%) by the use of increased doses of ascorbate (1–4 µg/kg) intravenously or intraperitoneally. The supply of vitamin C was also effective in inhibiting the formation of metastases (50–90%) [110]. In combination with immunotherapy, vitamin C increased the immunogenicity of effector T cells in murine models [111,112]. Complete regression was observed in several mice, and immunity persisted after re-injecting the tumor cells. Influenced by vitamin C, increased tumor infiltration by CD8+ T cells (including cytotoxic T cells) and macrophages was demonstrated, and increased production of IL-12 by antigen-presenting cells was observed. Vitamin C contributes to the transformation of "cold tumors" insensitive to immunotherapy into "hot tumors" susceptible to treatment [110].

8.4. Vitamin D

Recent studies show that vitamin D can directly affect the intestinal and respiratory tract microbiome and alleviate dysbiosis [113]. In animal models, C57BL/6 mice reared on a vitamin D-rich diet had 50 times more bacteria in the colon and greater microbial diversity, as well as increased production of SCFAs per gram of dry weight, compared to those fed a low-vitamin D diet [114]. Butyrate increases the expression of the vitamin D receptor (VDR) in intestinal epithelial cells. A similar effect of VDR stimulation occurs after administration of the probiotic strains *Lactobacillus rhamnosus* GG ATCC 53,103 and *L. plantarum* [115]. The intestinal microbiota of mice deficient in VDR shows loss of *Lactobacillus spp.* and an increase in *Proteobacteria spp.* and *Bacteroidetes spp.* [115]. In humans, in a group of 3188 IBD patients, it was observed that higher plasma 25(OH)D3 concentration (27.1 ng/mL) was associated with a significantly reduced risk of *Clostridium difficile* infection [114,116]. In studies of patients with multiple sclerosis (MS), it has been shown that supplementation with 5000 IU of vitamin D3 daily for 90 days increased the number of *Akkermansia* as well as *Faecalibacterium* and *Coprococcus*, which produce butyrate and anti-inflammatory SCFA [117]. A study of MS patients treated with vitamin D3 showed that the supply of this vitamin caused changes in the levels of *Firmicutes, Actinobacteria* and *Proteobacteria* and an increase in the number of *Enterobacteria* compared to those who were not treated with vitamin D3 [118]. The daily intake of 60 µg of cholecalciferol resulted in an enrichment of *Bifidobacterium longum* in stool samples [119]. The use of high doses of 50,000 IU cholecalciferol weekly for 9 weeks reduced the amount of *Bacteroidetes* and *Lactobacillus*, whilst *Firmicutes* and *Bifidobacterium* increased after supplementation [120]. Subsequent studies confirm that high serum vitamin D levels can be correlated with high abundance of several *Firmicutes* such as *Ruminococcus, Coprococcus, Mogibacterium* and *Blautia* [121]. In another study, vitamin D supplementation (300,000 IU over 4 weeks) modified the composition of the gut microbiome resulting in the growth of beneficial bacteria such as *Alistipes, Faecalibacterium, Roseburia* and *Parabacteroides* [122,123]. A correlation was also observed between changes in the composition of the intestinal microbiome and the season of the year. In the summer–autumn period, when sun exposure and serum level of vitamin D are the highest, abundance of *Pediococcus spp., Clostridium* spp.and *Escherichia/Shigella spp.* is increased [124]. A randomized study of 23 patients with confirmed vitamin D deficiency revealed that 50,000 IU of oral vitamin D3 once weekly supplementation caused *Lactococcus* to increase, whereas *Veillonella* and *Erysipelotrichaceae* were substantially decreased after 12 weeks [113]. Vitamin D controls the expression of antimicrobial peptides, contributing to a protective effect on the intestinal and bronchial mucosa, it maintains the integrity of the mucosal barrier and it promotes epithelial healing [125].

Vitamin D develops a suppressive effect on the immune system. VDR receptors are found on the surface of dendritic cells, macrophages, T and B cells. Vitamin D inhibits the activity of the immune cells, the proliferation of B and T cells and the production of pro-inflammatory cytokines, IL-2, IL-12, IL-17, IFN-γ and TNF-α [126]. The influence of vitamin D on the development and growth of NKT cells was noted. Numerous observational studies have shown the impact of vitamin D deficiencies on the risk of autoimmune diseases such as type I diabetes, Hashimoto's thyroiditis, inflammatory bowel disease, systemic lupus erythematosus, multiple sclerosis, vitiligo, psoriasis and rheumatoid arthritis. Supplementation of high dose vitamin D could improve the clinical course of vitiligo. Since vitamin D deficiency affects the development of autoimmune diseases, its supplementation may prevent other serious adverse events during immunotherapy of cancer [108].

On the other hand, vitamin D increases the production of IL-10 by DCs and cathelicidin by macrophages, and it activates Tregs as well as induces the production of IL-4 by Th2 cells together with a downregulation of the pro-inflammatory Th1, Th17 and Th9 lymphocytes. In mice, the effect of high concentrations of vitamin D on the decreased level of IL-22 was also observed. Vitamin D inhibits inflammatory cytokine production by monocytes, and suppresses dendritic cell differentiation and maturation, which helps to maintain immune tolerance [125].

8.5. Vitamin E

Vitamin E influences the gut microbiome and correlates with an increase in *Firmicutes* [127,128] and a significant decrease in the *Bacteroidetes cluster* [127]. In a study comparing a group with supplementation of iron and vitamin E with a group with only iron supplementation, a marked decrease in *Bacteroides* and an increase in *Firmicutes* (especially *Roseburia*) was observed. Supplementation has been positively associated with SCFA production. Thus, the addition of vitamin E to therapeutic iron supplementation may create a more favorable profile of the gut microbiome by promoting the growth of butyrate-producing bacteria [129]. Higher levels of vitamin E have also been associated with greater abundance of *Akkermansia* and other health-promoting taxa such as *Lactobacillus*, *Bifidobacterium* and *Faecalibacterium* [102,130]. The research results are interesting, but there are too few of them and further analysis is needed.

Vitamin E has an antioxidant effect and participates in immune regulation by inhibiting the NF-kB and STAT3 signaling pathways. It affects the proliferation of cells through the phosphoinositide 3-kinase (PI3K) pathway and the process of apoptosis [101]. It was shown that the level of vitamin E in the blood was significantly lower in patients with prostate cancer (n = 32, mean concentration—5.2 µg/mL) than in healthy subjects (n = 40, mean concentration—14.2 µg/mL) [131]. Zhang et al. reported that vitamin E intake could reduce colorectal cancer risk [132]. A study involving 278 cases of lung cancer and 205 cases of prostate cancer presented a significantly lower concentration of α-tocopherol in cancer patients than in healthy volunteers [133]. Recent studies indicated the importance of vitamin E in immunotherapy with immune checkpoints inhibitors. Cancer patients with vitamin E supplementation during ICIs treatment had a prolongation of survival. Vitamin E acts on DCs through the SCARB1 receptor and inhibits the protein tyrosine phosphatase SHP1, the internal checkpoint of dendritic cells [134]. Cross-presentation of antigen triggered systemic, antigen-specific T-cell antitumor immunity. Combining immunotherapy with vitamin E supplementation could significantly increase the effectiveness of oncological treatment.

8.6. Vitamin K

Vitamin K supports the diversity of bacteria in the gut microbiome. In a group of Japanese women whose diets were poor in vitamin K, a high relative abundance of *Ruminococcaceae* and *Bacteroides* was demonstrated, while in a group of women on a vitamin-K-rich diet, a high relative abundance of *Bifidobacterium* and *Lactobacillales* was found [135]. The cytotoxic and antitumor properties of vitamin K result from the reactivity of the quinone moiety of this molecule, which generates oxygen free radicals. This effect is also associated with a change in the cell cycle at the transcriptional level and a disturbance in carboxylation biochemistry [94]. Vitamin K influences cell proliferation by enhancing the expression of protein kinase A and inhibiting NF-κB by suppressing IκB kinase. The anti-tumor activity of the vitamin K analog—PPM-18 has also been demonstrated in a group of bladder cancer patients [136]. PPM-18 activated AMP-activated protein kinase (AMPK) and inhibited the PI3K/AKT and mTORC1 pathways in bladder cancer cells, inducing autophagy and apoptosis of cancer cells. There are no studies analyzing the efficacy of combination therapy with anticancer drugs and vitamin K supplementation.

8.7. Iron

In vivo and in vitro studies have shown adverse effects of oral Fe supplementation on the composition of the gut microflora, gut metabolism and gut health. Changes in the bacterial composition caused by the administration of iron influenced the bacterial pathway of *Staphylococcus aureus*, suggesting a reduced protective gut microbiota response to bacterial infections and carcinogenesis [137]. Paganini and co-authors demonstrated a relationship between higher iron concentration and a decline in the amount of lactic acid bacteria—*Bifidobacterium* and *Lactobacillus* and an increase in enteropathogenic strains such as *Escherichia coli* [138]. In a group of 35 children in Kenya, after 4 months of Fe using, there was a lower number of the genus *Lactobacillus* ($p = 0.048$) and *Bifidobacterium* ($p = 0.058$), and a higher number of *Clostridiales* ($p = 0.015$) and *Enterobacteriaceae* family ($p = 0.086$), compared to the control group. Moreover, the number of *Ruminococcaceae*, *Lachnospiraceae* (mainly *Dorea*, *Blautia* and *Coprococcus*) and *Erysipelotrichaceae* was significantly higher in the group with Fe supplementation compared to the control group ($p < 0.05$ for all of the listed ones). Another study, involving 139 children aged 6–14 years, showed that after 6 months of iron supplementation, there was a significant increase in the number of *Enterobacteriaceae* ($p < 0.005$) and a decrease in the number of *Lactobacillus* ($p < 0.0001$). Moreover, an increase in concentration of fecal calprotectin ($p < 0.01$), which is a marker of enteritis, has been observed [139]. Simonyte et al. confirmed the above observations. Their study assessed the effect of various doses of supplemented iron on the microbiota and it was found that the consumption of a high dose of iron for 45 days reduced the amount of *Bifidobacterium* ($p < 0.001$, 60% vs. 78%) and *Lactobacillus* ($p < 0.007$, 8% vs. 42%), while no increase in pathogenic bacteria was observed [137]. It was also observed that an increase in SCFAs enhances iron absorption. In infants with iron deficiency, a reduction in the abundance of butyrate-producing species such as *Butyricicoccus*, *Roseburia* and *Coprococcus* was shown [35].

High iron level is associated with high risk of colorectal cancer by increasing the activity of bacterial enzymes involved in carcinogenesis of the large intestine. *Bifidobacteriaceae* are able to bind Fe in the large intestine and reduce the formation of free radicals. *Lactobacillus fermentum* reduces Fe (III) to Fe (II) and increases its absorption [140]. A very interesting discovery regarding the use of iron oxide nanoparticles (IONP) in cancer immunotherapy was described by Chung et al. [141]. IONPs can be used to stimulate immune cells to increase their activity at the tumor site and improve the response to cancer immunotherapy. Iron from IONPs is widely present in the organism, it is used by various cellular processes and it is biodegradable, which are advantages over other nanoparticles. IONPs can be converted to exhibit specific physicochemical properties, such as, for example, surface charge. By these modifications, the surface of the IONPs can be tailored to conjugate therapeutic agents as well as antibodies that are selective and specific for a particular cell type. The modified surface enables the delivery of antigens, adjuvants and therapeutic agents to immune cells, and the conjugation of antigens to IONPs protects them from degradation in vivo. IONPs' labeling of immune cells, such as DCs, macrophages and lymphocytes, increases the number of cells in the vicinity of the tumor. The magnetic properties of IONPs in MRI enable the targeting of molecules to specific tumor sites. Labeling with antibodies against immune checkpoints (e.g., anti-PD-L1) could increase the effectiveness of immunotherapy. In tumor-bearing C57BL/6 mice with anti-PD-L1 antibodies on the IONPs' surface, higher tumor growth suppression and survival rate were observed. IONPs can also be used in photothermal therapy to induce an immune response in tumors and provide immunostimulants to strengthen the effect.

8.8. Zinc

Dietary zinc deficiency affects the gut microbiota, and the gut microbiota affects the absorption of zinc in the intestines. Numerous studies indicate that prophylactic doses of zinc oxide (ZnO) in various animal models reduced the presence of anaerobic Gram-negative bacteria [142]. The supply of zinc caused a decrease in *Enterobacteriaceae*, mainly *Escherichia coli* and *Clostriudium spp.*, in pigs. Coated ZnO nanoparticles increased the microbial richness of *Ruminococcus flavefaciens* and *Prevotella* [143,144]. Data on changes in the number of *Lactobacillus* are inconsistent. Recent studies have shown a decrease in the level of *Lactobacillus* after zinc supplementation [144–146]; however, there are reports of an increase in the level of this bacterium after the use of Zn [147]. In studies carried out on chicks, it was shown that in the caecum of individuals with Zn deficiency a higher number of *Proteobacteria* and a smaller number of *Firmicutes* were observed compared to the group with iron supplementation. The *Firmicutes:Proteobacteria* ratio was significantly lower in the Zn-deficient group [148]. Moreover, in the Zn-deficient group, the number of *Bacteroidetes* increased while the *Actinobacteria* decreased. Zn-deficient chicks had a significantly higher relative abundance of *Enterococcus*, *Enterobacteriaceae* and *Ruminococcaceae*, and a significantly lower relative abundance of *Clostridiales* and *Peptostreptococcaceae*, compared to the Zn-supplemented group.

Zinc improved the function of the immune system by increasing the level of pro-inflammatory cytokines such as IL-1β, IL-2, IL-6, TNF-α and IFN-γ and reducing IL-10 in the serum, confirming the central role of Zn for cytokine production and immunoregulation [148,149]. Zinc supplementation in combination with the probiotic *Lactobacillus plantarum IS-10506* for 90 days resulted in a significantly increased humoral immune response [147]. Evidence from several studies showed that abnormal zinc metabolism has been closely associated with the development of various types of malignancies including breast, pancreatic, lung, liver, stomach, cervical and prostate cancer [150]. Cells of prostate cancer contained 62–85% less zinc than cells from normal tissues. Low zinc level has been correlated with a higher tendency to cancer progression and the advancement of the neoplastic process. In the treatment of prostate cancer, zinc can induce a strong necrotic response by activating ERK1/2 and protein kinase C (PKC) in tumor cells [150]. Similar to the above-mentioned iron, research is underway on the use of zinc in the form of nanoclusters in combination with bovine serum albumin (ZnS@BSA) [151]. Zinc ions are released in the tumor's acid microenvironment and activate the signaling pathway of cyclic guanosine monophosphate-adenosine monophosphate synthase/stimulator of interferon genes (cGAS/STING). This causes an influx of CD8+ T cells to the tumor and dendritic cells, leading to improved immunotherapy efficacy, what has been proven in mice with hepatocellular carcinoma.

8.9. Magnesium

Little research has been done on the effects of magnesium on the gut microbiome. It has been shown so far that low doses of magnesium in the diet (30 mg/kg) resulted in a greater abundance of selected bacterial species in mice and a higher presence of rare species than in a high magnesium supplementation diet (4000 mg/kg) [152]. The intestinal microbiota of hypo-Mg mice showed a lower relative abundance of *Actinomycetes* and *Proteobacteria* while a higher abundance of *Bacteroidetes, Clostridiales* and *Clostridiaceae*. In hyper-Mg mice, a higher abundance of *Bifidobacterium, Adlercreutzia* and *Lachnospiraceae* was observed. In studies on liver damage caused by methotrexate therapy, it was shown that magnesium Isoglycyrrhizinate (MgIG) changed the composition of the intestinal microbes by increasing the level of probiotic *Lactobacillus* and reducing the level of *Muribaculaceae* [153]. Another study demonstrated that mice on a low-magnesium diet showed a lowered number of *Bifidobacterium* in the gut and high levels of TNF-α and IL-6 [154].

Table 2. The relationship between micronutrients and microbiome.

Micronutrient	Influence on Microbiome	Reference
Vitamin A	*Akkermansia* ↑	[83]
	Bifidobacterium ↑	[83,85]
	Proteobacteria to *Actinobacteria* ratio ↑ *Proteobacteria* to *Firmicutes* ratio ↑	[84]
	Bacteroidetes ↑ *Proteobacteria* ↑ *Actinobacter* ↑ *Enterobacter* ↑	[85]
Vitamin B1	*Bacteroides* ↑, *Faecalibacterium* ↑, *Prevotella* ↑	[99]
Vitamin B2	*Faecalibacterium* ↑, *Roseburia* ↑, *Enterobacteriaceae* ↓	[101,102]
	Alistipes shahii ↑	[103]
Vitamin B3	*Bacteroidetes* ↑	[103]
Vitamin B12	*Akkermansia* ↑	[107]

Table 2. *Cont.*

Micronutrient	Influence on Microbiome	Reference
Vitamin C	*Collinsella* ↑	[103]
	Bacteroides ↑, *Roseburia* ↑, *Faecalibacterium* ↑, *Akkermansia* ↑, *Bifidobacterium* ↑	[109]
Vitamin D	*Lactobacillus rhamnosus* ↑, *Lactobacillus plantarum* ↑	[115]
	Clostridium difficile ↓	[114,116]
	Akkermansia ↑, *Faecalibacterium* ↑, *Coprococcus* ↑	[117]
	Enterobacteria ↑	[118]
	Bifidobacterium longum ↑	[119,120]
	Ruminococcus ↑, *Mogibacterium* ↑, *Blautia* ↑	[121]
	Alistipes ↑, *Roseburia* ↑, *Parabacteroides* ↑	[122,123]
	Pediococcus ↑, *Clostridium* ↑, *Escherichia* ↑, *Shigella* ↑	[124]
Vitamin E	*Firmicutes* ↑	[127,128]
	Bacteroidetes cluster ↓	[127]
	Akkermansia ↑, *Lactobacillus* ↑, *Bifidobacterium* ↑, *Faecalibacterium* ↑	[102,130]
Vitamin K	*Bifidobacterium* ↑, *Lactobacillales* ↑	[135]
Iron	*Bifidobacterium* ↓, *Escherichia coli* ↑, *Ruminococcaceae* ↑, *Lachnospiraceae* ↑, *Erysipelotrichaceae* ↑	[138]
	Enterobacteriaceae ↑	[139]
	Lactobacillus ↓	[138,139]
Zinc	*Escherichia coli* ↓, *Clostriudium* ↓	[142]
	Ruminococcus flavefaciens ↑, *Prevotella* ↑	[143,144]
	Lactobacillus ↓	[144–146]
Magnesium	*Bifidobacterium* ↑, *Adlercreutzia* ↑, *Lachnospiraceae* ↑	[152]
	Lactobacillus ↑, *Muribaculaceae* ↓	[153]
Selenium	*Lachnospiraceae* ↑, *Ruminococcaceae* ↑, *Christensenellaceae* ↑, *Lactobacillus* ↑	[155]

↑-increase in the number of bacteria; ↓-decrease in the number of bacteria.

8.10. Selenium

Selenium supplementation determined an increase in the number of families *Lachnospiraceae*, *Ruminococcaceae*, *Christensenellaceae* and *Lactobacillus* in the gut microbiome [155]. Selenium stimulates the functionality of NK cells, macrophages and neutrophils as well as the production of IFN-γ, TNF-α and IL-6 [155]. Selenium supplementation enhances the cytotoxic functions of NK cells in mice by increasing the expression of IL-2 receptors (IL-2R) on their surface. Consumption of Se-enriched foods (200 mg per serving) over 3 days increased the levels of IL-2, IL-4, IL-5, IL-13 and IL-22, indicating that selenium promotes the immune response of Th1 and Th2 cells. Selenium is anti-cancerous in the tumor microenvironment, inhibiting the proliferation of cancer cells. In leukemia, sodium selenite (200 mg/day for 8 weeks) increased the CD8+ T cells-mediated tumor cytotoxicity and NK cell activity. Similar observations have been made in different neoplasms [156]. It strengthens the immune system by regulating the production of antibodies. Immunomodulating functions of selenium could reduce immunorelated adverse events (irAEs) of cancer immunotherapy [157].

8.11. Omega-3

Studies comparing the effects of different doses of omega-3 polyunsaturated fatty acids (PUFAs) showed that supplementation with low doses of PUFAs (30 mg) was associated with a higher concentration of *Bacteroidales, Clostridium, Eubacterium* and *Planococcaceae* and with a lower abundance of *Lactobacillus, Helicobacter* and *Ruminococcus* than supplementation with 60 mg or 90 mg of the omega-3 PUFAs [158]. *Firmicutes, Clostridiales, Lactobacillus* and *Bifidobacterium* were relatively more abundant in the group with supplementation of 60 mg of PUFAs, while *Bacteroidetes* were less abundant in this group. However, in the group treated with 90 mg omega-3 PUFAs, there was a much higher concentration of *Helicobacter, Jeotgalicoccus, Staphylococcus, Ruminococcus* and *Alcaligenaceae* than in remaining groups. A higher percentage of *Lactobacillus, Helicobacter* and *Ruminococcus* and a lower percentage of *Bacteroides, Clostridium* and *Prevotella* was observed in groups receiving higher dose of PUFAs (60 and 90 mg). Studies on mice showed that omega-3 supplementation resulted in enrichment of the intestinal microbiome in *Bifidobacterium spp., Bacteroidetes, Lactobacillus spp.* (Firmicutes), Enterobacteriales (Proteobacteria), *Lactococcus, Eubacterium, Lachnospermaceae, Ruminococcansiaae* and *Akkermansia* [159].

The effects of omega-3 PUFAs on the immune system is manifested by the inhibition of release of pro-inflammatory cytokines: tumor necrosis factor-α (TNF-α), IL-1, IL-6, IL-8 and IL-12, as well as by activation of nuclear factor kappa B [159]. In addition, omega-3 PUFAs modulate the activity of immune cells, primarily neutrophil function, including migration and phagocytic capacity, as well as the production of reactive oxygen species and cytokines. It stimulates macrophages to produce and secrete cytokines and chemokines, and increases the ability to phagocytose. Moreover, PUFAs modulate the activation of T cells.

9. Conclusions

The effectiveness of immunotherapy depends on the activity of the host's immune system and its ability to defeat tumor escape mechanisms from immune surveillance. The transformation of "cold tumors" into "hot tumors" is associated with an increased number of immune cells and cytokines in the tumor microenvironment, an increased tumor cells apoptosis and a greater effectiveness of immunotherapy. The intestinal microbiome is a proven immune system modulating factor, which positive role has been observed in numerous cancers. An increase in the level of Th CD4+ and CD8+ cells and a decrease in Tregs in the tumor microenvironment correlate with the abundance of *Bifidobacterium, Faecalibacterium* genus *Ruminococcaceae* family and *Clostridiales* order in the gut. Increased TNF-α production is correlated with greater abundance of *Bacteroidetes*, especially *Alistipes*. A higher percentage of peripheral blood NK cells and memory CD8+ T cells have been associated with higher numbers of *Alistipes putredinis, Prevotella copri* and *Bifidobacterium longum*. Richness of *Bifidobacterium spp., Akkermanisa muciniphila* and *Enterococcus hire* improves anti-tumor specific immunity and the response to anti-PD-1 or anti-PD-L1 immunotherapy by activating antigen-presenting cells and cytotoxic T cells within the tumor. Moreover, *Bifidobacterium spp. Bacteroides*, especially *B. fragilis* and *B. thetaiotamicron*, may affect the IL-12- and IFN-γ-dependent Th1 immune response and enhance the efficacy of immunotherapy.

Micronutrients affect directly the activities of the immune system or regulate their function by influencing the composition of the microbiome. Therefore, micronutrients can significantly influence the effectiveness of immunotherapy and the development of irEAs. This may become an interesting direction for further research on the predictors of immunotherapy.

Vitamin A supplementation may contribute to the growth of *Bifidobacterium, Akkermansia, Proteobacteria* and *Firmicutes*, the richness of which have been correlated with the greater effectiveness of immunotherapy in NSCLC, RCC, hepatocellular and colorectal cancer patients. Retinol is required for B-cell stimulation, thymocyte growth and NK cell activation, leading to inhibition of tumor cell proliferation and tumor growth arrest. B vitamins affect the increased level of TNF-α and IL-6 in the tumor microenvironment, the activation of NF-κB factor in macrophages and the increased abundance of *Bacteroides*,

Faecalibacterium and *Prevotella*, which stimulate the response to immunotherapy in NSCLC and melanoma patients. Vitamin B2 stimulates T cell activation and enriches the overall microbiome diversity, especially in *Alistipes*, which may increase the effectiveness of NSCLC, RCC, sarcoma and melanoma immunotherapy. Vitamin B12 particularly stimulates growth of *Akkermansia muciniphila* and *Eubacterium halli* and the immune response mediated by NK and T cells. Vitamin C supplementation enriches the microbiome in *Roseburia, Faecalibacterium, Akkermansia, Bifidobacterium* and *Bacteroides* and may increase the effectiveness of the treatment of numerous neoplastic diseases, including leukemia, colorectal cancer, melanoma, pancreatic cancer, prostate cancer, NSCLC, breast cancer and ovarian cancer. Vitamin C increases the immunogenicity of effector T cells in murine models and inhibits tumor growth. Vitamin D and E stimulate the growth of *Lactobacillus, Akkermansia, Faecalibacterium, Firmicutes, Actinobacteria, Proteobacteria* and *Bifidobacterium*, which enhance the effectiveness of immunotherapy in melanoma patients. Zinc enriches the microbiome in *Prevotella, Proteobacteria* and *Actinobacteria* and improves the function of the immune system by increasing the level of pro-inflammatory cytokines such as IL-1β, IL-2, IL-6, TNF-α and IFN-γ in the tumor environment. Moreover, zinc has been studied as a drug transporter directly to the tumor. Magnesium promotes the growth of *Bifidobacterium* in the intestines and increases the level of TNF-α and IL-6. Selenium enriches the microbiome in *Lachnospiraceae, Ruminococcaceae, Christensenellaceae* and *Lactobacillus*, which may favor the therapy in hepatocellular carcinoma patients.

Author Contributions: Conception and design of the study: M.F., P.K. Administrative support: E.K., J.M. All authors were involved in data collection and assembly of data. Data analysis and interpretation: M.F., A.G., P.K. Manuscript writing: M.F., A.G., P.K. All authors have read and agreed to the published version of the manuscript.

Funding: This research received no external funding.

Conflicts of Interest: The authors declare no conflict of interest.

References

1. Sekirov, I.; Russell, S.L.; Antunes, L.C.; Finlay, B.B. Gut microbiota in health and disease. *Physiol. Rev.* **2010**, *90*, 859–904. [CrossRef] [PubMed]
2. Gasmi, A.; Tippairote, T.; Mujawdiya, P.K.; Peana, M.; Menzel, A.; Dadar, M.; Benahmed, A.G.; Bjørklund, G. The microbiota-mediated dietary and nutritional interventions for COVID-19. *Clin. Immunol.* **2021**, *226*, 108725. [CrossRef] [PubMed]
3. Mathieu, E.; Escribano-Vazquez, U.; Descamps, D.; Cherbuy, C.; Langella, P.; Riffault, S.; Remot, A.; Thomas, M. Paradigms of lung microbiota functions in health and disease, particularly, in asthma. *Front. Physiol.* **2018**, *9*, 1168. [CrossRef] [PubMed]
4. Brandi, G.; Frega, G. Microbiota: Overview and Implication in Immunotherapy-Based Cancer Treatments. *Int. J. Mol. Sci.* **2019**, *20*, 2699. [CrossRef]
5. Hugon, P.; Dufour, J.C.; Colson, P.; Fournier, P.E.; Sallah, K.; Raoult, D. A comprehensive repertoire of prokaryotic species identified in human beings. *Lancet Infect. Dis.* **2015**, *15*, 1211–1219. [CrossRef]
6. Huttenhower, C.; Gevers, D.; Knight, R.; Abubucker, S.; Badger, J.H.; Chinwalla, A.T.; Creasy, H.H.; Earl, A.M.; FitzGerald, M.G.; Fulton, R.S.; et al. Structure, function and diversity of the healthy human microbiome. *Nature* **2012**, *486*, 207–214. [CrossRef]
7. Szczyrek, M.; Bitkowska, P.; Chunowski, P.; Czuchryta, P.; Krawczyk, P.; Milanowski, J. Diet, Microbiome, and Cancer Immunotherapy-A Comprehensive Review. *Nutrients* **2021**, *13*, 2217. [CrossRef]
8. LeBlanc, J.G.; Milani, C.; de Giori, G.S.; Sesma, F.; van Sinderen, D.; Ventura, M. Bacteria as vitamin suppliers to their host: A gut microbiota perspective. *Curr. Opin. Biotechnol.* **2013**, *24*, 160–168. [CrossRef]
9. Scott, K.P.; Antoine, J.M.; Midtvedt, T.; van Hemert, S. Manipulating the gut microbiota to maintain health and treat disease. *Microb. Ecol. Health Dis.* **2015**, *26*, 25877. [CrossRef]
10. Ley, R.E.; Bäckhed, F.; Turnbaugh, P.; Lozupone, C.A. Knight RD, Gordon JI. Obesity alters gut microbial ecology. *Proc. Natl. Acad. Sci. USA* **2005**, *102*, 11070–11075. [CrossRef]
11. de Vos, W.M.; de Vos, E.A. Role of the intestinal microbiome in health and disease: From correlation to causation. *Nutr. Rev.* **2012**, *70* (Suppl. 1), S45–S56. [CrossRef] [PubMed]
12. Ferreira, C.M.; Vieira, A.T.; Vinolo, M.A.; Oliveira, F.A.; Curi, R.; Martins, F.d.S. The central role of the gut microbiota in chronic inflammatory diseases. *J. Immunol. Res.* **2014**, *2014*, 689492. [CrossRef] [PubMed]
13. Kennedy, P.J.; Cryan, J.F.; Dinan, T.G.; Clarke, G. Irritable bowel syndrome: A microbiome-gut-brain axis disorder? *World J Gastroenterol.* **2014**, *m20*, 14105–14125. [CrossRef] [PubMed]

14. Agus, A.; Clément, K.; Sokol, H. Gut microbiota-derived metabolites as central regulators in metabolic disorders. *Gut* **2021**, *70*, 1174–1182. [CrossRef]
15. Cheng, B.; Wen, Y.; Yang, X.; Cheng, S.; Liu, L.; Chu, X.; Ye, J.; Liang, C.; Yao, Y.; Jia, Y.; et al. Gut microbiota is associated with bone mineral density: An observational and genome-wide environmental interaction analysis in the UK Biobank cohort. *Bone Joint Res.* **2021**, *10*, 734–741. [CrossRef]
16. Tinkov, A.A.; Martins, A.C.; Avila, D.S.; Gritsenko, V.A.; Skalny, A.V.; Santamaria, A.; Lee, E.; Bowman, A.B.; Aschner, M. Gut Microbiota as a Potential Player in Mn-Induced. *Neurotoxicity. Biomol.* **2021**, *11*, 1292. [CrossRef]
17. Jia, W.; Rajani, C.; Xu, H.; Zheng, X. Gut microbiota alterations are distinct for primary colorectal cancer and hepatocellular carcinoma. *Protein Cell.* **2021**, *12*, 374–393. [CrossRef]
18. Sepich-Poore, G.D.; Zitvogel, L.; Straussman, R.; Hasty, J.; Wargo, J.A.; Knight, R. The microbiome and human cancer. *Science* **2021**, *371*, eabc4552. [CrossRef]
19. Levy, M.; Thaiss, C.A.; Elinav, E. Metabolites: Messengers between the microbiota and the immune system. *Genes Dev.* **2016**, *30*, 1589–1597. [CrossRef]
20. Sommer, F.; Bäckhed, F. The gut microbiota–masters of host development and physiology. *Nat. Rev. Microbiol.* **2013**, *11*, 227–238. [CrossRef]
21. Spiljar, M.; Merkler, D.; Trajkovski, M. The Immune System Bridges the Gut Microbiota with Systemic Energy Homeostasis: Focus on TLRs, Mucosal Barrier, and SCFAs. *Front. Immunol.* **2017**, *8*, 1353. [CrossRef] [PubMed]
22. Marinelli, L.; Tenore, G.C.; Novellino, E. Probiotic species in the modulation of the anticancer immune response. *Semin. Cancer Biol.* **2017**, *46*, 182–190. [CrossRef] [PubMed]
23. Gopalakrishnan, V.; Helmink, B.A.; Spencer, C.N.; Reuben, A.; Wargo, J.A. The Influence of the Gut Microbiome on Cancer, Immunity, and Cancer Immunotherapy. *Cancer Cell* **2018**, *33*, 570–580. [CrossRef]
24. Medzhitov, R. Toll-like receptors and innate immunity. *Nat. Rev. Immunol.* **2001**, *1*, 135–145. [CrossRef] [PubMed]
25. Akira, S.; Takeda, K. Toll-like receptor signalling. *Nat. Rev. Immunol.* **2004**, *4*, 499–511. [CrossRef] [PubMed]
26. Askenase, P.W.; Itakura, A.; Leite-de-Moraes, M.C.; Lisbonne, M.; Roongapinun, S.; Goldstein, D.R.; Szczepanik, M. TLR-4 dependent IL-4 production by invariant Valpha14+Jalpha18+ NKT cells to initiate contact sensitivity in vivo. *J. Immunol.* **2005**, *175*, 6390–6401. [CrossRef]
27. Caramalho, I.; Lopes-Carvalho, T.; Ostler, D.; Zelenay, S.; Haury, M.; Demengeot, J. Regulatory T cells selectively express toll-like receptors and are activated by lipopolysaccharide. *J. Exp. Med.* **2003**, *197*, 403–411. [CrossRef]
28. Shimizu, H.; Matsuguchi, T.; Fukuda, Y.; Nakano, I.; Hayakawa, T.; Takeuchi, O.; Akira, S.; Umemura, M.; Suda, T.; Yoshikai, Y. Toll-like receptor 2 contributes to liver injury by Salmonella infection through Fas ligand expression on NKT cells in mice. *Gastroenterology* **2002**, *123*, 1265–1277. [CrossRef]
29. Macpherson, A.J.; Harris, N.L. Interactions between commensal intestinal bacteria and the immune system. *Nat. Rev. Immunol.* **2004**, *4*, 478–485. [CrossRef]
30. Yi, M.; Yu, S.; Qin, S.; Liu, Q.; Xu, H.; Zhao, W.; Chu, Q.; Wu, K. Gut microbiome modulates efficacy of immune checkpoint inhibitors. *J. Hematol. Oncol.* **2018**, *11*, 47. [CrossRef]
31. Singh, R.K.; Chang, H.W.; Yan, D.; Lee, K.M.; Ucmak, D.; Wong, K.; Abrouk, M.; Farahnik, B.; Nakamura, M.; Zhu, T.H.; et al. Influence of diet on the gut microbiome and implications for human health. *J. Transl. Med.* **2017**, *15*, 73. [CrossRef] [PubMed]
32. Beam, A.; Clinger, E.; Hao, L. Effect of Diet and Dietary Components on the Composition of the Gut Microbiota. *Nutrients* **2021**, *13*, 2795. [CrossRef] [PubMed]
33. Makki, K.; Deehan, E.C.; Walter, J.; Bäckhed, F. The Impact of Dietary Fiber on Gut Microbiota in Host Health and Disease. *Cell Host Microbe* **2018**, *23*, 705–715. [CrossRef] [PubMed]
34. Slavin, J. Fiber and Prebiotics: Mechanisms and Health Benefits. *Nutrients* **2013**, *5*, 1417–1435. [CrossRef]
35. Zakrzewska, Z.; Zawartka, A.; Schab, M.; Martyniak, A.; Skoczeń, S.; Tomasik, P.J.; Wędrychowicz, A. Prebiotics, Probiotics, and Postbiotics in the Prevention and Treatment of Anemia. *Microorganisms* **2022**, *10*, 1330. [CrossRef]
36. Wrzosek, L.; Miquel, S.; Noordine, M.L.; Bouet, S.; Curt, M.J.C.; Robert, V.; Philippe, C.; Bridonneau, C.; Cherbuy, C.; Robbe-Masselot, C.; et al. Bacteroides thetaiotaomicron and Faecalibacterium prausnitzii influence the production of mucus glycans and the development of goblet cells in the colonic epithelium of a gnotobiotic model rodent. *BMC Biol.* **2013**, *11*, 61. [CrossRef]
37. Furusawa, Y.; Obata, Y.; Fukuda, S.; Endo, T.A.; Nakato, G.; Takahashi, D.; Nakanishi, Y.; Uetake, C.; Kato, K.; Kato, T.; et al. Commensal microbe-derived butyrate induces the differentiation of colonic regulatory T cells. *Nature* **2013**, *504*, 446–450. [CrossRef]
38. Smith, P.M.; Howitt, M.R.; Panikov, N.; Michaud, M.; Gallini, C.A.; Bohlooly, Y.M.; Glickman, J.N.; Garrett, W.S. The microbial metabolites, short-chain fatty acids, regulate colonic Treg cell homeostasis. *Science* **2013**, *341*, 569–573. [CrossRef]
39. Tan, T.G.; Sefik, E.; Geva-Zatorsky, N.; Kua, L.; Naskar, D.; Teng, F.; Pasman, L.; Ortiz-Lopez, A.; Jupp, R.; Wu, H.-J.J.; et al. Identifying species of symbiont bacteria from the human gut that, alone, can induce intestinal Th17 cells in mice. *Proc. Natl. Acad. Sci. USA* **2016**, *113*, E8141–E8150. [CrossRef]
40. Neff, C.P.; Rhodes, M.E.; Arnolds, K.L.; Collins, C.B.; Donnelly, J.; Nusbacher, N.; Jedlicka, P.; Schneider, J.M.; McCarter, M.D.; Shaffer, M.; et al. Diverse Intestinal Bacteria Contain Putative Zwitterionic Capsular Polysaccharides with Anti-inflammatory Properties. *Cell Host Microbe* **2016**, *20*, 535–547. [CrossRef]

41. Morrison, D.J.; Preston, T. Formation of short chain fatty acids by the gut microbiota and their impact on human metabolism. *Gut Microbes* **2016**, *7*, 189–200. [CrossRef] [PubMed]
42. Remely, M.; Aumueller, E.; Merold, C.; Dworzak, S.; Hippe, B.; Zanner, J.; Pointner, A.; Brath, H.; Haslberger, A.G. Effects of short chain fatty acid producing bacteria on epigenetic regulation of FFAR3 in type 2 diabetes and obesity. *Gene* **2014**, *537*, 85–92. [CrossRef] [PubMed]
43. Velikonja, A.; Lipoglavšek, L.; Zorec, M.; Orel, R.; Avguštin, G. Alterations in gut microbiota composition and metabolic parameters after dietary intervention with barley beta glucans in patients with high risk for metabolic syndrome development. *Anaerobe* **2019**, *55*, 67–77. [CrossRef]
44. Connolly, M.L.; Tzounis, X.; Tuohy, K.; Lovegrove, J. Hypocholesterolemic and Prebiotic Effects of a Whole-Grain Oat-Based Granola Breakfast Cereal in a Cardio-Metabolic "At Risk" Population. *Front. Microbiol.* **2016**, *7*, 1755. [CrossRef] [PubMed]
45. Vanegas, S.M.; Meydani, M.; Barnett, J.B.; Goldin, B.; Kane, A.; Rasmussen, H.; Brown, C.; Vangay, P.; Knights, D.; Jonnalgadda, S.; et al. Substituting whole grains for refined grains in a 6-wk randomized trial has a modest effect on gut microbiota and immune and inflammatory markers of healthy adults. *Am. J. Clin. Nutr.* **2017**, *105*, 635–650. [CrossRef] [PubMed]
46. Kovatcheva-Datchary, P.; Nilsson, A.C.; Akrami, R.; Lee, Y.S.; De Vadder, F.; Arora, T.; Hallén, A.; Martens, E.; Björck, I.; Bäckhed, F. Dietary fiber-induced improvement in glucose metabolism is associated with increased abundance of prevotella. *Cell Metab.* **2015**, *22*, 971–982. [CrossRef] [PubMed]
47. Costabile, A.; Klinder, A.; Fava, F.; Napolitano, A.; Fogliano, V.; Leonard, C.; Gibson, G.R.; Tuohy, K. Whole-grain wheat breakfast cereal has a prebiotic effect on the human gut microbiota: A double-blind, placebo-controlled, crossover study. *Br. J. Nutr.* **2007**, *99*, 110–120. [CrossRef]
48. Zhao, L.; Zhang, F.; Ding, X.; Wu, G.; Lam, Y.Y.; Wang, X.; Fu, H.; Xue, X.; Lu, C.; Ma, J.; et al. Gut bacteria selectively promoted by dietary fibers alleviate type 2 diabetes. *Science* **2018**, *359*, 1151–1156. [CrossRef]
49. Routy, B.; Le Chatelier, E.; Derosa, L.; Duong, C.P.M.; Alou, M.T.; Daillère, R.; Fluckiger, A.; Messaoudene, M.; Rauber, C.; Roberti, M.P.; et al. Gut microbiome influences efficacy of PD-1-based immunotherapy against epithelial tumors. *Science* **2018**, *359*, 91–97. [CrossRef]
50. Sivan, A.; Corrales, L.; Hubert, N.; Williams, J.B.; Aquino-Michaels, K.; Earley, Z.M.; Benyamin, F.W.; Lei, Y.M.; Jabri, B.; Alegre, M.; et al. Commensal Bifidobacterium promotes antitumor immunity and facilitates anti-PD-L1 efficacy. *Science* **2015**, *350*, 1084–1089. [CrossRef]
51. Li, W.; Deng, Y.; Chu, Q.; Zhang, P. Gut microbiome and cancer immunotherapy. *Cancer Lett.* **2019**, *447*, 41–47. [CrossRef] [PubMed]
52. Vétizou, M.; Pitt, J.M.; Daillère, R.; Lepage, P.; Waldschmitt, N.; Flament, C.; Rusakiewicz, S.; Routy, B.; Roberti, M.P.; Duong, C.P.; et al. Anticancer immunotherapy by CTLA-4 blockade relies on the gut microbiota. *Science* **2015**, *350*, 1079–1084. [CrossRef] [PubMed]
53. Reed, J.P.; Devkota, S.; Figlin, R.A. Gut microbiome, antibiotic use, and immunotherapy responsiveness in cancer. *Ann. Transl. Med.* **2019**, *7*, S309. [CrossRef] [PubMed]
54. Hakozaki, T.; Okuma, Y.; Omori, M.; Hosomi, Y. Impact of prior antibiotic use on the efficacy of nivolumab for non-small cell lung cancer. *Oncol. Lett.* **2019**, *17*, 2946–2952. [CrossRef]
55. Ahmed, J.; Kumar, A.; Parikh, K.; Anwar, A.; Knoll, B.M.; Puccio, C.; Chun, H.; Fanucchi, M.; Lim, S.H. Use of broad-spectrum antibiotics impacts outcome in patients treated with immune checkpoint inhibitors. *OncoImmunology* **2018**, *7*, e1507670. [CrossRef]
56. Villéger, R.; Lopès, A.; Carrier, G.; Veziant, J.; Billard, E.; Barnich, N.; Gagnière, J.; Vazeille, E.; Bonnet, M. Intestinal Microbiota: A Novel Target to Improve Anti-Tumor Treatment? *Int. J. Mol. Sci.* **2019**, *20*, 4584. [CrossRef] [PubMed]
57. Huemer, F.; Rinnerthaler, G.; Westphal, T.; Hackl, H.; Hutarew, G.; Gampenrieder, S.P.; Weiss, L.; Greil, R. Impact of antibiotic treatment on immune-checkpoint blockade efficacy in advanced non-squamous non-small cell lung cancer. *Oncotarget* **2018**, *9*, 16512–16520. [CrossRef]
58. Desai, M.S.; Seekatz, A.M.; Koropatkin, N.M.; Kamada, N.; Hickey, C.A.; Wolter, M.; Pudlo, N.A.; Kitamoto, S.; Terrapon, N.; Muller, A.; et al. A Dietary Fiber-Deprived Gut Microbiota Degrades the Colonic Mucus Barrier and Enhances Pathogen Susceptibility. *Cell* **2016**, *167*, 1339–1353. [CrossRef]
59. Yan, X.; Zhang, S.; Deng, Y.; Wang, P.; Hou, Q.; Xu, H. Prognostic Factors for Checkpoint Inhibitor Based Immunotherapy: An Update with New Evidences. *Front. Pharmacol.* **2018**, *9*, 1050. [CrossRef]
60. Pitt, J.M.; Vétizou, M.; Waldschmitt, N.; Kroemer, G.; Chamaillard, M.; Boneca, I.G.; Zitvogel, L. Fine-Tuning Cancer Immunotherapy: Optimizing the Gut Microbiome. *Cancer Res.* **2016**, *76*, 4602–4607. [CrossRef]
61. Frankel, A.E.; Deshmukh, S.; Reddy, A.; Lightcap, J.; Hayes, M.; McClellan, S.; Singh, S.; Rabideau, B.; Glover, T.G.; Roberts, B.; et al. Cancer Immune Checkpoint Inhibitor Therapy and the Gut Microbiota. *Integr. Cancer Ther.* **2019**, *18*, 1–10. [CrossRef] [PubMed]
62. Gopalakrishnan, V.; Spencer, C.N.; Nezi, L.; Reuben, A.; Andrews, M.C.; Karpinets, T.V.; Prieto, P.A.; Vicente, D.; Hoffman, K.; Wei, S.C.; et al. Gut microbiome modulates response to anti-PD-1 immunotherapy in melanoma patients. *Science* **2018**, *359*, 97–103. [CrossRef] [PubMed]
63. Chaput, N.; Lepage, P.; Coutzac, C.; Soularue, E.; Le Roux, K.; Monot, C.; Boselli, L.; Routier, E.; Cassard, L.; Collins, M.; et al. Baseline gut microbiota predicts clinical response and colitis in metastatic melanoma patients treated with ipilimumab. *Ann. Oncol.* **2017**, *28*, 1368–1379. [CrossRef] [PubMed]

64. Dubin, K.; Callahan, M.K.; Ren, B.; Khanin, R.; Viale, A.; Ling, L.; No, D.; Gobourne, A.; Littmann, E.; Huttenhower, C.; et al. Intestinal microbiome analyses identify melanoma patients at risk for checkpoint-blockade-induced colitis. *Nat. Commun.* **2016**, *7*, 10391. [CrossRef]
65. Matson, V.; Fessler, J.; Bao, R.; Chongsuwat, T.; Zha, Y.; Alegre, M.L.; Luke, J.J.; Gajewski, T.F. The commensal microbiome is associated with anti–PD-1 efficacy in metastatic melanoma patients. *Science* **2018**, *359*, 104–108. [CrossRef]
66. Chen, P.L.; Roh, W.; Reuben, A.; Cooper, Z.A.; Spencer, C.N.; Prieto, P.A.; Miller, J.P.; Bassett, R.L.; Gopalakrishnan, V.; Wani, K.; et al. Analysis of immune signatures in longitudinal tumor samples yields insight into biomarkers of response and mechanisms of resistance to immune checkpoint blockade. *Cancer Discov.* **2016**, *6*, 827–837. [CrossRef]
67. Tumeh, P.C.; Harview, C.L.; Yearley, J.H.; Shintaku, I.P.; Taylor, E.J.M.; Robert, L.; Chmielowski, B.; Spasic, M.; Henry, G.; Ciobanu, V.; et al. PD-1 blockade induces responses by inhibiting adaptive immune resistance. *Nature* **2014**, *515*, 568–571. [CrossRef]
68. Tsujikawa, T.; Kumar, S.; Borkar, R.N.; Azimi, V.; Thibault, G.; Chang, Y.H.; Balter, A.; Kawashima, R.; Choe, G.; Sauer, D.; et al. Quantitative multiplex immunohistochemistry reveals myeloid-inflamed tumor-immune complexity associated with poor prognosis. *Cell Rep.* **2017**, *19*, 203–217. [CrossRef]
69. Tanoue, T.; Morita, S.; Plichta, D.R.; Skelly, A.N.; Suda, W.; Sugiura, Y.; Narushima, S.; Vlamakis, H.; Motoo, I.; Sugita, K.; et al. A defined commensal consortium elicits CD8 T cells and anti-cancer immunity. *Nature* **2019**, *565*, 600–605. [CrossRef]
70. Song, P.; Yang, D.; Wang, H.; Cui, X.; Si, X.; Zhang, X.; Zhang, L. Relationship between intestinal flora structure and metabolite analysis and immunotherapy efficacy in Chinese NSCLC patients. *Thorac. Cancer* **2020**, *11*, 1621–1632. [CrossRef]
71. Jin, Y.; Dong, H.; Xia, L.; Yang, Y.; Zhu, Y.; Shen, Y.; Zheng, H.; Yao, C.; Wang, Y.; Lu, S. The Diversity of Gut Microbiome is Associated With Favorable Responses to Anti-Programmed Death 1 Immunotherapy in Chinese Patients With NSCLC. *J. Thorac. Oncol.* **2019**, *14*, 1378–1389. [CrossRef] [PubMed]
72. Lee, S.H.; Cho, S.Y.; Yoon, Y.; Park, C.; Sohn, J.; Jeong, J.J.; Jeon, B.N.; Jang, M.; An, C.; Lee, S.; et al. Bifidobacterium bifidum strains synergize with immune checkpoint inhibitors to reduce tumour burden in mice. *Nat. Microbiol.* **2021**, *6*, 277–288. [CrossRef] [PubMed]
73. Wojas-Krawczyk, K.; Kalinka, E.; Grenda, A.; Krawczyk, P.; Milanowski, J. Beyond PD-L1 Markers for Lung Cancer Immunotherapy. *Int. J. Mol. Sci.* **2019**, *20*, 1915. [CrossRef]
74. Carbone, C.; Piro, G.; Di Noia, V.; D'Argento, E.; Vita, E.; Ferrara, M.G.; Pilotto, S.; Milella, M.; Cammarota, G.; Gasbarrini, A.; et al. Lung and gut microbiota as potential hidden driver of immunotherapy efficacy in lung cancer. *Mediat. Inflamm.* **2019**, *2019*, 1–10. [CrossRef]
75. Zheng, Y.; Wang, T.; Tu, X.; Huang, Y.; Zhang, H.; Tan, D.; Jiang, W.; Cai, S.; Zhao, P.; Song, R.; et al. Gut microbiome affects the response to anti-PD-1 immunotherapy in patients with hepatocellular carcinoma. *J. Immunother. Cancer.* **2019**, *7*, 193. [CrossRef] [PubMed]
76. Grenda, A.; Iwan, E.; Chmielewska, I.; Krawczyk, P.; Giza, A.; Bomba, A.; Frąk, M.; Rolska, A.; Szczyrek, M.; Kieszko, R.; et al. Presence of Akkermansiaceae in gut microbiome and immunotherapy effectiveness in patients with advanced non-small cell lung cancer. *AMB Express* **2022**, *12*, 86. [CrossRef]
77. Cekikj, M.; Jakimovska Özdemir, M.; Kalajdzhiski, S.; Özcan, O.; Sezerman, O.U. Understanding the Role of the Microbiome in Cancer Diagnostics and Therapeutics by Creating and Utilizing ML Models. *Appl. Sci.* **2022**, *12*, 4094. [CrossRef]
78. Sarao, L.K.; Arora, M. Probiotics, prebiotics, and microencapsulation: A review. *Crit. Rev. Food Sci. Nutr.* **2017**, *57*, 344–371. [CrossRef]
79. Fan, S.; Breidt, F.; Price, R.; Pérez-Díaz, I. Survival and Growth of Probiotic Lactic Acid Bacteria in Refrigerated Pickle Products. *J. Food Sci.* **2017**, *82*, 167–173. [CrossRef]
80. Ganesan, B.; Weimer, B.C.; Pinzon, J.; Dao Kong, N.; Rompato, G.; Brothersen, C.; McMahon, D.J. Probiotic bacteria survive in Cheddar cheese and modify populations of other lactic acid bacteria. *J. Appl. Microbiol.* **2014**, *116*, 1642–1656. [CrossRef]
81. Schab, M.; Skoczen, S. The Role of Nutritional Status, Gastrointestinal Peptides, and Endocannabinoids in the Prognosis and Treatment of Children with Cancer. *Int. J. Mol. Sci.* **2022**, *23*, 5159. [CrossRef] [PubMed]
82. Huda, M.N.; Ahmad, S.M.; Kalanetra, K.M.; Taft, D.H.; Alam, M.J.; Khanam, A.; Raqib, R.; Underwood, M.A.; Mills, D.A.; Stephensen, C.B. Neonatal Vitamin A Supplementation and Vitamin A Status Are Associated with Gut Microbiome Composition in Bangladeshi Infants in Early Infancy and at 2 Years of Age. *J. Nutr.* **2019**, *149*, 1075–1088. [CrossRef] [PubMed]
83. Lv, Z.; Wang, Y.; Yang, T.; Zhan, X.; Li, Z.; Hu, H.; Li, T.; Chen, J. Vitamin A deficiency impacts the structural segregation of gut microbiota in children with persistent diarrhea. *J. Clin. Biochem. Nutr.* **2016**, *59*, 113–121. [CrossRef] [PubMed]
84. Mandal, S.; Godfrey, K.; McDonald, D.; Treuren, W.; Bjørnholt, J.; Midtvedt, T.; Moen, B.; Rudi, K.; Knight, R.; Brantsaeter, A.L.; et al. Fat and Vitamin Intakes during Pregnancy Have Stronger Relations with a Pro-Inflammatory Maternal Microbiota than Does Carbohydrate Intake. *Microbiome* **2016**, *4*, 1–11. [CrossRef] [PubMed]
85. Liu, J.; Liu, X.; Xiong, X.Q.; Yang, T.; Cui, T.; Hou, N.L.; Lai, X.; Liu, S.; Guo, M.; Liang, X.H.; et al. Effect of vitamin A supplementation on gut microbiota in children with autism spectrum disorders—A pilot study. *BMC Microbiol.* **2017**, *17*, 204. [CrossRef] [PubMed]
86. Lu, M.S.; Fang, Y.J.; Chen, Y.M.; Luo, W.P.; Pan, Z.Z.; Zhong, X.; Zhang, C.X. Higher intake of carotenoid is associated with a lower risk of colorectal cancer in Chinese adults: A case-control study. *Eur. J. Nutr.* **2015**, *54*, 619–628. [CrossRef]
87. Jung, S.; Wu, K.; Giovannucci, E.; Spiegelman, D.; Willett, W.C.; Smith-Warner, S.A. Carotenoid intake and risk of colorectal adenomas in a cohort of male health professionals. *Cancer Causes Control* **2013**, *24*, 705–717. [CrossRef]

88. Jin, Y.; Teh, S.S.; Lau, H.L.N.; Xiao, J.; Mah, S.H. Retinoids as anti-cancer agents and their mechanisms of action. *Am. J. Cancer Res.* **2022**, *12*, 938–960.
89. Pastorino, U.; Infante, M.; Maioli, M.; Chiesa, G.; Buyse, M.; Firket, N.; Rosmentz, P.; Clerici, M.; Soresi, E.; Valente, M. Adjuvant treatment of stage I lung cancer with high-dose vitamin A. *J. Clin. Oncol.* **1993**, *11*, 1216–1222. [CrossRef]
90. Mamede, A.C.; Tavares, S.D.; Abrantes, A.M.; Trindade, J.; Maia, J.M.; Botelho, M.F. The role of vitamins in cancer: A review. *Nutr. Cancer* **2011**, *63*, 479–494. [CrossRef]
91. Kim, J.A.; Jang, J.H.; Lee, S.Y. An Updated Comprehensive Review on Vitamin A and Carotenoids in Breast Cancer: Mechanisms, Genetics, Assessment, Current Evidence, and Future Clinical Implications. *Nutrients* **2021**, *13*, 3162. [CrossRef] [PubMed]
92. Park, E.Y.; Pinali, D.; Lindley, K.; Lane, M.A. Hepatic vitamin A preloading reduces colorectal cancer metastatic multiplicity in a mouse xenograft model. *Nutr. Cancer* **2012**, *64*, 732–740. [CrossRef] [PubMed]
93. Weinzweig, J.; Tattini, C.; Lynch, S.; Zienowicz, R.; Weinzweig, N.; Spangenberger, A.; Edstrom, L. Investigation of the growth and metastasis of malignant melanoma in a murine model: The role of supplemental vitamin A. *Plast. Reconstr. Surg.* **2003**, *112*, 152–158;159–161. [CrossRef] [PubMed]
94. Venturelli, S.; Leischner, C.; Helling, T.; Burkard, M.; Marongiu, L. Vitamins as Possible Cancer Biomarkers: Significance and Limitations. *Nutrients* **2021**, *13*, 3914. [CrossRef] [PubMed]
95. Craft, N.E.; Furr, H.C. Methods for assessment of vitamin A (retinoids) and carotenoids. *Lab. Assess Vitam.* **2018**, *2*, 23–55.
96. Tobin, R.P.; Jordan, K.R.; Robinson, W.A.; Davis, D.; Borges, V.F.; Gonzalez, R.; Lewis, K.D.; McCarter, M.D. Targeting myeloid-derived suppressor cells using all-trans retinoic acid in melanoma patients treated with Ipilimumab. *Int. Immunopharmacol.* **2018**, *63*, 282–291. [CrossRef]
97. Kunisawa, J.; Sugiura, Y.; Wake, T.; Nagatake, T.; Suzuki, H.; Nagasawa, R.; Shikata, S.; Honda, K.; Hashimoto, E.; Suzuki, Y.; et al. Mode of Bioenergetic Metabolism during B Cell Differentiation in the Intestine Determines the Distinct Requirement for Vitamin B1. *Cell Rep.* **2015**, *13*, 122–131. [CrossRef]
98. Hu, S.; He, W.; Du, X.; Huang, Y.; Fu, Y.; Yang, Y.; Hu, C.; Li, S.; Wang, Q.; Wen, Q.; et al. Vitamin B1 Helps to Limit Mycobacterium tuberculosis Growth via Regulating Innate Immunity in a Peroxisome Proliferator-Activated Receptor-γ-Dependent Manner. *Front. Immunol.* **2018**, *9*, 1778. [CrossRef]
99. Park, J.; Hosomi, K.; Kawashima, H.; Chen, Y.A.; Mohsen, A.; Ohno, H.; Konishi, K.; Tanisawa, K.; Kifushi, M.; Kogawa, M.; et al. Dietary Vitamin B1 Intake Influences Gut Microbial Community and the Consequent Production of Short-Chain Fatty Acids. *Nutrients* **2022**, *14*, 2078. [CrossRef]
100. Rouxel, O.; Da Silva, J.; Beaudoin, L.; Nel, I.; Tard, C.; Cagninacci, L.; Kiaf, B.; Oshima, M.; Diedisheim, M.; Salou, M.; et al. Cytotoxic and regulatory roles of mucosal-associated invariant T cells in type 1 diabetes. *Nat. Immunol.* **2017**, *18*, 1321–1331. [CrossRef]
101. von Martels, J.Z.; Bourgonje, A.R.; Klaassen, M.A.; Alkhalifah, H.A.; Sadaghian Sadabad, M.; Vich Vila, A.; Gacesa, R.; Gabriëls, R.Y.; Steinert, R.E.; Jansen, B.H.; et al. Riboflavin supplementation in patients with Crohn's disease [the RISE-UP study]. *J. Crohns Colitis* **2020**, *14*, 595–607. [CrossRef] [PubMed]
102. Barone, M.; D'Amico, F.; Brigidi, P.; Turroni, S. Gut microbiome-micronutrient interaction: The key to controlling the bioavailability of minerals and vitamins? *Biofactors* **2022**, *48*, 307–314. [CrossRef] [PubMed]
103. Pham, V.T.; Dold, S.; Rehman, A.; Bird, J.K.; Steinert, R.E. Vitamins, the gut microbiome and gastrointestinal health in humans. *Nutr. Res.* **2021**, *95*, 35–53. [CrossRef] [PubMed]
104. Fangmann, D.; Theismann, E.M.; Türk, K.; Schulte, D.M.; Relling, I.; Hartmann, K.; Keppler, J.K.; Knipp, J.R.; Rehman, A.; Heinsen, F.A.; et al. Targeted Microbiome Intervention by Microencapsulated Delayed-Release Niacin Beneficially Affects Insulin Sensitivity in Humans. *Diabetes Care* **2018**, *41*, 398–405. [CrossRef] [PubMed]
105. Shibata, N.; Kunisawa, J.; Kiyono, H. Dietary and Microbial Metabolites in the Regulation of Host Immunity. *Front. Microbiol.* **2017**, *8*, 2171. [CrossRef]
106. Yoshii, K.; Hosomi, K.; Sawane, K.; Kunisawa, J. Metabolism of Dietary and Microbial Vitamin B Family in the Regulation of Host Immunity. *Front. Nutr.* **2019**, *6*, 48. [CrossRef]
107. Belzer, C.; Chia, L.W.; Aalvink, S.; Chamlagain, B.; Piironen, V.; Knol, J.; de Vos, W.M. Microbial metabolic networks at the mucus layer lead to diet-independent butyrate and vitamin B12 production by intestinal symbionts. *MBio* **2017**, *8*, e00770-17. [CrossRef]
108. Yuen, R.C.; Tsao, S.Y. Embracing cancer immunotherapy with vital micronutrients. *World J. Clin. Oncol.* **2021**, *12*, 712–724. [CrossRef]
109. Mach, N.; Clark, A. Micronutrient deficiencies and the human gut microbiota. *Trends Microbiol.* **2017**, *25*, 607–610. [CrossRef]
110. Böttger, F.; Vallés-Martí, A.; Cahn, L.; Jimenez, C.R. High-dose intravenous vitamin C a promising multi-targeting agent in the treatment of cancer. *J. Exp. Clin. Cancer Res.* **2021**, *40*, 343. [CrossRef]
111. Luchtel, R.A.; Bhagat, T.; Pradhan, K.; Jacobs, W.R.; Levine, M.; Verma, A.; Shenoy, N. High-dose ascorbic acid synergizes with anti-PD1 in a lymphoma mouse model. *Proc. Natl. Acad. Sci. USA* **2020**, *117*, 1666–1677. [CrossRef] [PubMed]
112. Magrì, A.; Germano, G.; Lorenzato, A.; Lamba, S.; Chilà, R.; Montone, M.; Amodio, M.; Ceruti, T.; Sassi, F.; Arena, S.; et al. High-dose vitamin C enhances cancer immunotherapy. *Sci. Transl. Med.* **2020**, *12*, eaay8707. [CrossRef] [PubMed]
113. Kanhere, M.; He, J.; Chassaing, B.; Ziegler, T.R.; Alvarez, J.A.; Ivie, E.A.; Hao, L.; Hanfelt, J.; Gewirtz, A.T.; Tangpricha, V. Bolus Weekly Vitamin D3 Supplementation Impacts Gut and Airway Microbiota in Adults With Cystic Fibrosis: A Double-Blind, Randomized, Placebo-Controlled Clinical Trial. *J. Clin. Endocrinol. Metab.* **2018**, *103*, 564–574. [CrossRef] [PubMed]

114. Clark, A.; Mach, N. Role of Vitamin D in the Hygiene Hypothesis: The Interplay between Vitamin D, Vitamin D Receptors, Gut Microbiota, and Immune Response. *Front. Immunol.* **2016**, *7*, 627. [CrossRef] [PubMed]
115. Celiberto, L.S.; Graef, F.A.; Healey, G.R.; Bosman, E.S.; Jacobson, K.; Sly, L.M.; Vallance, B.A. Inflammatory bowel disease and immunonutrition: Novel therapeutic approaches through modulation of diet and the gut microbiome. *Immunology* **2018**, *155*, 36–52. [CrossRef]
116. Ananthakrishnan, A.N.; Cagan, A.; Gainer, V.S.; Cheng, S.-C.; Cai, T.; Szolovits, P.; Shaw, S.Y.; Churchill, S.; Kralson, E.W.; Murphy, S.N.; et al. Higher plasma 25(OH)D is associated with reduced risk of Clostridium difficile infection in patients with inflammatory bowel diseases. *Aliment Pharmacol. Ther.* **2014**, *39*, 1136–1142. [CrossRef]
117. Cantarel, B.L.; Waubant, E.; Chehoud, C.; Kuczynski, J.; DeSantis, T.Z.; Warrington, J.; Venkatesan, A.; Fraser, C.M.; Mowry, E.M. Gut microbiota in MS: Possible influence of immunomodulators. *J. Investig. Med.* **2015**, *63*, 729–734. [CrossRef]
118. Mielcarz, D.W.; Kasper, L.H. The gut microbiome in multiple sclerosis. *Curr. Treat. Options. Neurol.* **2015**, *17*, 344. [CrossRef]
119. Cole, E.T.; Scott, R.A.; Connor, A.L.; Wilding, I.R.; Petereit, H.U.; Schminke, C.; Beckert, T.; Cadé, D. Enteric coated HPMC capsules designed to achieve intestinal targeting. *Int. J. Pharm.* **2002**, *231*, 83–95. [CrossRef]
120. Tabatabaeizadeh, S.A.; Fazeli, M.; Meshkat, Z.; Khodashenas, E.; Esmaeili, H.; Mazloum, S.; Ferns, G.A.; Abdizadeh, M.F.; Ghayour-Mobarhan, M. The effects of high doses of vitamin D on the composition of the gut microbiome of adolescent girls. *Clin. Nutr. ESPEN* **2020**, *35*, 103–108. [CrossRef]
121. Pham, V.T.; Fehlbaum, S.; Seifert, N.; Richard, N.; Bruins, M.J.; Sybesma, W.; Rehman, A.; Steiner, R.E. Effects of colon-targeted vitamins on the composition and metabolic activity of the human gut microbiome-A pilot study. *Gut Microbes* **2021**, *13*, 1–20. [CrossRef] [PubMed]
122. Vernia, F.; Valvano, M.; Longo, S.; Cesaro, N.; Viscido, A.; Latella, G. Vitamin D in Inflammatory Bowel Diseases. Mechanisms of Action and Therapeutic Implications. *Nutrients* **2022**, *14*, 269. [CrossRef] [PubMed]
123. Schaffler, H.; Herlemann, D.P.; Klinitzke, P.; Berlin, P.; Kreikemeyer, B.; Jaster, R.; Lamprecht, G. Vitamin D administration leads to a shift of the intestinal bacterial composition in Crohn's disease patients, but not in healthy controls. *J. Dig. Dis.* **2018**, *19*, 225–234. [CrossRef] [PubMed]
124. Soltys, K.; Stuchlikova, M.; Hlavaty, T.; Gaalova, B.; Budis, J.; Gazdarica, J.; Krajcovicova, A.; Zelinkova, Z.; Szemes, T.; Kuba, D.; et al. Seasonal changes of circulating 25-hydroxyvitamin D correlate with the lower gut microbiome composition in inflammatory bowel disease patients. *Sci. Rep.* **2020**, *10*, 6024. [CrossRef] [PubMed]
125. Qiu, F.; Zhang, Z.; Yang, L.; Li, R.; Ma, Y. Combined effect of vitamin C and vitamin D3 on intestinal epithelial barrier by regulating notch signaling pathway. *Nutr. Metab.* **2021**, *18*, 49. [CrossRef]
126. Cantorna, M.T.; Snyder, L.; Lin, Y.D.; Yang, L. Vitamin D and 1,25(OH)2D regulation of T cells. *Nutrients* **2015**, *7*, 3011–3021. [CrossRef]
127. Li, L.; Krause, L.; Somerset, S. Associations between micronutrient intakes and gut microbiota in a group of adults with cystic fibrosis. *Clin. Nutr.* **2017**, *36*, 1097–1104. [CrossRef]
128. Carrothers, J.M.; York, M.A.; Brooker, S.L.; Lackey, K.A.; Williams, J.E.; Shafii, B.; Price, W.J.; Settles, M.L.; McGuire, M.A.; McGuire, M.K. Fecal microbial community structure is stable over time and related to variation in macronutrient and micronutrient intakes in lactating women. *J. Nutr.* **2015**, *145*, 2379–2388. [CrossRef]
129. Tang, M.; Frank, D.N.; Sherlock, L.; Ir, D.; Robertson, C.E.; Krebs, N.F. Effect of Vitamin E with Therapeutic Iron Supplementation on Iron Repletion and Gut Microbiome in US Iron Deficient Infants and Toddlers. *J. Pediatr. Gastroenterol. Nutr.* **2016**, *63*, 379–385. [CrossRef]
130. Choi, Y.; Lee, S.; Kim, S.; Lee, J.; Ha, J.; Oh, H.; Lee, Y.; Kim, Y.; Yoon, Y. Vitamin E (α-tocopherol) consumption influences gut microbiota composition. *Int. J. Food Sci. Nutr.* **2020**, *71*, 221–225. [CrossRef]
131. Nomura, A.M.; Stemmermann, G.N.; Lee, J.; Craft, N.E. Serum micronutrients and prostate cancer in Japanese Americans in Hawaii. *Cancer Epidemiol Biomark. Prev.* **1997**, *6*, 487–491.
132. Zhang, Q.; Meng, Y.; Du, M.; Li, S.; Xin, J.; Ben, S.; Zhang, Z.; Gu, D.; Wang, M. Evaluation of common genetic variants in vitamin E-related pathway genes and colorectal cancer susceptibility. *Arch. Toxicol.* **2021**, *95*, 2523–2532. [CrossRef]
133. Goodman, G.E.; Schaffer, S.; Omenn, G.S.; Chen, C.; King, I. The association between lung and prostate cancer risk, and serum micronutrients: Results and lessons learned from beta-carotene and retinol efficacy trial. *Cancer Epidemiol. Biomark. Prev.* **2003**, *12*, 518–526.
134. Yuan, X.; Duan, Y.; Xiao, Y.; Sun, K.; Qi, Y.; Zhang, Y.; Ahmed, Z.; Moiani, D.; Yao, J.; Li, H.; et al. Vitamin E Enhances Cancer Immunotherapy by Reinvigorating Dendritic Cells via Targeting Checkpoint SHP1. *Cancer Discov.* **2022**, *12*, 1742–1759. [CrossRef] [PubMed]
135. Seura, T.; Yoshino, Y.; Fukuwatari, T. The Relationship between Habitual Dietary Intake and Gut Microbiota in Young Japanese Women. *J. Nutr. Sci. Vitam.* **2017**, *63*, 396–404. [CrossRef]
136. Lu, H.; Mei, C.; Yang, L.; Zheng, J.; Tong, J.; Duan, F.; Liang, H.; Hong, L. PPM-18, an Analog of Vitamin K Induces Autophagy and Apoptosis in Bladder Cancer Cells Through ROS and AMPK Signaling Pathways. *Front. Pharmacol.* **2021**, *12*, 684915. [CrossRef] [PubMed]
137. Simonyté Sjödin, K.; Domellöf, M.; Lagerqvist, C.; Hernell, O.; Lönnerdal, B.; Szymlek-Gay, E.A.; Sjödin, A.; West, C.E.; Lind, T. Administration of ferrous sulfate drops has significant effects on the gut microbiota of iron-sufficient infants: A randomised controlled study. *Gut* **2019**, *68*, 2095–2097. [CrossRef] [PubMed]

138. Paganini, D.; Zimmermann, M.B. The effects of iron fortification and supplementation on the gut microbiome and diarrhea in infants and children: A review. *Am. J. Clin. Nutr.* **2017**, *106*, 1688S–1693S. [CrossRef] [PubMed]
139. Zimmermann, M.B.; Chassard, C.; Rohner, F.; N'goran, E.K.; Nindjin, C.; Dostal, A.; Utzinger, J.; Ghattas, H.; Lacroix, C.; Hurrell, R.F. The effects of iron fortification on the gut microbiota in African children: A randomized controlled trial in Cote d'Ivoire. *Am. J. Clin. Nutr.* **2010**, *92*, 1406–1415. [CrossRef] [PubMed]
140. González, A.; Gálvez, N.; Martín, J.; Reyes, F.; Pérez-Victoria, I.; Dominguez-Vera, J.M. Identification of the key excreted molecule by Lactobacillus fermentum related to host iron absorption. *Food Chem.* **2017**, *228*, 374–380. [CrossRef]
141. Chung, S.; Revia, R.A.; Zhang, M. Iron oxide nanoparticles for immune cell labeling and cancer immunotherapy. *Nanoscale Horiz.* **2021**, *6*, 696–717. [CrossRef] [PubMed]
142. Pieper, R.; Vahjen, W.; Neumann, K.; VanKessel, A.G.; Zentek, J. Dose-dependent effects of dietary zinc oxide on bacterial communities and metabolic profiles in the ileum of weaned pigs. *J. Anim. Physiol. Anim. Nutr.* **2012**, *96*, 825–833. [CrossRef] [PubMed]
143. Liu, H.; Bai, M.; Xu, K.; Zhou, J.; Zhang, X.; Yu, R.; Huang, R.; Yin, Y. Effects of different concentrations of coated nano zinc oxide material on fecal bacterial composition and intestinal barrier in weaned piglets. *J. Sci. Food Agric.* **2021**, *101*, 735–745. [CrossRef]
144. Satessa, G.D.; Kjeldsen, N.J.; Mansouryar, M.; Hansen, H.H.; Bache, J.K.; Nielsen, M.O. Effects of alternative feed additives to medicinal zinc oxide on productivity, diarrhoea incidence and gut development in weaned piglets. *Animal* **2020**, *26*, 1–9. [CrossRef]
145. Starke, I.C.; Pieper, R.; Neumann, K.; Zentek, J.; Vahjen, W. The impact of high dietary zinc oxide on the development of the intestinal microbiota in weaned piglets. *FEMS Microbiol. Ecol.* **2014**, *87*, 416–427. [CrossRef] [PubMed]
146. Højberg, O.; Canibe, N.; Poulsen, H.D.; Hedemann, M.S.; Jensen, B.B. Influence of dietary zinc oxide and copper sulfate on the gastrointestinal ecosystem in newly weaned piglets. *Appl. Environ. Microbiol.* **2005**, *71*, 2267–2277. [CrossRef]
147. Vahjen, W.; Pieper, R.; Zentek, J. Increased dietary zinc oxide changes the bacterial core and enterobacterial composition in the ileum of piglets. *J. Anim. Sci.* **2011**, *89*, 2430–2439. [CrossRef]
148. Reed, S.; Neuman, H.; Moscovich, S.; Glahn, R.P.; Koren, O.; Tako, E. Chronic Zinc Deficiency Alters Chick Gut Microbiota Composition and Function. *Nutrients* **2015**, *7*, 9768–9784. [CrossRef]
149. Surono, I.S.; Martono, P.D.; Kameo, S.; Suradji, E.W.; Koyama, H. Effect of probiotic L. plantarum IS-10506 and zinc supplementation on humoral immune response and zinc status of Indonesian pre-school children. *J. Trace Elem. Med. Biol.* **2014**, *28*, 465–469. [CrossRef]
150. Li, D.; Stovall, D.B.; Wang, W.; Sui, G. Advances of Zinc Signaling Studies in Prostate Cancer. *Int. J. Mol. Sci.* **2020**, *21*, 667. [CrossRef]
151. Cen, D.; Ge, Q.; Xie, C.; Zheng, Q.; Guo, J.; Zhang, Y.; Wang, Y.; Li, X.; Gu, Z.; Cai, X. ZnS@BSA Nanoclusters Potentiate Efficacy of Cancer Immunotherapy. *Adv. Mater.* **2021**, *33*, e2104037. [CrossRef] [PubMed]
152. Del Chierico, F.; Trapani, V.; Petito, V.; Reddel, S.; Pietropaolo, G.; Graziani, C.; Masi, L.; Gasbarrini, A.; Putignani, L.; Scaldaferri, F.; et al. Dietary Magnesium Alleviates Experimental Murine Colitis through Modulation of Gut Microbiota. *Nutrients* **2021**, *13*, 4188. [CrossRef] [PubMed]
153. Xia, Y.; Shi, H.; Qian, C.; Han, H.; Lu, K.; Tao, R.; Gu, R.; Zhao, Y.; Wei, Z.; Lu, Y. Modulation of Gut Microbiota by Magnesium Isoglycyrrhizinate Mediates Enhancement of Intestinal Barrier Function and Amelioration of Methotrexate-Induced Liver Injury. *Front. Immunol.* **2022**, *13*, 874878. [CrossRef] [PubMed]
154. Schiopu, C.; Ștefănescu, G.; Diaconescu, S.; Bălan, G.G.; Gimiga, N.; Rusu, E.; Moldovan, C.A.; Popa, B.; Tataranu, E.; Olteanu, A.V.; et al. Magnesium Orotate and the Microbiome-Gut-Brain Axis Modulation: New Approaches in Psychological Comorbidities of Gastrointestinal Functional Disorders. *Nutrients* **2022**, *14*, 1567. [CrossRef]
155. Ramírez-Acosta, S.; Selma-Royo, M.; Collado, M.C.; Navarro-Roldán, F.; Abril, N.; García-Barrera, T. Selenium supplementation influences mice testicular selenoproteins driven by gut microbiota. *Sci. Rep.* **2022**, *12*, 4218. [CrossRef]
156. Razaghi, A.; Poorebrahim, M.; Sarhan, D.; Björnstedt, M. Selenium stimulates the antitumour immunity: Insights to future research. *Eur. J. Cancer* **2021**, *155*, 256–267. [CrossRef]
157. Saeed, F.; Nadeem, M.; Ahmed, R.S.; Tahir Nadeem, M.; Arshad, M.S.; Ullah, A. Studying the impact of nutritional immunology underlying the modulation of immune responses by nutritional compounds–A review. *Food Agric. Immunol.* **2016**, *27*, 205–229. [CrossRef]
158. Zhu, X.; Bi, Z.; Yang, C.; Guo, Y.; Yuan, J.; Li, L.; Guo, Y. Effects of different doses of omega-3 polyunsaturated fatty acids on gut microbiota and immunity. *Food Nutr. Res.* **2021**, *65*. [CrossRef]
159. Zorgetto-Pinheiro, V.A.; Machate, D.J.; Figueiredo, P.S.; Marcelino, G.; Hiane, P.A.; Pott, A.; Guimarães, R.C.; Bogo, D. Omega-3 Fatty Acids and Balanced Gut Microbiota on Chronic Inflammatory Diseases: A Close Look at Ulcerative Colitis and Rheumatoid Arthritis Pathogenesis. *J. Med. Food.* **2022**, *25*, 341–354. [CrossRef]

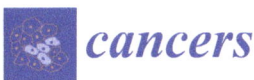

Review

Recent Advances in Bacteria-Based Cancer Treatment

Xianyuan Wei [1,2], Meng Du [3], Zhiyi Chen [3] and Zhen Yuan [1,2,*]

1. Faculty of Health Sciences, University of Macau, Taipa, Macau 999078, China
2. Centre for Cognitive and Brain Sciences, University of Macau, Taipa, Macau 999078, China
3. Institute of Medical Imaging, Hengyang Medical School, University of South China, Hengyang 421200, China
* Correspondence: zhenyuan@um.edu.mo; Tel.: +86-853-8822-4989

Simple Summary: Cancer refers to a disease involving abnormal cells that proliferate uncontrollably and can invade normal body tissue. It was estimated that at least 9 million patients are killed by cancer annually. Recent studies have demonstrated that bacteria play a significant role in cancer treatment and prevention. Owing to its unique mechanism of abundant pathogen-associated molecular patterns in antitumor immune responses and preferentially accumulating and proliferating within tumors, bacteria-based cancer immunotherapy has recently attracted wide attention. We aim to illustrate that naïve bacteria and their components can serve as robust theranostic agents for cancer eradication. In addition, we summarize the recent advances in efficient antitumor treatments by genetically engineering bacteria and bacteria-based nanoparticles. Further, possible future perspectives in bacteria-based cancer immunotherapy are also inspected.

Abstract: Owing to its unique mechanism of abundant pathogen-associated molecular patterns in antitumor immune responses, bacteria-based cancer immunotherapy has recently attracted wide attention. Compared to traditional cancer treatments such as surgery, chemotherapy, radiotherapy, and phototherapy, bacteria-based cancer immunotherapy exhibits the versatile capabilities for suppressing cancer thanks to its preferentially accumulating and proliferating within tumors. In particular, bacteria have demonstrated their anticancer effect through the toxins, and other active components from the cell membrane, cell wall, and dormant spores. More importantly, the design of engineering bacteria with detoxification and specificity is essential for the efficacy of bacteria-based cancer therapeutics. Meanwhile, bacteria can deliver the cytokines, antibody, and other anticancer theranostic nanoparticles to tumor microenvironments by regulating the expression of the bacterial genes or chemical and physical loading. In this review, we illustrate that naïve bacteria and their components can serve as robust theranostic agents for cancer eradication. In addition, we summarize the recent advances in efficient antitumor treatments by genetically engineering bacteria and bacteria-based nanoparticles. Further, possible future perspectives in bacteria-based cancer immunotherapy are also inspected.

Keywords: tumor therapy; engineered bacteria; bacteria-based cancer treatment

1. Introduction

Cancer refers to a disease involving abnormal cells that proliferate uncontrollably and can invade normal body tissue. According to the World Health Organization (WHO), cancer is the second leading cause of death worldwide [1]. It was estimated that at least 9 million patients are killed by cancer annually. Conventional therapies for cancer include surgery, chemotherapy, and radiotherapy. However, the downside of these traditional cancer treatment methods is that patients often suffer from various side effects during treatment. In particular, conventional treatment exhibits low specificity, leading to drug resistance in cancer cells.

Meanwhile, bacteria also have played an important role in maintaining good health and preventing diseases from healthier environments for millions of years. It is estimated that the human body contains trillions of bacteria [2]. The human gastrointestinal tract is the largest reservoir of commensal bacteria [3]. Intestinal bacteria such as Firmicutes, Bacteroides, Actinomycetes, and Enterobacteriaceae promote human health by synthesizing vitamin K, preventing colonization of pathogens, and maintaining the homeostasis of intestines [4]. There are more than 500 strains of bacteria such as *Streptococcus* and *Actinomycetes* in the mouth, which forms a protective biofilm on the surface of the teeth [5–7]. Additionally, Lactobacillus is dominant in the human vagina, maintaining the pH homeostasis of the environment by secreting lactic acid and inhibiting the interaction of other bacteria with epithelial cells [8]. By contrast, *Lactobacillus, Staphylococcus, Streptococcus*, etc., exist in the skin and nasal cavity, protecting the human body from other pathogens [7,9]. More importantly, recent studies have demonstrated that bacteria play a significant role in cancer treatment and prevention. In this review, we will firstly introduce the naïve bacteria and bacterial components of anticancer activity. We then summarize the recent work on efficient antitumor treatments that combine bacteria and nanoparticles. Further, we demonstrate that bacteria can be equipped with anticancer properties through gene editing technology, which provides a new insight into cancer therapy.

2. Bacterial Components of Antitumor Treatment

To date, bacterial toxins produced by bacterial cells, such as the Coley toxin, diphtheria toxin, Clostridium perfringens enterotoxin, bacterial enzymes L-asparaginase and arginine deaminase, and biosurfactant, such as surface and prodigiosin-like pixels, is able to effectively inhibit tumor growth through cell-cycle arrest, tumor-cell signal-pathway interruption, and other mechanisms. In addition, the components of bacteria, bacterial outer surface, the bacterial membrane, bacterial wall, and biofilm can also specifically activate the immune response to kill tumor cells.

2.1. Bacterial Toxins

In 1891, Dr. Coley successfully cured cancer patients with a mixture of live bacteria and "Coley toxin" heat-inactivated bacteria *Streptococcus pyogenes* and *Bacillus mirabilis*, opening the door to bacterial treatment of cancer [10,11]. Subsequent studies illustrated that Coley toxins include exotoxins produced by *Streptococcus pyogenes* and *Serratia marcescens*. In addition, *S. pyogenes* can produce pyrogenic exotoxins SpeA, SpeB, and SpeC, which have the ability to nonspecifically stimulate CD4+ lymphocytes, resulting in stronger secretion of different cytokines [12]. Similarly, prodigiosin, produced by *S. marcescens*, is a low molecular weight, red pigment, and heterocyclic tripyrrole toxin with antitumor activity, causing fever and potential antitumor immune response when combined with other components in the preparation [13].

Diphtheria toxin is a toxic protein produced by *Corynebacterium diphtheria*, while DTAT is its modified form, which targets the vascular endothelium of the tumor, results in the regression of cancer tissues in mice [14]. Clostridium difficile toxin includes two subtypes of cytotoxin (TcdB) and enterotoxin (TadA), which can kill cancer cells by recruiting proinflammatory factors to activate immune response [15]. Clostridium perfringens enterotoxin produced by *C. perfringens* also has anticancer activity, which leads to dose-dependent acute toxicity by binding to the overexpressed claudin-4 receptor on pancreatic cancer cells [16]. In addition, Verotoxin 1 (vt-1) is produced by pathogenic *Escherichia coli* and its function is to arrest the cancer cell cycle. Exotoxin A (PE) synthesized by *Pseudomonas aeruginosa* inhibits protein synthesis through ADP ribosylation, leading to cancer cell apoptosis [17,18]. The recombinant protein has better anticancer activity by modifying the cell structure recognition domain of the protein and preserving the membrane translocation domain and ADP ribosylation domain [15]. Hemolysin produced by bacteria, such as hemolysin A produced by *E. coli clyA* gene and hemolysin O produced by *Listeria monocytogenes*, is toxic to cancer cells. As a bacterial virulence factor, *Listeria monocytogenes* is released from phagocytes by perforating the phagocyte membrane. This phagosome escape mechanism enables *Listeria monocytogenes* to finally induce the immune response through MHC class

I molecules in the cytoplasm with the protein expressed by the vector as an endogenous antigen [19].

2.2. Bacterial Enzymes

Bacterial enzyme L-asparaginase from *Escherichia coli* is an effective cancer therapeutic agent, which can inhibit the progression of malignant cells by activating asparagine hydrolysis and reducing its blood concentration, thereby causing toxicity to the MCF-7, HepG2, and SK-LU-1 cell lines. Bacterial-derived asparaginase has been approved for the treatment of acute lymphoblastic leukemia and non-Hodgkin's lymphoma [20]. In addition, Fiedler et al. demonstrated that *Streptococcus pyogenes* produces arginine deaminase, which can consume arginine in tumor cells, resulting in decreased proliferation of arginine-deficient tumor glioblastoma multiforme [21].

2.3. Biosurfactant

Cyclic lipopeptide is an example of a biosurfactant with extensive antibacterial and antitumor activities that is produced by *Bacillus subtilis natto TK-1*. Xiaohong Cao et al. demonstrated that cyclic lipopeptide inhibited proliferation of human breast cancer MCF-7 cells by inducing apoptosis and increasing ion calcium concentration in the cytoplasm. Flow cytometric analysis revealed that cyclic lipopeptide caused dose- and time-dependent apoptosis through cell arrest at G(2)/M phase [22]. Another lipopeptide such as surfactin, have also been demonstrated their potential antitumor activity against several cancer cell lines. [23]. Surfactin induces the increase in calcium ions in human breast cancer MCF-7 cells and the accumulation of tumor suppressor p53 and cyclin kinase inhibitor p21, leading to cell-cycle arrest and apoptosis [22]. The same genus *Marine Bacillus subtilis* sp., can also produce an L-lysine biopolymer Epsilon-poly-L-lysine with antibacterial and anticancer activity. Studies have shown that Epsilon-poly-L-lysinet has obvious cytotoxicity on the cervical adenocarcinoma cell HeLaS3 and liver cancer cell HepG2 [24]. *Pseudomonas libanensis m9-3* produces a cyclic lipopeptide named viscosin with extensive antibacterial and antitumor activities. The MTT results indicated that viscosin inhibited the proliferation of MDA-MB-231 in breast cancer at 15 uM concentration. Moreover, viscosin also inhibited the migration of the prostate cancer cell line PC-3M [25,26]. The cyclic peptide AT514 (serratamolide) from *Serratia marcescens* is cytotoxic to B-cell chronic lymphocytic leukemia and induces endogenous apoptosis by activating the release of caspase-3, the antitumor function of which was confirmed in mouse experiments [27]. A variety of secondary metabolites, prodigiosin-like fragments, BE18591 and roseophilin with antitumor activity were isolated from *Streptomyces* sp. BE18591 inhibited the growth of the human Thomas cancer cell MKN-45 [28]. Roseophilin binds to the intracellular antiapoptotic receptor Mcl-1 and induces apoptosis of cancer cells [29,30]. Prodigiosin-like fragments showed significant cytotoxic activity against the colon cancer cell line HCT-116, liver cancer cell line HepG-2, and breast cancer cell line MCF-7. Table 1 lists biosurfactants with cancer cell proliferation, which are known as antitumor agents and inhibit some cancer progression processes. Biosurfactants show promising application in microemulsion-based drug formulations. Microemulsion comprises an aqueous phase, an oil phase, and a surfactant, which can encapsulate or solubilize a hydrophobic or hydrophilic drug for antitumor therapy. The combination of biosurfactant and liposome also demonstrates specific targeting to cancer cell. Shim, Ga Yong et al. revealed that surfactin enhanced cellular delivery of liposome siRNA in Hela cells. In this way, it was possible to improve the antitumor effectiveness of those nanoparticles [31]. Biosurfactants have application in broad-spectrum antitumor treatments and are viewed as safe vehicles or ingredients in drug-delivery systems.

Table 1. Biosurfactants with antitumor activity against cancer cells.

Biosurfactant		Cancer Type	References
Cyclic lipopeptide	*Bacillus subtilis natto TK-1*	Breast cancer	[22]
Surfactin	*Bacillus subtilis natto T-2*	Breast cancer	[23]
L-lysine biopolymer Epsilon-poly-L-lysine	*Marine Bacillus subtilis* sp.	Liver carcinoma Cervix adenocarcinoma	[24]
viscosin	*Pseudomonas libanensis m9-3*	Breast cancer	[25]
AT514	*Serratia marcescens*	B-cell chronic lymphocytic leukemia	[27]
BE18591	*Streptomyces* sp.	Gastric cancer	[28]
Roseophilin	*Streptomyces* sp.	Hematologic cancer Colon cancer	[29]

2.4. Extracellular Surface

Exopolysaccharides (EPS) are carbohydrate compounds secreted by Gram-positive *Lactobacillus* bacteria outside the cell wall and usually infiltrated into the culture medium in the process of growth and metabolism. Some adhere to the microbial cell wall to form a capsule, which are called capsular polysaccharides. They have a dose-dependent and time-dependent antitumor effect of antiproliferation, and they promote apoptosis in anticancer activity [32]. The S-layer that is composed of protein and glycoprotein on the outermost cell surface of Gram-positive bacteria also has antitumor activity. Studies have shown that the S-layer protein of *Lactobacillus acidophilus* CICC 6074 can be regarded as a potential antitumor drug [33].

2.5. Bacterial Cell Membrane

The bacterial membrane components used in anticancer treatment include the cytoplasmic membrane vesicles of Gram-positive bacteria and the outer membrane vesicles of negative bacteria, as well as membrane fragments. Because of its rich pathogen-associated molecular patterns (PAMPs), the bacterial membrane is recognized by antigen-presenting cells (APCs) and activates the immune activity of T cells. It can also bind and activate the toll-like receptor (TLR), which regulates the production of proinflammatory cytokines, such as IL-12, and other constituent molecules, such as CD40. Subsequently, these mediators produce interferon (IFN)-γ and start the Th1-dependent immune response, mainly mediated by CD8+ effector cells, which induces a strong immune response against cancer cells in the tumor microenvironment [34,35].

The results of Min Li et al. showed that the PAMP on *E. coli* outer membrane vesicles (OMVs) was effectively recognized and internalized by neutrophils in revascularization. Neutrophils then crossed the blood vessels and guided OMVs to target inflammatory tumors (Figure 1) [36].

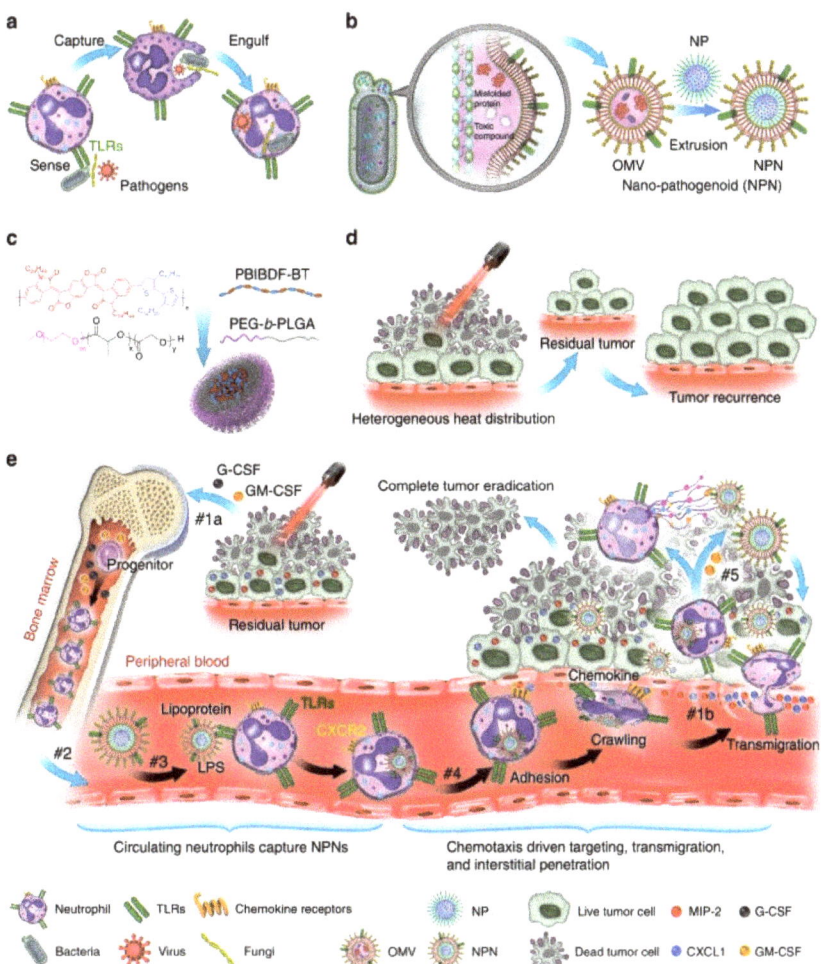

Figure 1. Schematic illustration showing the chemotaxis-driven delivery of NPNs for complete eradication of tumors post-phototherapy. (**a**) Neutrophils sense, capture, and engulf pathogens by recognizing the PAMPs with toll-like receptors (TLRs). (**b**) Preparation of NPNs by coating the OMVs on NPs, which inherit PAMPs from the OMVs. (**c**) Preparation of PEG-b-PLGA NPs encapsulating PBIBDF-BT (PBT) as a photothermal transducer. (**d**) The limited penetration of laser light used in PTT causes heterogeneous heat distribution within the tumor tissue and incomplete eradication of tumors, thus leading to tumor recurrence. (**e**) Treatment-induced cell death creates an inflammatory environment of the residual tumor and induces the production of granulocyte colony-stimulating factor (G-CSF), granulocyte–macrophage colony-stimulating factor (GM-CSF), and chemokines CXCL1 and MIP-2. #1a The released G-CSF and GM-CSF increase neutrophil production from bone marrow. #1b The released CXCL1 and MIP-2 broadcast the location of the inflamed tumor. #2 Neutrophils enter the blood circulation and encounter the injected NPNs. #3 Neutrophils sense NPNs with the recognition of LPS and lipoprotein by TLRs and subsequently engulf them. #4 Neutrophils laden with NPNs are recruited into the tumor site in response to the chemokine gradient through the following cascade: adhesion, crawling, and transmigration. #5 NPNs are released from neutrophils to kill tumor cells along with the formation of NETs in the inflamed tumor (Adapted from reference [36] with permission).

The OMVs of Gram-negative bacteria are mostly used in anticancer research and are composed of a lipopolysaccharide (LPS), outer membrane protein (OMP), and PG similar to the outer membrane. β-Barrel assembly machine (BamA) protein guides and inserts the outer membrane protein of the OMV into the outer membrane of newly produced PG to induce the outer membrane maturation of cells [37]. Knocking out the phospholipid transporter vacj/yrb increases the production of OMVs in two Gram-negative bacteria: *Haemophilus influenzae* and *Vibrio cholerae* [38]. RNA binding protein L7ae and lysosomal escape protein listeriolysin O are modified on the surface of bacterial OMVs. L7ae specifically binds to the mRNA vaccine to deliver antigens to dendritic cells (DCs). Listeriolysin O mediates the phagosome escape mechanism. This OMV-based mRNA tumor vaccine delivery platform can significantly inhibit the growth of melanoma and colon cancer cells [39]. OMVs of Gram-negative bacteria hybridize with tumor-derived cell membranes (MTs) to form new functional vesicles. In vivo experiments showed that MT-OMVs can induce adaptive immune response and then inhibit lung metastasis of the tumor [40].

As a tool for the delivery of nanomaterial and vaccines, the bacterial membrane plays not only the role of antitumor cells, but also a role in antivirus and antibacterial infection. Hydrophobic drugs can be loaded through the incubation method with convenient operation, and common drugs can be loaded through electroporation, ultrasonic method, extrusion method, freezing cycle, and saponin treatment method. The bacterial membrane can be loaded with anticancer compounds, functional small RNA molecules, cancer cell antibodies, and cytokines, and can jointly eliminate cancer cells through chemotherapy, gene silencing or mutation, immunity, photothermal therapy, photodynamic therapy, and other methods. Bacterial extracellular vesicles (BEVs) existing in the tumor microenvironment can be engulfed by cells through antigen–antibody-specific binding or membrane fusion. The BEV then releases the cargo in the cytoplasmic space, allowing its nanomaterials to play a role leading to apoptosis, necrosis, or autophagy of cancer cells. For example, RNA drugs and antisense oligonucleotides were loaded into extracellular vesicles by ultrasound, which played a role in the mouse breast cancer model [41].

Different pathogens will prefer colonization of specific tissues, such as *Klebsiella pneumonia* infecting the lungs, *Neisseria meningitidis* and *Listeria monocytogenes* infecting brain nerves, which means specific bacterial membranes can be used to target the corresponding cancer sites. After incubating the OMV of *Klebsiella pneumonia* with doxorubicin, a broad-spectrum chemotherapy drug, and then mixing in PBS and removing the free doxorubicin, it quickly reached the vicinity of the lung tumor in A549 BALB/c nude mice, and TUNEL results indicated that it significantly induced tumor cell apoptosis (Figure 2) [42].

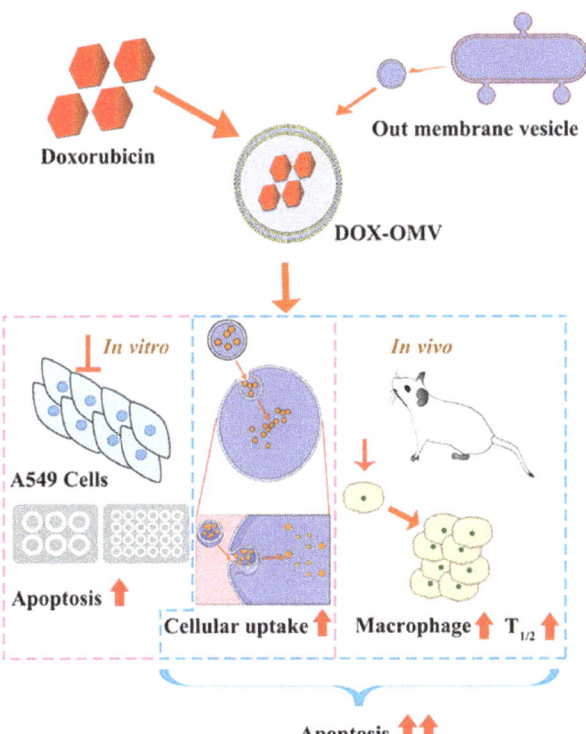

Figure 2. The attenuated *Klebsiella pneumonia* derived outer-membrane vesicles (OMVs), as a kind of biological drug-delivery carriers, are highly effective in transporting the chemotherapy drug doxorubicin (DOX) into nonsmall-cell lung cancer (NSCLC) A549 cells. Moreover, they can elicit appropriate immune responses, thereby enhancing the anti-NSCLC effect of DOX with no obvious toxicity in vivo (Adapted from reference [42] with permission).

2.6. Cell Wall

The bacterial cell wall is mainly composed of peptidoglycans. In addition to maintaining the shape of bacterial cells, peptide aggregation was also found to be related to regulating immune response, stimulating the production of tumor necrosis factor, interferon, and interleukin (IL-1, IL-6, IL-8, IL-12) [43].

2.7. Biofilm

Biofilm formed by bacteria also plays a role in tumor treatment. Biofilm is a glycoprotein lipid layer spontaneously formed by bacteria in the process of growth and attached to abiotic or biological surfaces including protein, DNA, metabolites, and so on. Biofilm forms in the tumor microenvironment and inhibits the growth, metastasis, and diffusion of tumor cells. The anticancer metabolites secreted by different bacteria are released in the biofilm, which can be accumulated and retained, so that they can be transferred to play a role in tumor cells [44,45].

2.8. Dormant Spores

In a harsh environment, bacteria will produce dormant spores. The spores of Clostridium can resist the harsh external environment and only revive when targeting the hypoxic tumor microenvironment. These advantages make anaerobic spores one way to target cancer cells. Studies have shown that *Clostridium novyi NT* spores do not contain lethal toxins, will not cause any systemic side effects in the injected host, and are an effective therapeutic agent for experimental tumors in mice [46]. The spores of *Clostridium* spp. are transformed into the active state in the tumor microenvironment only because of their strict anaerobic nature and are used in cancer treatment [47].

2.9. Magnetosomes

Magnetosomes are unique prokaryotic organelles containing 35 and 120 nm sized magnetite (Fe_3O_4) or cinerite (Fe_3S_4) magnetic iron mineral crystals surrounded by phospholipid bilayers. Mature magnetosomes are arranged in chains in the bacterial cytoplasm to form magnetosome chains, which cause magnetotactic bacteria to swim in the direction of the Earth's magnetic field line [48,49]. Magnetotropic bacteria (MTB) are natural biomineralized bacteria that synthesize multiple magnetic nanoparticle chains in their own cytoplasm and can sense external magnetic fields. In order to detect and treat cancer, the bacteria can be combined with chemotherapy or radiotherapy drugs to target their delivery through magnetic force [50].

3. Naïve Living Bacteria for Anticancer

Compared with the extracted bacterial components, anaerobic or facultative anaerobic naïve living bacteria have better tumor targeting. When naïve living bacteria enter the host body, they can actively target the tumor microenvironment, which includes the characteristics of hypoxia, high purine, and low acid content. They can deliver the anticancer bacterial components more efficiently. The bacteria with anticancer activity that have been verified by animal experiments include probiotics: *Lactobacillus* [51–58] and *Escherichia coli* [59], *Streptococcus, Lactococcus lactis, Lactobacillus casei, Lactobacillus casei Zhang, Bifidobacterium longum,* and *Clostridium butyricum,* etc.; general toxic bacteria include *Mycobacterium tuberculosis* [60], *Salmonella typhimurium* [61], and *Listeria monocytogenes* [62]; and pathogenic bacteria such as *Vibrio parahaemolyticus, Pseudomonas aeruginosa* [63], etc.

3.1. Mycobacterium tuberculosis

The first bacterial agent approved by the FDA was *Bacillus Calmette–Guerin* (BCG). The Pasteur strain was obtained by Calmette and Guérin after 231 passages in cultures as a vaccine for the prevention of tuberculosis. After entering the host, APC macrophages selectively ingest *Mycobacterium tuberculosis* and activate the powerful ability of the innate T-like effector cell group CD4+/CD8+ T cell. Weakened *Mycobacterium tuberculosis* is used to treat superficial nonmuscle invasive bladder cancer (NMIBC), which eventually leads to tumor cell apoptosis by activating the toll-related caspase-8 signaling pathway-like receptor 7 (TLR7). So far, this vaccine is still the most effective treatment for the disease [60,64,65].

3.2. Listeria monocytogenes

As a Gram-positive bacterium, *Listeria monocytogenes* is a superior carrier for cancer cell antigen delivery. It is absorbed by macrophages in the process of infection and synthesizes Listeria hemolysin O as a bacterial virulence factor, which destroys the integrity of the phagosome together with bacterial phospholipase. Listeria monocytogenes are released from phagocytes. This phagosome escape mechanism uses the *Listeria monocytogenes* protein as an endogenous antigen to finally induce CD4+ and CD8+ T-cell immune responses against tumors through MHC class I molecules [62,66,67].

3.3. Salmonella typhimurium

It was first reported in 1935 that *Salmonella typhimurium* has a high-efficiency antitumor effect. With in-depth study, it was found to enhance innate and adaptive anticancer immune responses through an inflammatory response. The specific enrichment ability of *Salmonella typhimurium* in the tumor hypoxic microenvironment is 1000 times greater than in normal tissues [61]. After *Salmonella typhimurium* is phagocytized by immune cells in vivo, because it lacks a phagosome escape mechanism, its surface protein is presented by

MHC class II molecules as an exogenous antigen to induce CD8+ T cells and CD4+ T-cell cancer immune response (Figure 3).

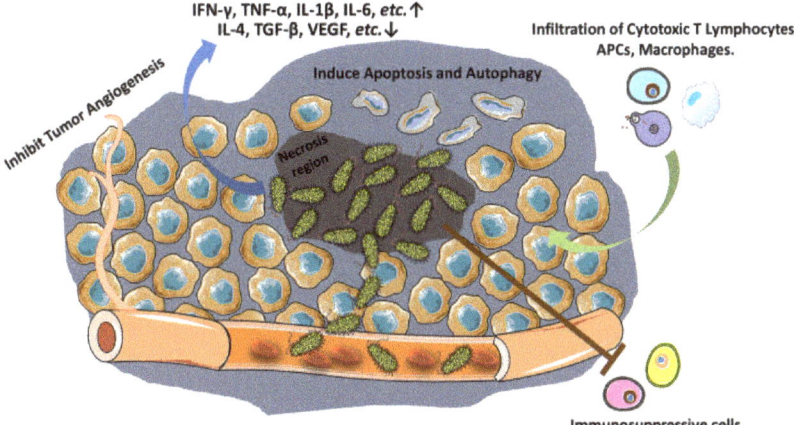

Figure 3. *Salmonella* stimulates host immune response against tumors. *Salmonella* accumulates in tumors (especially in necrosis region), inhibits tumor angiogenesis, and induces apoptosis and autophagy in tumor cells. *Salmonella* increases and activates cytotoxic T lymphocytes, antigen presenting cells (APCs) and macrophages against tumor cells, reduces tumor infiltration of Treg cells, and ablates the immunosuppressive capacity of myeloid-derived suppressor cells (MDSCs) and tumor-associated macrophages (Adapted from reference [61] with permission).

3.4. Lactic Acid Bacteria

Lactic acid bacteria are a kind of probiotic Gram-positive bacteria that include *Lactococcus* and *Lactobacillus*. Spherical lactic acid bacteria include *Streptococcus*, *Lactococcus lactis*, and *Pediococcus*. Lactobacilli include *Lactobacillus rhamnosus*, *Lactobacillus casei*, and *Bifidobacterium longum*. *Streptococcus* is a probiotic that kills tumor cells by activating host immunity and has been verified in animal experiments and clinical experiments [51]. *Lactococcus lactis* produces Nisin A, inhibits the growth of colon cancer tumors, and stops the cell division cycle [52]. *Lactobacillus casei* produces antimicrobial peptide kl15; interleukin (IL)-22 cytokines are downregulated, and caspase-7 and caspase-9 are upregulated, inducing apoptosis of colon cancer cells and the host immune response [52]. The oral probiotics *Lactobacillus casei Zhang* increase the levels of short-chain fatty acids and nicotinamide in the serum and kidney, which reduces the damage to kidney cells [53]. *Lactococcus lactis* and *Streptococcus bovis* produce Nisin A and bovicin HC5, respectively, which kill breast cancer cells. In addition, antimutagenic and anti-inflammatory effects from lactic acid bacteria were also found [54,55].

Bifidobacterium longum is a facultative anaerobic probiotic strain. After intravenous injection of mice, it was found to specifically locate solid tumors and slow tumor growth. Anticancer treatment seems to increase TNF-α Cytokine and nitric oxide synthesis [56–58].

Spores-dex is prepared by the chemical reaction between *Clostridium butyricum* and glucan. The spores-dex can specifically target colon cancer after oral administration. In the tumor microenvironment, *Clostridium butyricum* ferments glucan to produce anticancer short-chain fatty acids. In the subcutaneous tumor model of mice, the high-efficiency tumor inhibition ability of drug-loaded spores-dex was verified [68].

3.5. Escherichia coli

Escherichia coli is a model organism of Gram-negative bacteria. The bacteria mainly used for antitumor treatment are probiotic strains *Escherichia coli* Nissle 1917 (ECN) and wild-type MG1655, rather than serotype therapeutic strains. Genome analysis showed that ECN lacked virulence factors, such as α-. The expression of hemolysin, p-fimbriae adhesin, and adaptive factors do not produce any enterotoxins or cytotoxins related to pathogenic *Escherichia coli* strains, and it is an excellent targeted tumor vector [59].

3.6. Pseudomonas aeruginosa

Pseudomonas aeruginosa strain 1409 is a Gram-negative, pathogenic clinical strain that induces TC-1 cell necrosis by activating the TLR4 receptor, phosphorylation of RIP3, and activation of MLKl. Moreover, the necrotic tumor cells release HMGB1 to further induce the maturation and migration of DC cells. DC promotes the immune response of T cells by presenting tumor-related antigens, resulting in the large-scale death of tumor cells. *Pseudomonas aeruginosa* 1409 exerted a good therapeutic effect in the mouse TC-1 tumor model. However, it is worth noting that this bacterium is highly pathogenic, and it is resistant to three basic antibiotics. Thus, it is difficult to remove the colonization in the body, so it is not suitable for direct treatment of cancer [63].

4. Engineered Bacteria for Cancer Treatment

Engineered bacteria refer to expression exogenous protein in precise period and position. Despite the advantages of this, it is still limited by a few shortcomings that need to be urgently solved. The most important issue to be aware of is safety. Engineered bacterial therapeutics based on engineered bacteria refer to obtention of antibiotic resistance cassettes and ethical issues with transgenes, which presses challenges for the future of engineered bacteria therapy. Although direct injection of bacteria has an obvious killing effect on cancer cells, its side effects cannot be ignored. The research has shown that too high or too low a number of bacteria cause bacterial ecological imbalance [69], and the toxicity of bacteria is also harmful to normal tissues. The study by Cayetano Pleguezuelos-Manzano found that the occurrence of CRC in colorectal cancer was related to colistin produced by pathogenic *PKS* + *E. coli*. It is a toxin encoded and synthesized by a *PKS* island, which induces DNA double bond breakage and the death of host cells [70]. Bacteria are known as an autonomously disorganized and proliferating species. Its unique PAMPs and virulence factors induce an immune response in the human body, which promotes the killing of cancer cells by the human immune system. When the immune response is excessive, it threatens the patient's life. In short, safe and reliable attenuated targeted bacteria, gene editing to express endogenous bacterial toxins, pigment proteases, etc., or exogenous drug precursor enzymes, antigen immune fragments, cytokines, anti-immune checkpoints, and noncoding RNA, among others, are used. It can push the bacterial treatment of cancer to a new level of low dose and high efficiency. The clinical trials for bacterial cancer treatments are summarized in Table 2. The *S. typhimurium* VNP20009 strain and *Clostridium novyi*-NT spores have entered a phase I clinical trial, which all revealed a promising antitumor effect. The famous *S. typhimurium* VNP20009 strain achieved the purpose of constructing attenuated and purine-deficient strains through *msbB* and *purL* deletion. After intravenously injecting 1×10^6–1×10^9 CFU/mL of *S. typhimurium* VNP20009 in 24 patients with metastatic melanoma, bacteria target purine-rich tumor regions and reduce the host's nitric oxide and proinflammatory cytokines such as TNF-α and IL-1β. Unfortunately, no objective antitumor effect was observed. Engineering bacteria to specifically target tumors or the combinations of bacteria-based with antitumor protein will be applied in the future for therapeutic effect on tumors.

Table 2. Ongoing and previous clinical trial details on bacterial strain alone or in combination for cancer treatment (Adapted from reference [71] with permission).

Bacterial Strain	Phase	Cancer Type	Number of Patients	References
Salmonella typhimurium VNP20009 (attenuated Salmonella typhimurium)	I	Metastatic melanoma; metastatic renal cell carcinoma	25	[72]
S. typhimurium VNP20009 (live genetically modified S. typhimurium)	I	Melanoma	4	[73]
S. typhimurium VNP20009 (attenuated Salmonella bacterium expressing the E. coli cytosine deaminase gene)	I	Head and neck or esophageal adenocarcinoma	3	[74]
S. typhimurium VNP20009 (live, genetically modified Salmonella typhimurium	I	Patients with advanced or metastatic solid tumors	Not provided	NCT00004216 [75]
S. typhimurium VNP20009 (live, genetically modified Salmonella typhimurium)	I	Unspecified adult solid tumors	Not provided	NCT00006254 [76]
S. typhimurium VNP20009 (live, genetically modified Salmonella typhimurium)	I	Neoplasm or neoplasm metastatic tumors	45	NCT00004988 [77]
S. typhimurium (IL-2 expressing, attenuated S. typhimurium)	I	Liver cancer	22	NCT01099631 [78]
S. typhimurium Ty21a VXM01 (live attenuated S. typhi carrying an expression plasmid encoding VEGFR)	I	Pancreatic cancer	26	[79]
Clostridium Novyi-NT spores	I	Colorectal cancer	2	NCT00358397 [80]
Clostridium Novyi-NT spores	I	Solid tumor malignancies	5	NCT01118819 [81]
Clostridium novyi-NT	I	Solid tumor malignancies	24	NCT01924689 [82]
C. novyi-NT spores	Ib	Refractory advanced solid tumors	18	NCT03435952 [83]
Listeria monocytogenes	II	Metastatic pancreatic tumors	90	[84]
L. monocytogenes	II	Cervical cancer	109	[85]
L. monocytogenes	III	Cervical cancer	450-	NCT02853604 [86]

4.1. Engineered Bacteria to Achieve Detoxification

4.1.1. Modify the Bacterial Outer Membrane

The surface of Gram-negative bacteria is wrapped by an outer membrane rich in a variety of PAMP pathogen recognition molecules, which is a source of bacterial virulence. Through recombination or covering the outer membrane structure, the bacterial immune response to the human body can be reduced, and the dose tolerated by the human body can be increased to fight cancer cells. Specifically, the structure of lipid A, the main component of the outer membrane, is underacetylated by knocking out the *msbB* gene [87]. The synthase of the LPS such as *rfaG* and *rfaD* [88] is knocked out, resulting in the production of a truncated LPS with incomplete structure and overexpression of MSHA flagellin and bacterial surface capsular polysaccharide CAP to reduce the exposure of outer membrane surface virulence factors.

In *Salmonella typhimurium* and *Escherichia coli*, gene editing to knockout the *msbB* gene is a common method of detoxification. *msbB* encodes the catalytic enzyme of the acylation process of lipid A, the main component of the outer membrane, and converts the acylation of the pentaacylated lipopolysaccharide into a complete hexaacylated lipopolysaccharide. The *msbB* gene was knocked out to produce underage-type pentaacylated lipopolysaccharide and endotoxic lipid A [89]. The famous *S. typhimurium* VNP20009 strain achieved the purpose of constructing attenuated and purine-deficient strains through *msbB* and *purL* deletion. Ultimately, it targets purine-rich tumor regions and reduces the host's nitric oxide and proinflammatory cytokines such as TNF-α. This was verified in tumor experiments in mice and pigs and has been safely used in patients with metastatic melanoma and renal cancer in phase I clinical trials. However, no efficacy was observed [72].

To this day, PAMPs can also effectively reduce toxicity by covering the surface of bacteria. *Pseudomonas aeruginosa* mannose-sensitive hemagglutinin (PA-MSHA) is a Gram-negative bacterium that overexpresses MSHA flagella after gene editing. It weakens the toxicity of Pseudomonas aeruginosa by minimizing the exposure of surface virulence factors. Engineered PA-MSHA can inactivate the EGFR epidermal growth factor pathway signal in cancer cells and induce apoptosis. In the mouse model of bladder cancer, an injection of PA-MSHA effectively inhibited the growth of the tumor [90].

Tetsuhiro Harimoto et al. established a programmable cap expression system for bacterial surface capsular polysaccharides. The system regulates the extracellular biopolymer through the external inducer IPTG, so that the extracellular membrane is wrapped, temporarily avoiding the immune attack of the host and prolonging the circulation time of bacteria in the body. Their conclusion was proven in a mouse tumor model. By overexpressing ICAP, they were able to increase the maximum tolerated dose of bacteria by 10 times. They encapsulated *E. coli* strains, enabling them to escape the immune system and reach tumors. Because they did not administer IPTG in vivo, *E. coli* ICAP lost its encapsulation through time and was easier to eliminate from other parts of the body, thereby minimizing toxicity [91].

4.1.2. Nutritional Deficiencies

Transforming bacteria into specific nutrition-dependent mutations can also effectively reduce toxicity and improve their antitumor activity. *Salmonella typhimurium* produces leucine and arginine synthesis-deficient trophic strain a1-r by knocking out *leu* and *arg* genes [92]. Attenuated and purine-deficient strain VNP2009 was constructed by *msbB* and *purL* deletion, targeting purine-rich tumor regions [93].

AroA gene mutation leads to the nutritional deficiency of aromatic amino acids in bacteria, which is considered safe and used widely in attenuated strains. The absence of *aroA* in *Pseudomonas aeruginosa* resulted in a tenfold increase in the safe dose of the bacterium compared with the wild-type [94]. Genetic engineering of *aroA* and *aroD* double mutant *Salmonella typhimurium* as reported by Yoon W.S. was used to treat mouse melanoma, resulting in 50% tumor regression [95]. M. Gabriela Kramer et al. constructed *Salmonella typhimurium* LVR01 of attenuated mice knockout *aroC* and virus vector particles expressing the IL-12 (sfv-IL-12) gene. When inoculated into the mouse model of advanced breast cancer metastasis, sfv-IL-12 showed an effective antiangiogenesis effect, and the combined effect of sfv-IL-12 and lvr01 could inhibit tumor growth and metastasis, finally prolonging the survival time. It is an effective antimetastasis therapy [96].

4.1.3. Reduce Toxin Expression

Bacterial toxins as the main virulence factors downregulate or knockout the expression and synthesis of related toxin genes, which can greatly reduce the virulence of bacteria and improve the dose tolerance of the human body.

So far, gene-editing knockout of the Ppgpp gene in *Salmonella typhimurium* led to a defect in the synthesis of guanosine 5′-diphosphate-3′-diphosphate. This signal molecule participates in the expression of bacterial toxin genes and changes the structure of lipid

A through the deletion of *relA* and *spoT*, which can achieve a 10^5-fold detoxification effect [97]. After the lethal toxin genes *toxA* and *toxB* were knocked out by heat shock in *Clostridium novyii*, the bacterium turned into a nontoxic and safe strain. After intravenous injection of the active bacterium, it targeted the tumor area and attacked the cancer cells through cytokine aggregation immune cells, which eventually led to the reduction in tumor growth and its disappearance in mice [98]. The toxicity to normal cells was reduced by knocking out the exotoxin genes *exoS*, *exoT*, *aroA*, and *lasI* of *Pseudomonas aeruginosa* [99].

4.2. Engineered Bacteria to Targeting

So far, increasing tumor-targeting by genetic engineering can reduce the injection concentration of antitumor bacteria and improve their safety and antitumor efficacy. According to the characteristics of hypoxia, high purine, and weak acidity in the tumor microenvironment, endogenous inducible promoters with specific responses can be designed. Moreover, the addition of the exogenous inducers arabinose, salicylic acid, Tet, IPTG, ultraviolet light, light, heat, etc., at specific time and space can accurately induce the expression of substances with anticancer activity. Drugs can also be delivered to specific cancer cells by targeted cancer cell aptamers or proteins, such as the RGD membrane-penetrating peptide, nuclear localization signal, secretory system signal peptide, antibody, etc.

4.2.1. Endogenous Inducible Promoter

It is well-known that inducible promoters exert precise spatiotemporal regulation of protein expression. Promoters responding to hypoxia, acidity, high purine, and bacterial density of the tumor microenvironment were designed based on their characteristics. This ensures that after the bacteria are enriched into the tumor microenvironment, they will express proteins with anticancer activity to reduce the toxicity to normal tissues.

Mitra Samadi et al. designed a hypoxia-inducible expression system using the *nirB* promoter of the hypoxia response of *E. coli* BW25133 to express anticancer protein, cardiac peptides, and GFP signal proteins. In vivo experiments, this inhibited the growth and metastasis of mouse breast cancer tumors and improved the survival rate of the mice [100]. In addition, the hypoxia-responsive *fdhF* promoter in *E. coli* mc1061 can be used to accurately regulate the expression of anticancer compounds [101].

The weak acidity of the tumor microenvironment enables acid response promoters to express active anticancer proteins. Kelly Flentie screened five genes—*adiY*, *yohJ*, STM1787, TM1791, and STM1793—related to the acidic environment of tumors by co-culturing the library of *Salmonella typhimurium* transposon insertion mutants with melanoma or colon cancer cells. The corresponding promoter, as an acidic promoter, seems to play a role in targeted tumors [102].

The construction of the nutrient-deficient strains mentioned in Section 4.1.2 enable acteria to specifically enrich within purine and amino acid tumor microenvironments. Purine-deficient strains were constructed by purI deletion to target purine-rich tumor regions [93]. AroA gene mutations can lead to nutritional deficiencies of aromatic amino acids in bacteria, targeting amino acid-rich tumor regions [95].

By controlling the expression of lysed proteins through the Luxi and LuxR quorum-sensing response system, the engineering flora can be lysed in microcapsules, and the expressed protein product can be released to the outside of the cell with the ova subunit vaccine using the bacterial microcomponent BMC as the carrier. A mouse subcutaneous tumor model was introduced to demonstrate the potential of nanoparticle delivery, successfully activate immunity in mice, and play a preventive role against b16-ova tumors [103]. The deletion of the quorum-sensing gene can reduce the toxicity of bacteria and increase their number at a mild dose. The *lasI* gene encodes the syntheses of the quorum-sensing homoserine lactones 3-oxo-c12-hsl and *rhlI* encodes C4-HSL occur in *Pseudomonas aeroginosa*. By deleting the *lasI* and *rhlI* genes, the number of bacteria in mild doses was increased 10 times compared with the wild-type [94].

4.2.2. Exogenous Inducible Promoter

L-arabinose induced the araC promoter, salicylic acid induced the PM promoter, tetracycline induced the TET promoter; T7 promoter was induced by Isopropyl-β-D-thiogalactoside, single-stranded DNA repair protein RecA promoter was induced by ultraviolet light, and so on [104]. Protein expression promoters commonly used in bacteria have the ability to accurately induce engineering bacteria to express active antitumor proteins by in situ injection into the tumor microenvironment as exogenous inducers [105].

The activity of heat-sensitive promoter HSB was activated by ultrasound or light source stimulation. In wild-type *Escherichia coli* Nissle 1917, the temperature-sensitive promoter (HSB-GFP) plasmid was constructed to express the tumor necrosis factor α (TNF-α). The growth of 4T1 tumor mice injected with the bacterium was significantly inhibited after three heat-stimulation treatments [106].

Chunli Han designed a photogenetic scavenging gene circuit based on blue light-responsive OptO proteins EL222. The circuit adopted the strategy of dark inducing the expression of detoxifying protein CcdA and blue light inducing the expression of toxin protein CcdB. When exposed to a 488 nm laser, the engineering bacteria died. A photosensitive promoter is used to ensure that the engineering bacteria can be removed after use and to further ensure the safety of subcutaneous administration of engineering bacteria microcapsules. The survival of engineering bacteria microcapsules carrying photogenetic scavenging gene circuits after exposure to blue light in vitro or in vivo can be reduced by about three orders of magnitude [103].

4.2.3. Signal Peptide

The reported signal peptides that improve the targeted effect of cancer cells include membrane-penetrating peptides, nuclear localization sequences, bacterial secretion system signal peptides, and so on.

By displaying RGD (Arg-Gly-ASP)-penetrating peptide on the surface of bacteria, the tumor was targeted and the therapeutic effects of attenuated Salmonella were enhanced [107]. Sujie Huang et al. linked the DNA toxin drug camptothecin (CPT) with the nuclear localization sequence to construct a nanomaterial with cancer nuclear localization ability. Experiments proved the enhancement of cytotoxicity and selectivity [108].

The special protein secretion system of bacteria delivers effector proteins to target eukaryotic cells through complex needle-like molecular machines. Type III and VI secretion systems have been used to secrete fusion proteins with anticancer activity owing to their widespread presence in bacteria [109,110]. In *Pseudomonas aeruginosa*, 54 amino acid fragments at the N-terminal of the ExoS protein for the Type III secretion system-mediated translocation were fused with fragments at the C-terminal of ovalbumin for antigen–antibody specific binding by genetic engineering. Then, based on the special Type III secretion system of *Pseudomonas aeruginosa*, it was injected into the host cells to induce the immune response of CD8+ T lymphocytes [94].

4.2.4. Targeted Proteins

Current means to improve targeting cancer cells include engineering the expression of proteins with a high affinity with cancer cells. These toxin proteins or antibodies can specifically recognize cancer cell antigens

OpcA protein can cross the blood–brain barrier and target nerve cells. Engineering expression of the outer membrane invasion protein OpcA of *Neisseria meningitidis* can guide the specific enrichment of *Neisseria meningitidis* in the central nervous system. Methotrexate, a chemotherapy drug, was loaded into manganese dioxide (MnO2) hollow nanoparticles with surface-modified *Neisseria meningitidis* OpcA protein to construct a bionic nanotreatment system with great potential for glioblastoma (MTX@MnO2-Opca) [111].

Through genetic engineering methods, 30 amino acids that specifically express the C-terminal of *Clostridium perfringens* enterotoxin (CPE) were constructed to specifically bind to cldn-4 antigen on the surface of cancer cells and induce apoptosis of cldn-4-positive cancer cells [112].

Engineering expression of cytolysin A (ClyA), located on the outer membrane surface, express with antibody fragmentof cancer cells can also improve targeting [113]. CD20 is a specific antigen that is overexpressed by lymphoma cells. The engineered single domain antibody expressing CD20 in Salmonella can significantly improve the tumor specificity of Salmonella [114].

4.2.5. Aptamer

Aptamer is a single-stranded oligonucleotide synthesized by artificial screening, which specifically targets substrates such as small molecules, peptides, proteins, cells, and tissues. Zhongmin Geng et al. anchored the aptamer AS1411 on the surface of attenuated *Salmonella typhimurium* VNP2009 by amidation, which can specifically target the nucleolin nucleus overexpressed on the cancer cell membrane (Figure 4). In the tumor-bearing mouse model inoculated subcutaneously with 4T1 cancer cells, the accumulation of bacteria in the tumor tissue after 12 h was nearly two times higher than that of the nonanchored aptamers. In addition, the aptamer TLs11a, which has a high binding affinity with the hepatocellular carcinoma cell line, was also tested. After injection into mice, aptamer bacteria showed high enrichment of H22 cells and better inhibition of tumor growth [115].

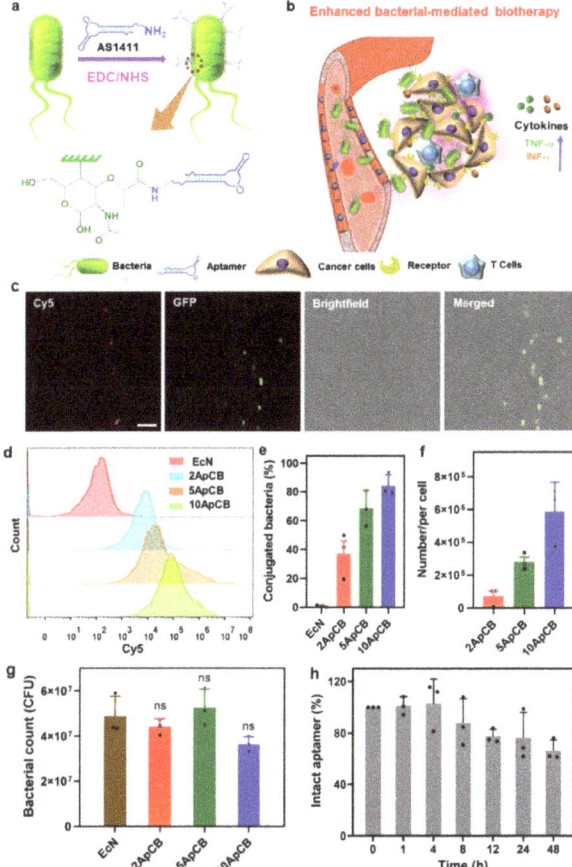

Figure 4. Design, preparation and characterization of ApCB. (**a**) Preparation of ApCB through amide condensation. (**b**) Aptamer-assisted tumor localization of bacteria for enhanced biotherapy. (**c**) Typical

LSCM images of aptamer-conjugated bacteria. The red and green channels indicate aptamers conjugated with Cy5- and EcN-producing GFP, respectively. Images are representative of three independent biological samples. Scale bar: 10 μm. (**d**) Flow cytometric analysis of EcN and EcN conjugated with Cy5-labeled AS1411. (**e**) Percentages of conjugated EcN under different feed ratios. Error bars represent the standard deviation (n = 3 independent experiments). Data are presented as mean values ± SD. (**f**) Average binding number of aptamers on each bacterial quantified by calculating the difference of fluorescent intensity of the aptamer solution after reaction. Error bars represent the standard deviation (n = 3 independent experiments). Data are presented as mean values ± SD. (**g**) Bacterial viabilities of EcN, 2ApCB, 5ApCB, and 10ApCB by LB agar plate counting. Plates were incubated at 37 °C for 24 h prior to enumeration (n = 3 independent experiments). Data are presented as mean values ± SD; significance was assessed using Student's t test (two-tailed); ns: no significance. (**h**) Degradation kinetics of the conjugated AS1411 in 90% phosphate-buffered serum solution at 37 °C. Error bars represent the standard deviation (n = 3 independent experiments). Original data are provided as a Source Data file. (Adapted from reference [115] with permission).

4.3. Engineered Bacteria to Anticancer

4.3.1. Drug Precursors and Drug Synthase

The gene of respiratory chain enzyme II NDH-2 was overexpressed in engineered *Escherichia coli* MG1655 to obtain a large amount of H_2O_2 (Figure 5.). The bacterial surface was covalently connected with magnetic Fe_3O_4 nanoparticles, which were then injected into animals to specifically colonize the tumor area and convert H_2O_2 into toxic hydroxyl radicals (OH) through the Fenton reaction, resulting in the increase in ROS and the induction of severe tumor cell apoptosis [116].

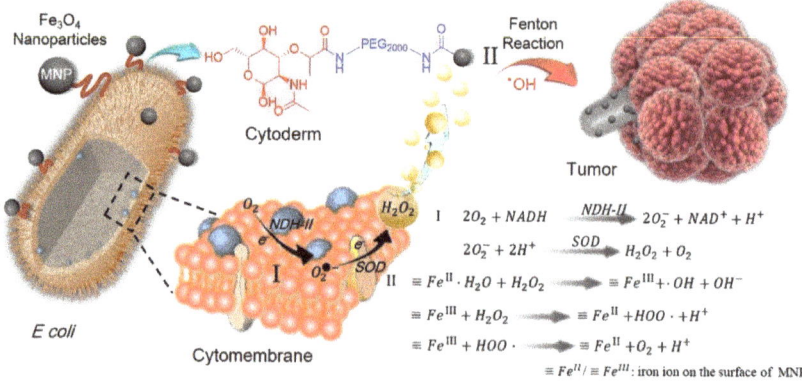

Figure 5. The scheme of bacteria-based Fenton-like bioreactor and its chemodynamic therapy process for antitumor therapy (Adapted from reference [116] with permission).

Cytosine deaminase has been successfully applied in two kinds of targeted pre-enzyme drug therapies in *Clostridium*. The first was gene editing *Clostridium* to overexpress cytosine deaminase and specifically convert the prodrug 5-fluorocytosine into the anticancer agent 5-fluorouracil at the tumor site. This anticancer effect was verified in tumor-bearing mice. The other was to overexpress the nitroreductase enzyme in Clostridium by gene editing. In the tumor microenvironment, CB1954 was converted into a DNA crosslinker with antibacterial and cancerous properties [117].

4.3.2. Antibodies

The expression of immune checkpoint PD-1/PD-L1 and CTLA-4 inhibitors can block checkpoints and induce immune cells to activate a strong immune response. In addition, highly specific antibodies expressing tumor antigens can inhibit the growth of cancer cells. After gene editing, *C. novyi* NT and *C. sporogenes* are used to express the heavy chain variable region of the highly specific antibody of tumor antigen. This protein binds and inhibits the activity of HIF cells, reduces the expression of transcription factor hypoxia-inducible factor 1alpha, leads to the transformation of the tumor microenvironment from hypoxia to oxygen enrichment, slows the growth of cancer cells, and reduces the risk of cancer cell metastasis [118].

The gene expresses tumor-specific antigen NY-ESO-1 in *Salmonella typhimurium*, secretes it through the Type III protein secretion system, and presents the antigen to CD8+ T cells and CD4+ T cells through the MHC class I pathway, specifically activating the immune pathway against NY-ESO-1-positive cancer cells [119]. *Salmonella typhimurium* is presented by MHC class II molecules as an exogenous antigen to induce the immune response of CD8+ T cells and CD4+ T cells [119]. *Listeria monocytogenes* has the phagosome escape mechanism mentioned above. As an endogenous antigen, it finally induces the immune response through MHC I class molecules. Both bacteria have been widely studied as vaccine carriers in popular cancer treatment [120].

4.3.3. Cytokines

Cell necrosis factor TNF-α is a double-edged sword, which can activate transcription factor nuclear factor NF-κb at a low dose. It can stimulate the proliferation of tumor cells, but it can also be used as a tumor suppressant at high doses. The gene-edited *Clostridium acetobutyricum* DSM792 expresses and secretes mouse TNF-α. The purpose of this experiment was to specifically target the tumor microenvironment and controllably regulate TNF-α secretion. Unfortunately, owing to the low level of bacterial colonization in the tumor microenvironment and the specific expression of TNF-α, a limited level failed to achieve the effect of tumor treatment [121]. The role of cytokine interleukin-2 (IL-2) is to kill tumor cells by activating natural killer cells and enhancing MHC-restricted T cells. However, high doses of IL-2 are toxic to normal tissues, so bacteria with active targeting are selected as carriers. The genetically edited *Clostridium acetobutyricum* DSM792 successfully slowed the growth of mouse tumors in animal experiments by specifically expressing mouse IL-2 [122]. Fas, a proapoptotic factor, can initiate apoptotic signals in cells and induce apoptosis of Fas-sensitive cells. Fas ligand FasL membrane protein was expressed in *Salmonella typhimurium* and injected intravenously into mouse d2f2 breast cancer or CT-26 colon cancer tumors. It was observed that the growth of primary tumors in mice was inhibited by 59% and 82%, respectively [123].

Hypoxia-inducible factor 1alpha is a transcription factor of genes responsible for cell survival triggered by hypoxia in the tumor microenvironment. Arjan J. Groot et al. inhibited tumor growth by expressing scFv of HIF-1α in *Clostridium* [118].

4.3.4. Noncoding RNA

siRNA that interferes with the expression of target genes or miRNA that affects the post-transcriptional function of genes is loaded into bacterial microcapsules using electro-transfer, chemotransfer, etc. It improves the specificity of noncoding RNA and protects RNA from degradation during delivery. So far, CRISPR cas9 protein and sgRNA have only been delivered in cell vesicles and liposomes. For example, delivery through bacterial vesicles can more conveniently engineer the membrane surface to improve targeting and protection during delivery [124,125].

At present, Mir-16 mimic coated by nonliving bacterial minicells has inhibited tumor growth in animal models by restoring miRNA levels in tumor cells in phase 1 clinical trials [126,127]. Kinesin spindle protein (KSP) is overexpressed in tumor tissues and is an ideal candidate for targeted cancer therapy. Vipul Gujrati et al. loaded small interfering RNA targeting KSP into attenuated OMV by electroporation. After injecting OMV-packaged siRNA into tumor mice, obviously targeted gene silencing and tumor inhibition were indicated [128].

4.3.5. Pigment Synthase and Fluorescent Protein

Vipul Gujrati et al. expressed rhizobium tyrosinase MelA protein in attenuated *E. coli*, which can metabolize tyrosine into natural melanin and accumulate, with bacteria obtaining an unexpected photothermal effect. It can monitor the distribution of bacteria in vivo under near-infrared light irradiation and photothermal treatment of 4T1 tumor-bearing mice [129]. Zhijuan Yang et al. expressed firefly luciferase in *Salmonella typhimurium* ΔppGpp (STΔppGpp) (Figure 6.). The bacterium and photosensitizer Ce6 were injected into large tumor rabbits, and D-fluorescein continuously produced light to stimulate Ce6 to produce exogenous ROS. Compared with the external 660 nm light excitation of Ce6 by traditional photodynamic therapy, the internal light source of D-fluorescein had better photodynamic effect to excite Ce6 and inhibit tumor growth [130].

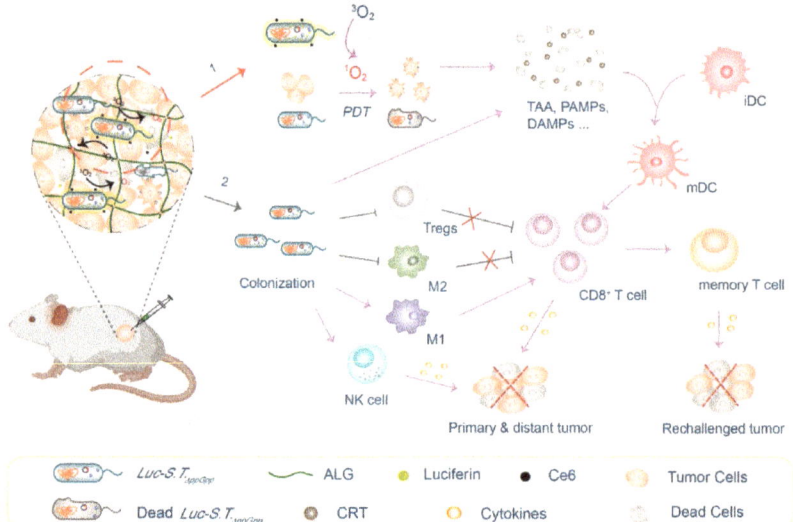

Figure 6. A scheme illustrating the engineering of bioluminescent bacteria to boost PDT and antitumor immunity for synergistic cancer treatment. Upon i.t. injection, engineered Luc-S.T.ΔppGpp would rapidly colonize and emit bioluminescence in the presence of substrate D-luciferin as the light source to boost PDT by activating Ce6, thereby causing cell death of both cancer cells and Luc-S.T.ΔppGpp itself to release tumor associate antigens (TAAs), DAMPs (e.g., CRT), and PAMPs (1). Meanwhile, such Luc-S.T.ΔppGpp colonization could also efficiently reverse the immunosuppressive tumor microenvironments (TMEs) by promoting intratumoral frequencies of M1 macrophages and NK cells, while suppressing intratumoral frequencies of M2 macrophages and Tregs (2). As the result, such Luc-S.T.ΔppGpp as both implantable light source (in the presence of D-luciferin) and immunostimulator could elicit potent innate and adaptive antitumor immunity to effectively suppress the growth of treated tumors, inhibit tumor metastasis, and prevent against tumor recurrence (Adapted from reference [130] with permission).

Engineered bacteria express luciferase fused with the human influenza hemagglutinin tag (Luc–HA) and bioluminescence detection technology is used to visualize the distribution of bacteria in organisms [131] to achieve Lux fluorescein and fluorescence tracing. In addition, *E. coli* was injected into mice with tumor colonization. When facultative anaerobic *E. coli* actively targeted the tumor microenvironment, 18F fluorodeoxysorbitol (FDS) positron emission tomography (PET), which can be used for specific binding with *E. coli*, was injected to image the distribution of *E. coli* in vivo. This method is expected to be used for semiquantitative visualization of tumor-targeted bacteria [132]. Engineering bacteria expressing GFP, YFP, mCherry, and other fluorescent proteins are injected into the body through microcapsules for in vivo imaging observation. The results indicate that the fluorescence can be maintained in the body for no less than 15 days [103].

4.3.6. Bacterial Toxins

Among the bacterial component anticancer 1.1 bacterial toxins, a variety that have been experimentally proven to have anticancer activity are listed, including the Coley toxin, diphtheria toxin, *Clostridium perfringens* enterotoxin, azurol, cyclic dipeptide, rhamnolipid, and cytochrome A.

Overexpression of high concentrations of cytolysin A (ClyA) in engineered bacteria can bind and form pores in eukaryotic cell membranes, triggering caspase-mediated programmed cell death [113]. Pei Pan et al. designed the engineering bacterium BAC to increase the tumor-targeted ability and overexpressed the cytolysin A (ClyA) protein to regulate the cell cycle from the antiradiation phase to the radiation-sensitive phase. It inhibited the growth of mouse breast cancer and reduced the side effects of radiotherapy [133].

Yale Yue et al. constructed a protein expression plasmid to fuse the tumor antigen (Ag) and Fc fragments of mouse immunoglobulin G (IgG) to the C-terminal of OMV (ClyA–Ag–MFC) surface protein ClyA. In situ controllable production of the OMV carrying the tumor antigen (OMV–Ag–MFC) was achieved in the intestine by oral administration of modified bacterial *E. coli* and expression-inducer L-arabinose. These OMV–Ag–MFCs effectively cross the intestinal epithelial barrier and are absorbed by DCS in the lamina propria, followed by lymph node drainage and tumor antigen presentation. In a variety of mouse cancer models, tumor antigen-specific immune activation significantly inhibited tumor growth and resisted tumor challenges [131].

5. Bacteria-Based Nanoparticles for Cancer Treatment

Bacteria and nanomaterials are directly antitumor through the covalent connection of chemical amide bonds and can also be adsorbed together through electrostatic interaction. In addition, bacterial membrane fragments and outer membrane vesicles can be fused with bacteria through repeated freezing and thawing, ultrasound, extrusion, and other methods. The new combination of nanomaterials and bacteria can inhibit the growth of tumors through the anticancer activities of nanomaterials such as photothermal and photodynamic therapy, which not only reduce the toxicity to normal cells, but also increase tumor specificity.

5.1. Chemical Bond Connection

So far, the way to a stable combination of bacteria and nanomaterials has been mainly through peptidoglycans of the bacterial cell wall or cell membrane liposomes to form stable amide bonds with nanomaterials. Through an amide condensation reaction, MnO_2 was modified on the surface of *Shewanella oneidensis* MR-1 bacterial cells, which can specifically decompose lactic acid. *Shewanella oneidensis* MR-1 (*S. oneidensis* MR-1) continuously decomposes lactic acid produced by the glucose metabolism in the tumor microenvironment by transferring electrons to the metallic mineral MnO_2 in an anaerobic environment. This inhibited the growth of CT26 tumor cells in mouse experiments [134].

Wencheng Wu et al. immobilized liposomes co-loaded with lactic acid oxidase (LOD) and prodrug tirapazamine (TPZ) on the surface of *lactic acid bacteria* (LA) through an amide condensation reaction (Figure 7). Tumor specificity by LA can effectively deliver drug substances to tumor tissues. Loaded lactic acid oxidase (LOD) catalyzes the oxidation of lactic acid to H_2O_2, increasing the level of oxidative stress, which further aggravates hypoxia in tumors, thereby activating the TPZ prodrug sensitive to hypoxia and inducing significant tumor cell apoptosis and immunogenic cell death ICD [135].

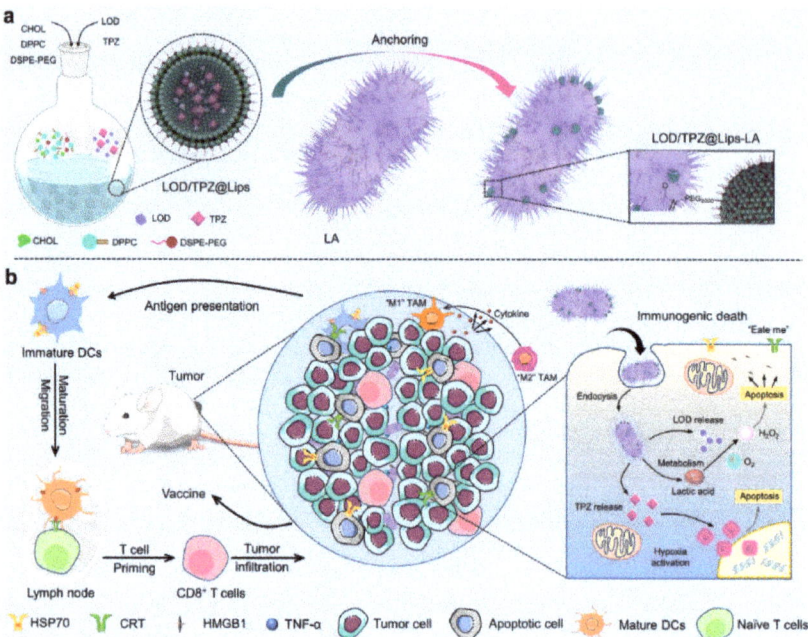

Figure 7. Schematic illustration of (**a**) the construction of LOD/TPZ@Lips-LA microbiotic nanomedicine by bonding LA and LOD co-loaded liposome onto the lactobacillus (LA) and (**b**) LOD/TPZ@Lips-LA triggered immunogenic cell death (ICD) and immune activation in tumor in synergy with the TZP-triggered chemotherapy (Adapted from reference [135] with permission).

5.2. Electrostatic Interaction

The cell walls of Gram-positive bacteria are crosslinked by negatively charged N-acetylglucosamine and N-acetyl cell wall acid. LPS, the outer membrane component of Gram-negative bacteria, is usually negatively charged. Therefore, stable binding bacterial nanomaterials can be obtained by incubating the positively charged nanomaterials with negatively charged bacteria.

Di Wei Zheng et al. assembled carbon-dot-doped carbon nitride (C_3N_4) on the surface of engineered *E. coli* carrying a nitric oxide (NO)-generating enzyme by electrostatic interaction. Under the light, the photoelectrons produced by C_3N_4 can be transferred to *E. coli* and promote endogenous NO_3^- metabolism to tumor cells. This method has achieved good therapeutic effects in mouse tumor models [136]. Shuaijie Ding connected black phosphorus quantum dots (BPQDs) to the surface of *E. coli* genetically engineered to express catalase by electrostatic adsorption, thereby producing an engineered *E. coli*/BPQD (EB) system (Figure 8). After intravenous injection into mice, EB can target hypoxic tumor tissues and produce reactive oxygen species to destroy bacterial membranes. The released catalase degrades hydrogen peroxide to produce oxygen to alleviate hypoxia in tumors, thereby enhancing BPQD-mediated photodynamic therapy. The system can effectively kill tumor cells in vivo [137].

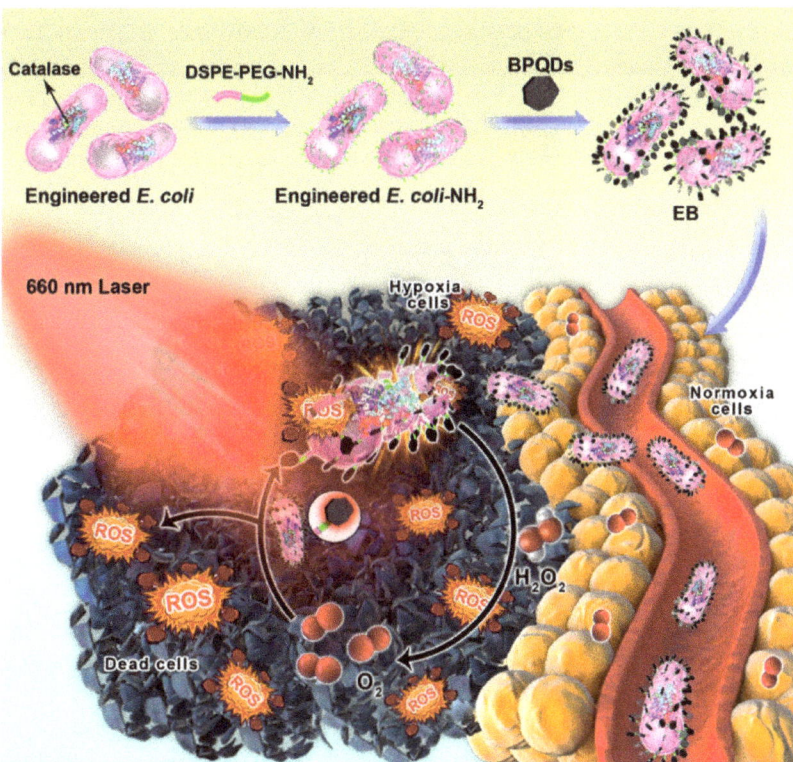

Figure 8. Schematic illustration of a novel engineered bacterium/black phosphorus quantum dot hybrid system for hypoxic tumor targeting and efficient photodynamic therapy (Adapted from reference [137] with permission).

5.3. Bacterial Loading Nanomaterials

So far, nanomaterials with antitumor activity have been combined with bacteria using liquid nitrogen through repeated heating, freezing and thawing, ultrasonic vibration, physical extrusion, buffer solution incubation, electroconversion, chemical conversion to form perforation, etc. The common feature is that nanomaterials are wrapped or wrapped to form biologically active nanomaterials. Yao Liu et al. constructed an immunotherapy system of a natural red blood cell (RBC) membrane wrapping *Listeria monocytogenes*, with virulence factors removed by the extrusion method (LMO@RBC) (Figure 9). The nanomaterial produces a low systemic inflammatory response, and its accumulation effect in tumors is also improved owing to the long-term blood circulation ability of RBCs and the tumor hypoxic microenvironment colonization ability of LMO. In the BALB/c solid tumor model, LMO@RBC reached the tumor microenvironment, promoted the release of ROS in the tumor area and the activation of caspase 8, inducing extensive porogen gasdermin C (GSDMC) and dependent pyroptosis, which showed a high inhibitory effect on the growth of primary tumors and distant tumors [138].

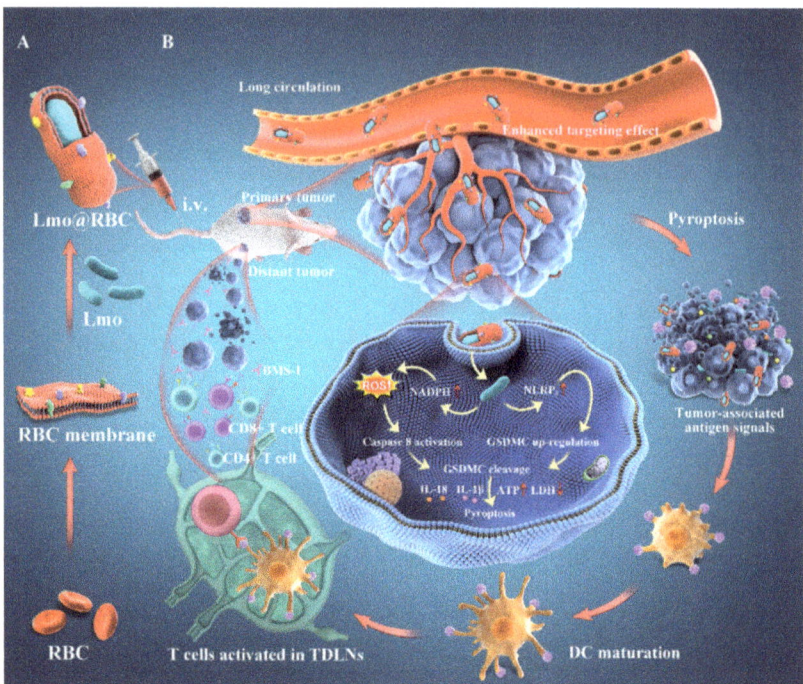

Figure 9. Schematic depiction of utilizing LMO@RBC to improve cancer immunotherapy. (**A**) Schematic illustration of RBC membranes extraction and the preparation of LMO@RBC. (**B**) Tumor-homing LMO@RBC effectively accumulated in primary tumor after intravenous administration and triggers cancer cell pyroptosis. Pyroptotic cancer cells in primary tumor release proinflammatory substances, which induce DC maturation and T cell activation in tumor-draining lymph nodes (TDLNs), resulting in efficient suppression of primary and remote tumors (Adapted from reference [138] with permission).

In addition, Jiayu Zhang et al. modified the PD-L1 antibody on the surface of a *Salmonella typhimurium* OMV by co-extrusion of a 200 nm polycarbonate membrane and added hydrophilic catalase CAT and hydrophobic photosensitizer Ce6 to the OMV. By alleviating tumor hypoxia and improving the photodynamic and immunotherapeutic effects, the tumor was significantly inhibited [139].

6. Conclusions

Bacteria function as mutually beneficial symbiotic partners with the human body. Great progress has been made in nearly a century since bacteria were first used to treat cancer in 1891, and some results have entered the stage of clinical evaluation.

In this review, we discussed the anticancer activity of bacterial cellular components, including bacterial specific virulence factors, bacterial toxins, bacterial enzymes, biosurfactant, the outer surface of Gram-positive bacteria, bacterial cell membranes, cell walls, biofilms formed by spontaneous aggregation, dormant spores formed by poor nutrition, and magnetosomes, among others. In addition, we discussed the direct anticancer effect of naïve living bacteria. For example, probiotic lactic acid bacteria and *Escherichia coli* are used to treat colon cancer, breast cancer, etc. The general pathogenic bacteria *Mycobacterium tuberculosis*, *Listeria monocytogenes*, and *Salmonella typhimurium* are used to treat nonmuscle invasive bladder cancer and breast cancer. The pathogen *Pseudomonas aeruginosa* inhibits tumor growth in the mouse TC-1 tumor model. However, the natural virulence factors in bacteria can activate relevant PAMP immune responses, and they are difficult to remove after colonization. Therefore, engineered bacteria after gene editing are more suitable for cancer treatment. Genetic engineering transformation methods are as follows: (1) Engineering bacteria that edit genes such as *msbB*, *rfaG*, and *rfaD* can modify the structure of the outer membrane of Gram-negative bacteria and reduce the toxicity to the host. (2) Through overexpression of MSHA flagella or ICAP capsular polysaccharide, the bacterial surface virulence factors are masked. (3) Transforming bacteria into specific nutrition-dependent mutations can also effectively reduce toxicity, such as *aroA* gene mutations that lead to bacterial aromatic amino acid nutritional deficiencies. (4) Downregulation or knockout of the expression and synthesis genes of bacterial toxin-related toxins, which are the main virulence factors, can greatly reduce the virulence of bacteria. (5) The expression of an inducible promoter has precise space–time regulation ability, which can improve the specificity of bacteria. Exogenous inducible promoters induce the expression of anticancer active ingredients such as environmental factors and endogenous inducible promoters. (6) Other ways to improve specificity are the expression of the membrane-penetrating peptide RGD by engineered bacteria and the secretion of the systemic effector protein signal peptide by bacteria. (7) Engineering bacteria-expressed antibodies with high affinity to cancer cell surface antigens or that connect with single-stranded oligonucleotide aptamers is one way to improve specificity. (8) Engineered bacteria can also treat tumors by expressing active anticancer ingredients, such as the expression of drug synthase, cancer cell antibodies, the immune checkpoint inhibition antibody anti-PD-L1, cytokines, siRNA, miRNA, Crispr-Cas9, pigment synthase, fluorescent protein, bacterial toxin, and so on. Bacteria and nanomaterials are combined through chemical bonds, amide bonds, electrostatic interaction, or extrusion ultrasound. This anticancer approach combines the active targeting by bacteria and the high-efficiency cancer cell lethality of nanomaterials, from the cellular components of bacteria to naïve living bacteria, and the combination of engineered bacteria and nanomaterials. The application of bacteria in cancer treatment has changed from weak specific and weak immune response to efficient specific and immune activation response, with significant anticancer activity.

Despite the advantages of bacteria-based antitumor therapy, it is still limited by a few shortcomings that need to be urgently resolved. The most important is effectiveness. Bacteria in anticancer treatment refer to precise targeting processes and complex human immune responses in tumor environments. Engineered bacteria need to cross complex blood vessels in high-speed blood flow to reach the tumor environment after intravenous injection. How to accumulate enough engineered bacteria to exert anticancer effects is an urgent consideration. Ensuring the highly efficient expression of proteins that exert anticancer effects for a long time has an important impact on bacteria-based anticancer therapy. Another issue to be aware of is safety. Bacteria are known as an autonomously disorganized and proliferating species. Their unique PAMPs and virulence factors induce an immune response in the human body, which promotes the killing of cancer cells by the human immune system. When the immune response is excessive, it threatens the patient's life. Genetic material based on engineered bacteria also refers to ethical issues with transgenes, which presses challenges for the future of engineered bacteria therapy. In general, future development directions of bacterial tumor therapy will be to combine nanomaterials and engineering bacteria and to explore the physical and functional relationship between bacteria and nanomaterials. The results will be a more specific, effective, and accurate tumor immune response together with a comprehensive and less toxic treatment system.

Funding: This research was funded by Science and Technology Development Fund: 0011/2018/A1; Science and Technology Development Fund: 025/2015/A1; University of Macau: MYRG2014-00093-FHS; University of Macau: MYRG 2015-00036-FHS; University of Macau: MYRG2016-00110-FHS; University of Macau: MYRG2018-00081; National Key R&D Plan of China: 2018YFB0407200; Shenzhen Science and Technology Innovation Commission: JCYJ20170307110157501; National Natural Science Foundation of China: 81771930.

Conflicts of Interest: The authors declare no conflict of interest.

References

1. de Martel, C.; Georges, D.; Bray, F.; Ferlay, J.; Clifford, G.M. Global burden of cancer attributable to infections in 2018: A worldwide incidence analysis. *Lancet Glob. Health* **2020**, *8*, E180–E190. [CrossRef]
2. Sender, R.; Fuchs, S.; Milo, R. Revised Estimates for the Number of Human and Bacteria Cells in the Body. *PLoS Biol.* **2016**, *14*, e1002533. [CrossRef] [PubMed]
3. van Schaik, W. The human gut resistome. *Philos. Trans. R. Soc. Lond. B Biol. Sci.* **2015**, *370*, 20140087. [CrossRef] [PubMed]
4. Dulal, S.; Keku, T.O. Gut Microbiome and Colorectal Adenomas. *Cancer J.* **2014**, *20*, 225–231. [CrossRef] [PubMed]
5. Arweiler, N.B.; Netuschil, L. The Oral Microbiota. *Adv. Exp. Med. Biol.* **2016**, *902*, 45–60. [PubMed]
6. Yamashita, Y.; Takeshita, T. The oral microbiome and human health. *J. Oral Sci.* **2017**, *59*, 201–206. [CrossRef]
7. Byrd, A.L.; Belkaid, Y.; Segre, J.A. The human skin microbiome. *Nat. Rev. Microbiol.* **2018**, *16*, 143–155. [CrossRef]
8. Mirmonsef, P.; Hotton, A.L.; Gilbert, D.; Burgad, D.; Landay, A.; Weber, K.M.; Cohen, M.; Ravel, J.; Spear, G.T. Free Glycogen in Vaginal Fluids Is Associated with Lactobacillus Colonization and Low Vaginal pH. *PLoS ONE* **2014**, *9*, e102467. [CrossRef]
9. De Boeck, I.; Broek, M.F.V.D.; Allonsius, C.N.; Spacova, I.; Wittouck, S.; Martens, K.; Wuyts, S.; Cauwenberghs, E.; Jokicevic, K.; Vandenheuvel, D.; et al. Lactobacilli Have a Niche in the Human Nose. *Cell Rep.* **2020**, *31*, 107674. [CrossRef]
10. Nauts, H.C.; E Swift, W.; Coley, B.L. The treatment of malignant tumors by bacterial toxins as developed by the late William B. Coley, M.D., reviewed in the light of modern research. *Cancer Res.* **1946**, *6*, 205–216.
11. McCarthy, E.F. The toxins of William B. Coley and the treatment of bone and soft-tissue sarcomas. *Iowa Orthop. J.* **2006**, *26*, 154–158.
12. Dmitrieva, N.F.; Trofimov, D.I.; Eshchina, A.S.; A Riapis, L.; Pavlova, O.G.; Petrova, T.V.; A Skorkina, I.; Gerasimov, A.N.; Alekseev, L.P.; Zhuravlev, M.V.; et al. Frequency of genes speA, speB, and speC in Streptococcus pyogenes strains and the identification of the infective agent by polymerase chain reaction. *J. Microbiol. Epidemiol. Immunobiol.* **2002**, 3–6.
13. Elahian, F.; Moghimi, B.; Dinmohammadi, F.; Ghamghami, M.; Hamidi, M.; Mirzaei, S.A. The Anticancer Agent Prodigiosin Is Not a Multidrug Resistance Protein Substrate. *DNA Cell Biol.* **2013**, *32*, 90–97. [CrossRef]
14. Lewis, D.J.; Dao, H.; Nagarajan, P.; Duvic, M. Primary cutaneous anaplastic large-cell lymphoma: Complete remission for 13 years after denileukin diftitox. *JAAD Case Rep.* **2017**, *3*, 501–504. [CrossRef]
15. Siegall, C.B.; Chaudhary, V.K.; Fitzgerald, D.J.; Pastan, I. Functional analysis of domains II, Ib, and III of Pseudomonas exotoxin. *J. Biol. Chem.* **1989**, *264*, 14256–14261. [CrossRef]
16. Michl, P.; Buchholz, M.; Rolke, M.; Kunsch, S.; Löhr, M.; McClane, B.; Tsukita, S.; Leder, G.; Adler, G.; Gress, T.M. Claudin-4: A new target for pancreatic cancer treatment using Clostridium perfringens enterotoxin. *Gastroenterology* **2001**, *121*, 678–684. [CrossRef]
17. Rommasi, F. Bacterial-Based Methods for Cancer Treatment: What We Know and Where We Are. *Oncol. Ther.* **2022**, *10*, 23–54. [CrossRef]
18. Michalska, M.; Wolf, P. Pseudomonas Exotoxin A: Optimized by evolution for effective killing. *Front. Microbiol.* **2015**, *6*, 963. [CrossRef]
19. Singh, R.; Dominiecki, M.E.; Jaffee, E.M.; Paterson, Y. Fusion to Listeriolysin O and delivery by Listeria monocytogenes enhances the immunogenicity of HER-2/neu and reveals subdominant epitopes in the FVB/N mouse. *J. Immunol.* **2005**, *175*, 3663–3673. [CrossRef]
20. Mayakrishnan, V.; Kannappan, P.; Tharmalingam, N.; Bose, R.J.C.; Madheswaran, T.; Ramasamy, M. Bacterial cancer therapy: A turning point for new paradigms. *Drug Discov. Today* **2022**, *27*, 2043–2050. [CrossRef]
21. Fiedler, T.; Strauss, M.; Hering, S.; Redanz, U.; William, D.; Rosche, Y.; Classen, C.F.; Kreikemeyer, B.; Linnebacher, M.; Maletzki, C. Arginine deprivation by arginine deiminase of Streptococcus pyogenes controls primary glioblastoma growth in vitro and in vivo. *Cancer Biol. Ther.* **2015**, *16*, 1047–1055. [CrossRef]
22. Cao, X.; Wang, A.H.; Jiao, R.Z.; Wang, C.L.; Mao, D.Z.; Yan, L.; Zeng, B. Surfactin induces apoptosis and G(2)/M arrest in human breast cancer MCF-7 cells through cell cycle factor regulation. *Cell Biochem. Biophys.* **2009**, *55*, 163–171. [CrossRef]
23. Gudiña, E.J.; Rangarajan, V.; Sen, R.; Rodrigues, L.R. Potential therapeutic applications of biosurfactants. *Trends Pharmacol. Sci.* **2013**, *34*, 667–675. [CrossRef]
24. El-Sersy, N.A.; Abdelwahab, A.E.; Abouelkhiir, S.S.; Abou-Zeid, D.M.; Sabry, S.A. Antibacterial and anticancer activity of epsilon-poly-L-lysine (epsilon-PL) produced by a marine *Bacillus subtilis* sp. *J. Basic Microbiol.* **2012**, *52*, 513–522. [CrossRef]
25. Saini, H.S.; Barragán-Huerta, B.E.; Lebrón-Paler, A.; Pemberton, J.E.; Vázquez, R.R.; Burns, A.M.; Marron, M.T.; Seliga, C.J.; Gunatilaka, A.A.L.; Maier, R.M. Efficient Purification of the Biosurfactant Viscosin from *Pseudomonas libanensis* Strain M9-3 and Its Physicochemical and Biological Properties. *J. Nat. Prod.* **2008**, *71*, 1011–1015. [CrossRef]
26. De Vleeschouwer, M.; Van Kersavond, T.; Verleysen, Y.; Sinnaeve, D.; Coenye, T.; Martins, J.C.; Madder, A. Identification of the Molecular Determinants Involved in Antimicrobial Activity of Pseudodesmin A, a Cyclic Lipopeptide From the Viscosin Group. *Front. Microbiol.* **2020**, *11*, 646. [CrossRef]
27. Escobar-Diaz, E.; Lopez-Martin, E.M.; Hernandez del Cerro, M.; Puig-Kroger, A.; Soto-Cerrato, V.; Montaner, B.; Giralt, E.; Garcia-Marco, J.A.; Perez-Tomas, R.; Garcia-Pardo, A. AT514, a cyclic depsipeptide from Serratia marcescens, induces apoptosis of B-chronic lymphocytic leukemia cells: Interference with the Akt/NF-kappaB survival pathway. *Leukemia* **2005**, *19*, 572–579. [CrossRef]

28. Kojiri, K.; Nakajima, S.; Suzuki, H.; Okura, A.; Suda, H. A new antitumor substance, BE-18591, produced by a streptomycete. I. Fermentation, isolation, physico-chemical and biological properties. *J. Antibiot.* **1993**, *46*, 1799–1803. [CrossRef]
29. Bracken, J.D.; Carlson, A.D.; Frederick, J.; Nguyen, M.; Shore, G.C.; Harran, P.G. Tailored fragments of roseophilin selectively antagonize Mcl-1 in vitro. *Tetrahedron Lett.* **2015**, *56*, 3612–3616. [CrossRef]
30. Kawasaki, T.; Sakurai, F.; Hayakawa, Y. A Prodigiosin from the Roseophilin Producer Streptomyces griseoviridis. *J. Nat. Prod.* **2008**, *71*, 1265–1267. [CrossRef]
31. Shim, G.Y.; Kim, S.H.; Han, S.-E.; Kim, Y.; Oh, Y.J.A.J.P.S. Cationic surfactin liposomes for enhanced cellular delivery of siRNA. *Asian J. Pharm. Sci.* **2009**, *4*, 207–214.
32. Garbacz, K. Anticancer activity of lactic acid bacteria. *Semin. Cancer Biol.* 2022; in press.
33. Zhang, T.; Pan, D.; Yang, Y.; Jiang, X.; Zhang, J.; Zeng, X.; Wu, Z.; Sun, Y.; Guo, Y. Effect of *Lactobacillus acidophilus* CICC 6074 S-Layer Protein on Colon Cancer HT-29 Cell Proliferation and Apoptosis. *J. Agric. Food Chem.* **2020**, *68*, 2639–2647. [CrossRef] [PubMed]
34. Moriyama, K.; Nishida, O. Targeting Cytokines, Pathogen-Associated Molecular Patterns, and Damage-Associated Molecular Patterns in Sepsis via Blood Purification. *Int. J. Mol. Sci.* **2021**, *22*, 8882. [CrossRef] [PubMed]
35. Eletto, D.; Mentucci, F.; Voli, A.; Petrella, A.; Porta, A.; Tosco, A. Helicobacter pylori Pathogen-Associated Molecular Patterns: Friends or Foes? *Int. J. Mol. Sci.* **2022**, *23*, 3531. [CrossRef]
36. Li, M.; Li, S.; Zhou, H.; Tang, X.; Wu, Y.; Jiang, W.; Tian, Z.; Zhou, X.; Yang, X.; Wang, Y. Chemotaxis-driven delivery of nano-pathogenoids for complete eradication of tumors post-phototherapy. *Nat. Commun.* **2020**, *11*, 1126. [CrossRef]
37. Mamou, G.; Corona, F.; Cohen-Khait, R.; Housden, N.G.; Yeung, V.; Sun, D.; Sridhar, P.; Pazos, M.; Knowles, T.J.; Kleanthous, C.; et al. Peptidoglycan maturation controls outer membrane protein assembly. *Nature* **2022**, *606*, 953–959. [CrossRef]
38. Roier, S.; Zingl, F.G.; Cakar, F.; Durakovic, S.; Kohl, P.; Eichmann, T.O.; Klug, L.; Gadermaier, B.; Weinzerl, K.; Prassl, R.; et al. A novel mechanism for the biogenesis of outer membrane vesicles in Gram-negative bacteria. *Nat. Commun.* **2016**, *7*, 10515. [CrossRef]
39. Li, Y.; Ma, X.; Yue, Y.; Zhang, K.; Cheng, K.; Feng, Q.; Ma, N.; Liang, J.; Zhang, T.; Zhang, L.; et al. Rapid Surface Display of mRNA Antigens by Bacteria-Derived Outer Membrane Vesicles for a Personalized Tumor Vaccine. *Adv. Mater.* **2022**, *34*, e2109984. [CrossRef]
40. Zou, M.-Z.; Li, Z.-H.; Bai, X.-F.; Liu, C.-J.; Zhang, X.-Z. Hybrid Vesicles Based on Autologous Tumor Cell Membrane and Bacterial Outer Membrane To Enhance Innate Immune Response and Personalized Tumor Immunotherapy. *Nano Lett.* **2021**, *21*, 8609–8618. [CrossRef]
41. Jayasinghe, M.K.; Pirisinu, M.; Yang, Y.; Peng, B.; Pham, T.T.; Lee, C.Y.; Tan, M.; Vu, L.T.; Dang, X.T.T.; Pham, T.C.; et al. Surface-engineered extracellular vesicles for targeted delivery of therapeutic RNAs and peptides for cancer therapy. *Theranostics* **2022**, *12*, 3288–3315. [CrossRef]
42. Kuerban, K.; Gao, X.; Zhang, H.; Liu, J.; Dong, M.; Wu, L.; Ye, R.; Feng, M.; Ye, L. Doxorubicin-loaded bacterial outer-membrane vesicles exert enhanced anti-tumor efficacy in non-small-cell lung cancer. *Acta Pharm. Sin. B* **2020**, *10*, 1534–1548. [CrossRef]
43. Hamann, L.; El-Samalouti, V.; Ulmer, A.J.; Flad, H.-D.; Rietschel, E.T. Components of gut bacteria as immunomodulators. *Int. J. Food Microbiol.* **1998**, *41*, 141–154. [CrossRef]
44. Divyashree, M.; Prakash, S.K.; Aditya, V.; Aljabali, A.A.; Alzahrani, K.J.; Azevedo, V.; Góes-Neto, A.; Tambuwala, M.M.; Barh, D. Bugs as drugs: Neglected but a promising future therapeutic strategy in cancer. *Future Oncol.* **2022**, *18*, 1609–1626. [CrossRef]
45. Adnan, M.; Khan, S.; Al-Shammari, E.; Patel, M.; Saeed, M.; Hadi, S. In pursuit of cancer metastasis therapy by bacteria and its biofilms: History or future. *Med. Hypotheses* **2017**, *100*, 78–81. [CrossRef]
46. Diaz, L.A.; Cheong, I.; Foss, C.A.; Zhang, X.; Peters, B.A.; Agrawal, N.; Bettegowda, C.; Karim, B.; Liu, G.; Khan, K.; et al. Pharmacologic and Toxicologic Evaluation of C. novyi-NT Spores. *Toxicol. Sci.* **2005**, *88*, 562–575. [CrossRef]
47. Umer, B.; Good, D.; Anné, J.; Duan, W.; Wei, M.Q. Clostridial Spores for Cancer Therapy: Targeting Solid Tumour Microenvironment. *J. Toxicol.* **2012**, *2012*, 862764. [CrossRef]
48. Lower, B.H.; Bazylinski, D.A. The Bacterial Magnetosome: A Unique Prokaryotic Organelle. *J. Mol. Microbiol. Biotechnol.* **2013**, *23*, 63–80. [CrossRef]
49. Uebe, R.; Schüler, D. Magnetosome biogenesis in magnetotactic bacteria. *Nat. Rev. Microbiol.* **2016**, *14*, 621–637. [CrossRef]
50. Gandia, D.; Gandarias, L.; Rodrigo, I.; Robles-Garcia, J.; Das, R.; Garaio, E.; Garcia, J.A.; Phan, M.H.; Srikanth, H.; Orue, I.; et al. Unlocking the Potential of Magnetotactic Bacteria as Magnetic Hyperthermia Agents. *Small* **2019**, *15*, e1902626. [CrossRef]
51. Marzhoseyni, Z.; Shojaie, L.; Tabatabaei, S.A.; Movahedpour, A.; Safari, M.; Esmaeili, D.; Mahjoubin-Tehran, M.; Jalili, A.; Morshedi, K.; Khan, H.; et al. Streptococcal bacterial components in cancer therapy. *Cancer Gene Ther.* **2022**, *29*, 141–155. [CrossRef]
52. Joo, N.E.; Ritchie, K.; Kamarajan, P.; Miao, D.; Kapila, Y.L. Nisin, an apoptogenic bacteriocin and food preservative, attenuates HNSCC tumorigenesis via CHAC 1. *Cancer Med.* **2012**, *1*, 295–305. [CrossRef]
53. Zhu, H.; Cao, C.; Wu, Z.; Zhang, H.; Sun, Z.; Wang, M.; Xu, H.; Zhao, Z.; Wang, Y.; Pei, G.; et al. The probiotic L. casei Zhang slows the progression of acute and chronic kidney disease. *Cell Metab.* **2021**, *33*, 1926–1942.e8. [CrossRef]
54. Rodrigues, G.; Silva, G.G.O.; Buccini, D.F.; Duque, H.M.; Dias, S.C.; Franco, O.L. Bacterial Proteinaceous Compounds With Multiple Activities Toward Cancers and Microbial Infection. *Front. Microbiol.* **2019**, *10*, 1690. [CrossRef]

55. Paiva, A.D.; de Oliveira, M.D.; de Paula, S.O.; Baracat-Pereira, M.C.; Breukink, E.; Mantovani, H.C. Toxicity of bovicin HC5 against mammalian cell lines and the role of cholesterol in bacteriocin activity. *Microbiology* **2012**, *158 Pt 11*, 2851–2858. [CrossRef]
56. Lee, D.K.; Jang, S.; Kim, M.J.; Kim, J.H.; Chung, M.J.; Kim, K.J.; Ha, N.J. Anti-proliferative effects of Bifidobacterium adolescentis SPM0212 extract on human colon cancer cell lines. *BMC Cancer* **2008**, *8*, 310. [CrossRef]
57. Yazawa, K.; Fujimori, M.; Amano, J.; Kano, Y.; Taniguchi, S. Bifidobacterium longum as a delivery system for cancer gene therapy: Selective localization and growth in hypoxic tumors. *Cancer Gene Ther.* **2000**, *7*, 269–274. [CrossRef]
58. Fujimori, M.; Amano, J.; Taniguchi, S. The genus Bifidobacterium for cancer gene therapy. *Curr. Opin. Drug Discov. Dev.* **2002**, *5*, 200–203.
59. Grozdanov, L.; Raasch, C.; Schulze, J.; Sonnenborn, U.; Gottschalk, G.; Hacker, J.; Dobrindt, U. Analysis of the Genome Structure of the Nonpathogenic Probiotic *Escherichia coli* Strain Nissle 1917. *J. Bacteriol.* **2004**, *186*, 5432–5441. [CrossRef]
60. Yu, D.; Wu, C.; Ping, S.; Keng, C.; Shen, K. Bacille Calmette-Guerin can induce cellular apoptosis of urothelial cancer directly through toll-like receptor 7 activation. *Kaohsiung J. Med. Sci.* **2015**, *31*, 391–397. [CrossRef]
61. Wang, D.; Wei, X.; Kalvakolanu, D.V.; Guo, B.; Zhang, L. Perspectives on Oncolytic Salmonella in Cancer Immunotherapy—A Promising Strategy. *Front. Immunol.* **2021**, *12*, 615930. [CrossRef]
62. Oladejo, M.; Paterson, Y.; Wood, L.M. Clinical Experience and Recent Advances in the Development of Listeria-Based Tumor Immunotherapies. *Front. Immunol.* **2021**, *12*, 642316. [CrossRef] [PubMed]
63. Qi, J.-L.; He, J.-R.; Jin, S.-M.; Yang, X.; Bai, H.-M.; Liu, C.-B.; Ma, Y.-B. *P. aeruginosa* Mediated Necroptosis in Mouse Tumor Cells Induces Long-Lasting Systemic Antitumor Immunity. *Front. Oncol.* **2020**, *10*, 610651. [CrossRef] [PubMed]
64. Pi, J.; Zhang, Z.; Yang, E.; Chen, L.; Zeng, L.; Chen, Y.; Wang, R.; Huang, D.; Fan, S.; Lin, W.; et al. Nanocages engineered from Bacillus Calmette-Guerin facilitate protective Vgamma2Vdelta2 T cell immunity against Mycobacterium tuberculosis infection. *J. Nanobiotechnol.* **2022**, *20*, 36. [CrossRef] [PubMed]
65. Gontero, P.; Bohle, A.; Malmstrom, P.-U.; O'Donnell, M.A.; Oderda, M.; Sylvester, R.; Witjes, F. The Role of Bacillus Calmette-Guérin in the Treatment of Non–Muscle-Invasive Bladder Cancer. *Eur. Urol.* **2010**, *57*, 410–429. [CrossRef]
66. Poussin, M.A.; Goldfine, H. Involvement of *Listeria monocytogenes* Phosphatidylinositol-Specific Phospholipase C and Host Protein Kinase C in Permeabilization of the Macrophage Phagosome. *Infect. Immun.* **2005**, *73*, 4410–4413. [CrossRef]
67. Brunt, L.M.; A Portnoy, D.; Unanue, E.R. Presentation of Listeria monocytogenes to CD8+ T cells requires secretion of hemolysin and intracellular bacterial growth. *J. Immunol.* **1990**, *145*, 3540–3546.
68. Zheng, D.; Li, R.; An, J.; Xie, T.; Han, Z.; Xu, R.; Fang, Y.; Zhang, X. Prebiotics-Encapsulated Probiotic Spores Regulate Gut Microbiota and Suppress Colon Cancer. *Adv. Mater.* **2020**, *32*, e2004529. [CrossRef]
69. Wang, L.; Zhou, J.; Xin, Y.; Geng, C.; Tian, Z.; Yu, X.; Dong, Q. Bacterial overgrowth and diversification of microbiota in gastric cancer. *Eur. J. Gastroenterol. Hepatol.* **2016**, *28*, 261–266. [CrossRef]
70. Pleguezuelos-Manzano, C.; Puschhof, J.; Rosendahl Huber, A.; Van Hoeck, A.; Wood, H.M.; Nomburg, J.; Gurjao, C.; Manders, F.; Dalmasso, G.; Stege, P.B.; et al. Mutational signature in colorectal cancer caused by genotoxic pks (+) *E. coli*. *Nature* **2020**, *580*, 269–273. [CrossRef]
71. Duong, M.T.-Q.; Qin, Y.; You, S.-H.; Min, J.-J. Bacteria-cancer interactions: Bacteria-based cancer therapy. *Exp. Mol. Med.* **2019**, *51*, 1–15. [CrossRef]
72. Toso, J.F.; Gill, V.J.; Hwu, P.; Marincola, F.M.; Restifo, N.P.; Schwartzentruber, D.J.; Sherry, R.M.; Topalian, S.L.; Yang, J.C.; Stock, F.; et al. Phase I study of the intravenous administration of attenuated Salmonella typhimurium to patients with metastatic melanoma. *J. Clin. Oncol.* **2002**, *20*, 142–152. [CrossRef]
73. Heimann, D.M.; Rosenberg, S.A. Continuous Intravenous Administration of Live Genetically Modified Salmonella Typhimurium in Patients With Metastatic Melanoma. *J. Immunother.* **2003**, *26*, 179–180. [CrossRef]
74. Nemunaitis, J.; Cunningham, C.; Senzer, N.; Kuhn, J.; Cramm, J.; Litz, C.; Cavagnolo, R.; Cahill, A.; Clairmont, C.; Sznol, M. Pilot trial of genetically modified, attenuated Salmonella expressing the E. coli cytosine deaminase gene in refractory cancer patients. *Cancer Gene Ther.* **2003**, *10*, 737–744. [CrossRef]
75. VNP20009 in Treating Patients with Advanced or Metastatic Solid Tumors That Have Not Responded to Previous Therapy. 2019. Available online: ClinicalTrials.gov (accessed on 3 October 2022).
76. VNP20009 in Treating Patients with Advanced Solid Tumors. 2019. Available online: ClinicalTrials.gov (accessed on 3 October 2022).
77. Treatment of Patients with Cancer with Genetically Modified Salmonella Typhimurium Bacteria. 2019. Available online: ClinicalTrials.gov (accessed on 3 October 2022).
78. IL-2 Expressing, Attenuated Salmonella Typhimurium in Unresectable Hepatic Spread. 2019. Available online: ClinicalTrials.gov (accessed on 3 October 2022).
79. Schmitz-Winnenthal, F.H.; Hohmann, N.; Schmidt, T.; Podola, L.; Friedrich, T.; Lubenau, H.; Springer, M.; Wieckowski, S.; Breiner, K.M.; Mikus, G.; et al. A phase 1 trial extension to assess immunologic efficacy and safety of prime-boost vaccination with VXM01, an oral T cell vaccine against VEGFR2, in patients with advanced pancreatic cancer. *OncoImmunology* **2018**, *7*, e1303584. [CrossRef]
80. One Time Injection of Bacteria to Treat Solid Tumors That Have Not Responded to Standard Therapy. 2019. Available online: ClinicalTrials.gov (accessed on 3 October 2022).

81. Safety Study of Clostridium Novyi-NT Spores to Treat Patients with Solid Tumors That Have Not Responded to Standard Therapies. 2019. Available online: ClinicalTrials.gov (accessed on 3 October 2022).
82. Safety Study of Intratumoral Injection of Clostridium Novyi-NT Spores to Treat Patients with Solid Tumors That Have Not Responded to Standard Therapies. 2019. Available online: ClinicalTrials.gov (accessed on 3 October 2022).
83. Pembrolizumab with Intratumoral Injection of Clostridium Novyi-NT. 2019. Available online: ClinicalTrials.gov (accessed on 3 October 2022).
84. Le, D.T.; Wang-Gillam, A.; Picozzi, V.; Greten, T.F.; Crocenzi, T.; Springett, G.; Morse, M.; Zeh, H.; Cohen, D.; Fine, R.L.; et al. Safety and Survival With GVAX Pancreas Prime and *Listeria Monocytogenes*–Expressing Mesothelin (CRS-207) Boost Vaccines for Metastatic Pancreatic Cancer. *J. Clin. Oncol.* **2015**, *33*, 1325–1333. [CrossRef]
85. Basu, P.; Mehta, A.; Jain, M.; Gupta, S.; Nagarkar, R.V.; John, S.; Petit, R. A Randomized Phase 2 Study of ADXS11-001 Listeria monocytogenes–Listeriolysin O Immunotherapy with or without Cisplatin in Treatment of Advanced Cervical Cancer. *Int. J. Gynecol. Cancer* **2018**, *28*, 764–772. [CrossRef]
86. Study of ADXS11–001 in Subjects with High Risk Locally Advanced Cervical Cancer. 2019. Available online: ClinicalTrials.gov (accessed on 3 October 2022).
87. Kong, Q.; Six, D.A.; Liu, Q.; Gu, L.; Roland, K.L.; Raetz, C.R.H.; Curtiss, R. Palmitoylation State Impacts Induction of Innate and Acquired Immunity by the Salmonella enterica Serovar Typhimurium *msbB* Mutant. *Infect. Immun.* **2011**, *79*, 5027–5038. [CrossRef]
88. Kong, Q.; Yang, J.; Liu, Q.; Alamuri, P.; Roland, K.L.; Curtiss, R. Effect of Deletion of Genes Involved in Lipopolysaccharide Core and O-Antigen Synthesis on Virulence and Immunogenicity of Salmonella enterica Serovar Typhimurium. *Infect. Immun.* **2011**, *79*, 4227–4239. [CrossRef]
89. Kocijancic, D.; Felgner, S.; Schauer, T.; Frahm, M.; Heise, U.; Zimmermann, K.; Erhardt, M.; Weiss, S. Local application of bacteria improves safety of *Salmonella*-mediated tumor therapy and retains advantages of systemic infection. *Oncotarget* **2017**, *8*, 49988–50001. [CrossRef]
90. Chang, L.; Xiao, W.; Yang, Y.; Li, H.; Xia, D.; Yu, G.; Guo, X.; Guan, W.; Hu, Z.; Xu, H.; et al. Pseudomonas aeruginosa-mannose–sensitive hemagglutinin inhibits epidermal growth factor receptor signaling pathway activation and induces apoptosis in bladder cancer cells in vitro and in vivo. *Urol. Oncol.* **2014**, *32*, 36.e11–36.e18. [CrossRef]
91. Harimoto, T.; Hahn, J.; Chen, Y.-Y.; Im, J.; Zhang, J.; Hou, N.; Li, F.; Coker, C.; Gray, K.; Harr, N.; et al. A programmable encapsulation system improves delivery of therapeutic bacteria in mice. *Nat. Biotechnol.* **2022**, *40*, 1259–1269. [CrossRef]
92. Zhao, M.; Yang, M.; Li, X.-M.; Jiang, P.; Baranov, E.; Li, S.; Xu, M.; Penman, S.; Hoffman, R.M. Tumor-targeting bacterial therapy with amino acid auxotrophs of GFP-expressing *Salmonella typhimurium*. *Proc. Natl. Acad. Sci. USA* **2005**, *102*, 755–760. [CrossRef]
93. Clairmont, C.; Lee, K.C.; Pike, J.; Ittensohn, M.; Low, K.B.; Pawelek, J.; Bermudes, D.; Brecher, S.M.; Margitich, D.; Turnier, J.; et al. Biodistribution and Genetic Stability of the Novel Antitumor Agent VNP20009, a Genetically Modified Strain of *Salmonella typhimurium*. *J. Infect. Dis.* **2000**, *181*, 1996–2002. [CrossRef]
94. Epaulard, O.; Derouazi, M.; Margerit, C.; Marlu, R.; Filopon, D.; Polack, B.; Toussaint, B. Optimization of a Type III Secretion System-Based *Pseudomonas aeruginosa* Live Vector for Antigen Delivery. *Clin. Vaccine Immunol.* **2008**, *15*, 308–313. [CrossRef]
95. Yoon, W.S.; Choi, W.C.; Sin, J.-I.; Park, Y.K. Antitumor therapeutic effects of Salmonella typhimurium containing Flt3 Ligand expression plasmids in melanoma-bearing mouse. *Biotechnol. Lett.* **2007**, *29*, 511–516. [CrossRef]
96. Kramer, M.G.; Masner, M.; Casales, E.; Moreno, M.; Smerdou, C.; Chabalgoity, J.A. Neoadjuvant administration of Semliki Forest virus expressing interleukin-12 combined with attenuated Salmonella eradicates breast cancer metastasis and achieves long-term survival in immunocompetent mice. *BMC Cancer* **2015**, *15*, 620. [CrossRef]
97. Na, H.S.; Kim, H.J.; Lee, H.-C.; Hong, Y.; Rhee, J.H.; E Choy, H. Immune response induced by Salmonella typhimurium defective in ppGpp synthesis. *Vaccine* **2006**, *24*, 2027–2034. [CrossRef] [PubMed]
98. Dang, L.H.; Bettegowda, C.; Huso, D.L.; Kinzler, K.W.; Vogelstein, B. Combination bacteriolytic therapy for the treatment of experimental tumors. *Proc. Natl. Acad. Sci. USA* **2001**, *98*, 15155–15160. [CrossRef] [PubMed]
99. Pang, Z.; Gu, M.-D.; Tang, T. Pseudomonas aeruginosa in Cancer Therapy: Current Knowledge, Challenges and Future Perspectives. *Front. Oncol.* **2022**, *12*, 891187. [CrossRef] [PubMed]
100. Samadi, M.; Majidzadeh-A, K.; Salehi, M.; Jalili, N.; Noorinejad, Z.; Mosayebzadeh, M.; Muhammadnejad, A.; Khatibi, A.S.; Moradi-Kalbolandi, S.; Farahmand, L. Engineered hypoxia-responding Escherichia coli carrying cardiac peptide genes, suppresses tumor growth, angiogenesis and metastasis in vivo. *J. Biol. Eng.* **2021**, *15*, 20. [CrossRef] [PubMed]
101. Anderson, J.C.; Clarke, E.J.; Arkin, A.P.; Voigt, C.A. Environmentally Controlled Invasion of Cancer Cells by Engineered Bacteria. *J. Mol. Biol.* **2006**, *355*, 619–627. [CrossRef]
102. Flentie, K.; Kocher, B.; Gammon, S.T.; Novack, D.V.; McKinney, J.S.; Piwnica-Worms, D. A Bioluminescent Transposon Reporter-Trap Identifies Tumor-Specific Microenvironment-Induced Promoters in *Salmonella* for Conditional Bacterial-Based Tumor Therapy. *Cancer Discov.* **2012**, *2*, 624–637. [CrossRef]
103. Han, H.; Zhang, X.; Pang, G.; Zhang, Y.; Pan, H.; Li, L.; Cui, M.; Liu, B.; Kang, R.; Xue, X.; et al. Hydrogel microcapsules containing engineered bacteria for sustained production and release of protein drugs. *Biomaterials* **2022**, *287*, 121619. [CrossRef]
104. Ganai, S.; Arenas, R.B.; Forbes, N.S. Tumour-targeted delivery of TRAIL using Salmonella typhimurium enhances breast cancer survival in mice. *Br. J. Cancer* **2009**, *101*, 1683–1691. [CrossRef]

105. Terpe, K. Overview of bacterial expression systems for heterologous protein production: From molecular and biochemical fundamentals to commercial systems. *Appl. Microbiol. Biotechnol.* **2006**, *72*, 211–222. [CrossRef]
106. Li, L.; Pan, H.; Pang, G.; Lang, H.; Shen, Y.; Sun, T.; Zhang, Y.; Liu, J.; Chang, J.; Kang, J.; et al. Precise Thermal Regulation of Engineered Bacteria Secretion for Breast Cancer Treatment In Vivo. *ACS Synth. Biol.* **2022**, *11*, 1167–1177. [CrossRef]
107. Park, S.-H.; Zheng, J.H.; Nguyen, V.H.; Jiang, S.-N.; Kim, D.-Y.; Szardenings, M.; Min, J.H.; Hong, Y.; Choy, H.E. RGD Peptide Cell-Surface Display Enhances the Targeting and Therapeutic Efficacy of Attenuated *Salmonella*-mediated Cancer Therapy. *Theranostics* **2016**, *6*, 1672–1682. [CrossRef]
108. Huang, S.; Zhu, Z.; Jia, B.; Zhang, W.; Song, J. Design of acid-activated cell-penetrating peptides with nuclear localization capacity for anticancer drug delivery. *J. Pept. Sci.* **2021**, *27*, e3354. [CrossRef]
109. Coulthurst, S.J. The Type VI secretion system—A widespread and versatile cell targeting system. *Res. Microbiol.* **2013**, *164*, 640–654. [CrossRef]
110. Galán, J.E.; Lara-Tejero, M.; Marlovits, T.C.; Wagner, S. Bacterial Type III Secretion Systems: Specialized Nanomachines for Protein Delivery into Target Cells. *Annu. Rev. Microbiol.* **2014**, *68*, 415–438. [CrossRef]
111. Dong, C.Y.; Huang, Q.X.; Cheng, H.; Zheng, D.W.; Hong, S.; Yan, Y.; Niu, M.T.; Xu, J.G.; Zhang, X.Z. Neisseria meningitidis Opca Protein/MnO$_2$ Hybrid Nanoparticles for Overcoming the Blood-Brain Barrier to Treat Glioblastoma. *Adv. Mater* **2022**, *34*, e2109213. [CrossRef]
112. Yao, Q.; Cao, S.; Li, C.; Mengesha, A.; Low, P.; Kong, B.; Dai, S.; Wei, M. Turn a diarrhoea toxin into a receptor-mediated therapy for a plethora of CLDN-4-overexpressing cancers. *Biochem. Biophys. Res. Commun.* **2010**, *398*, 413–419. [CrossRef]
113. Murase, K. Cytolysin A (ClyA): A Bacterial Virulence Factor with Potential Applications in Nanopore Technology, Vaccine Development, and Tumor Therapy. *Toxins* **2022**, *14*, 78. [CrossRef]
114. Massa, P.E.; Paniccia, A.; Monegal, A.; De Marco, A.; Rescigno, M. Salmonella engineered to express CD20-targeting antibodies and a drug-converting enzyme can eradicate human lymphomas. *Blood* **2013**, *122*, 705–714. [CrossRef]
115. Geng, Z.; Cao, Z.; Liu, R.; Liu, K.; Liu, J.; Tan, W. Aptamer-assisted tumor localization of bacteria for enhanced biotherapy. *Nat. Commun.* **2021**, *12*, 6584. [CrossRef]
116. Fan, J.X.; Peng, M.Y.; Wang, H.; Zheng, H.R.; Liu, Z.L.; Li, C.X.; Wang, X.N.; Liu, X.H.; Cheng, S.X.; Zhang, X.Z. Engineered Bacterial Bioreactor for Tumor Therapy via Fenton-Like Reaction with Localized H$_2$O$_2$ Generation. *Adv. Mater* **2019**, *31*, e1808278. [CrossRef]
117. Minton, N.P.; Mauchline, M.L.; Lemmon, M.J.; Brehm, J.K.; Fox, M.; Michael, N.P.; Giaccia, A.; Brown, J.M. Chemotherapeutic tumour targeting using clostridial spores. *FEMS Microbiol. Rev.* **1995**, *17*, 357–364. [CrossRef]
118. Groot, A.J.; Mengesha, A.; van der Wall, E.; van Diest, P.J.; Theys, J.; Vooijs, M. Functional antibodies produced by oncolytic clostridia. *Biochem. Biophys. Res. Commun.* **2007**, *364*, 985–989. [CrossRef]
119. Nishikawa, H.; Sato, E.; Briones, G.; Chen, L.-M.; Matsuo, M.; Nagata, Y.; Ritter, G.; Jäger, E.; Nomura, H.; Kondo, S.; et al. In vivo antigen delivery by aSalmonella typhimurium type III secretion system for therapeutic cancer vaccines. *J. Clin. Investig.* **2006**, *116*, 1946–1954. [CrossRef]
120. Shahabi, V.; Maciag, P.C.; Rivera, S.; Wallecha, A. Live, attenuated strains of Listeria and Salmonella as vaccine vectors in cancer treatment. *Bioeng. Bugs* **2010**, *1*, 237–245. [CrossRef] [PubMed]
121. McIntosh, J.K.; Mulé, J.J.; A Krosnick, J.; A Rosenberg, S. Combination cytokine immunotherapy with tumor necrosis factor alpha, interleukin 2, and alpha-interferon and its synergistic antitumor effects in mice. *Cancer Res.* **1989**, *49*, 1408–1414. [PubMed]
122. Barbe, S.; Van Mellaert, L.; Theys, J.; Geukens, N.; Lammertyn, E.; Lambin, P.; Anne, J. Secretory production of biologically active rat interleukin-2 by Clostridium acetobutylicum DSM792 as a tool for anti-tumor treatment. *FEMS Microbiol. Lett.* **2005**, *246*, 67–73. [CrossRef] [PubMed]
123. Loeffler, M.; Le'Negrate, G.; Krajewska, M.; Reed, J.C. Inhibition of Tumor Growth Using Salmonella Expressing Fas Ligand. *J. Natl. Cancer Inst.* **2008**, *100*, 1113–1116. [CrossRef]
124. Deng, H.; Tan, S.; Gao, X.; Zou, C.; Xu, C.; Tu, K.; Song, Q.; Fan, F.; Huang, W.; Zhang, Z. Cdk5 knocking out mediated by CRISPR-Cas9 genome editing for PD-L1 attenuation and enhanced antitumor immunity. *Acta Pharm. Sin. B* **2020**, *10*, 358–373. [CrossRef]
125. Meng, W.; He, C.; Hao, Y.; Wang, L.; Li, L.; Zhu, G. Prospects and challenges of extracellular vesicle-based drug delivery system: Considering cell source. *Drug Deliv.* **2020**, *27*, 585–598. [CrossRef]
126. Yan, Y.; Liu, X.-Y.; Lu, A.; Wang, X.-Y.; Jiang, L.-X.; Wang, J.-C. Non-viral vectors for RNA delivery. *J. Control Release* **2022**, *342*, 241–279. [CrossRef]
127. Reid, G.; Kao, S.C.; Pavlakis, N.; Brahmbhatt, H.; MacDiarmid, J.; Clarke, S.; Boyer, M.; van Zandwijk, N. Clinical development of TargomiRs, a miRNA mimic-based treatment for patients with recurrent thoracic cancer. *Epigenomics* **2016**, *8*, 1079–1085. [CrossRef]
128. Gujrati, V.; Kim, S.; Kim, S.-H.; Min, J.J.; E Choy, H.; Kim, S.C.; Jon, S. Bioengineered Bacterial Outer Membrane Vesicles as Cell-Specific Drug-Delivery Vehicles for Cancer Therapy. *ACS Nano* **2014**, *8*, 1525–1537. [CrossRef]
129. Gujrati, V.; Prakash, J.; Malekzadeh-Najafabadi, J.; Stiel, A.; Klemm, U.; Mettenleiter, G.; Aichler, M.; Walch, A.; Ntziachristos, V. Bioengineered bacterial vesicles as biological nano-heaters for optoacoustic imaging. *Nat. Commun.* **2019**, *10*, 1114. [CrossRef]

130. Yang, Z.; Zhu, Y.; Dong, Z.; Hao, Y.; Wang, C.; Li, Q.; Wu, Y.; Feng, L.; Liu, Z. Engineering bioluminescent bacteria to boost photodynamic therapy and systemic anti-tumor immunity for synergistic cancer treatment. *Biomaterials* **2022**, *281*, 121332. [CrossRef]
131. Yue, Y.; Xu, J.; Li, Y.; Cheng, K.; Feng, Q.; Ma, X.; Ma, N.; Zhang, T.; Wang, X.; Zhao, X.; et al. Antigen-bearing outer membrane vesicles as tumour vaccines produced in situ by ingested genetically engineered bacteria. *Nat. Biomed. Eng.* **2022**, *6*, 898–909. [CrossRef]
132. Kang, S.R.; Jo, E.J.; Nguyen, V.H.; Zhang, Y.; Yoon, H.S.; Pyo, A.; Kim, D.Y.; Hong, Y.; Bom, H.S.; Min, J.J. Imaging of tumor colonization by Escherichia coli using (18)F-FDS PET. *Theranostics* **2020**, *10*, 4958–4966. [CrossRef]
133. Pan, P.; Dong, X.; Chen, Y.; Zeng, X.; Zhang, X.-Z. Engineered Bacteria for Enhanced Radiotherapy against Breast Carcinoma. *ACS Nano* **2022**, *16*, 801–812. [CrossRef]
134. Chen, Q.; Wang, J.; Wang, X.; Fan, J.; Liu, X.; Li, B.; Han, Z.; Cheng, S.; Zhang, X. Inhibition of Tumor Progression through the Coupling of Bacterial Respiration with Tumor Metabolism. *Angew. Chem. Int. Ed.* **2020**, *59*, 21562–21570. [CrossRef]
135. Wu, W.; Pu, Y.; Yao, H.; Lin, H.; Shi, J. Microbiotic nanomedicine for tumor-specific chemotherapy-synergized innate/adaptive antitumor immunity. *Nano Today* **2022**, *42*, 101377. [CrossRef]
136. Zheng, D.-W.; Chen, Y.; Li, Z.-H.; Xu, L.; Li, C.-X.; Li, B.; Fan, J.-X.; Cheng, S.-X.; Zhang, X.-Z. Optically-controlled bacterial metabolite for cancer therapy. *Nat. Commun.* **2018**, *9*, 1680. [CrossRef]
137. Ding, S.; Liu, Z.; Huang, C.; Zeng, N.; Jiang, W.; Li, Q. Novel Engineered Bacterium/Black Phosphorus Quantum Dot Hybrid System for Hypoxic Tumor Targeting and Efficient Photodynamic Therapy. *ACS Appl. Mater. Interfaces* **2021**, *13*, 10564–10573. [CrossRef]
138. Liu, Y.; Lu, Y.; Ning, B.; Su, X.; Yang, B.; Dong, H.; Yin, B.; Pang, Z.; Shen, S. Intravenous Delivery of Living *Listeria monocytogenes* Elicits Gasdmermin-Dependent Tumor Pyroptosis and Motivates Anti-Tumor Immune Response. *ACS Nano* **2022**, *16*, 4102–4115. [CrossRef]
139. Zhang, J.; Li, Z.; Liu, L.; Li, L.; Zhang, L.; Wang, Y.; Zhao, J. Self-Assembly Catalase Nanocomplex Conveyed by Bacterial Vesicles for Oxygenated Photodynamic Therapy and Tumor Immunotherapy. *Int. J. Nanomed.* **2022**, *17*, 1971–1985. [CrossRef]

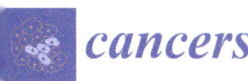

Review

Immunotherapy of Neuroendocrine Neoplasms: Any Role for the Chimeric Antigen Receptor T Cells?

Giuseppe Fanciulli [1,*,†], Roberta Modica [2,†], Anna La Salvia [3], Federica Campolo [4], Tullio Florio [5,6], Nevena Mikovic [7], Alice Plebani [8], Valentina Di Vito [4], Annamaria Colao [2,9] and Antongiulio Faggiano [7,‡] on behalf of NIKE Group

1. Neuroendocrine Tumour Unit, Department of Medicine, Surgery and Pharmacy, University of Sassari—Endocrine Unit, AOU Sassari, 07100 Sassari, Italy
2. Endocrinology, Diabetology and Andrology Unit, Department of Clinical Medicine and Surgery, Federico II University of Naples, 80131 Naples, Italy
3. Division of Medical Oncology 2, IRCCS Regina Elena National Cancer Institute, 00144 Rome, Italy
4. Department of Experimental Medicine, "Sapienza" University of Rome, 00161 Rome, Italy
5. Department of Internal Medicine, University of Genoa, 16132 Genoa, Italy
6. Scientific Institute for Research, Hospitalisation and Healthcare Ospedale Policlinico San Martino, 16132 Genoa, Italy
7. Endocrinology Unit, Department of Clinical and Molecular Medicine, Sant'Andrea Hospital, ENETS Center of Excellence, Sapienza University of Rome, 00189 Rome, Italy
8. Laboratory of Geriatric and Oncologic Neuroendocrinology Research, Istituto Auxologico Italiano IRCCS, Cusano Milanino, 20095 Milan, Italy
9. UNESCO Chair, Education for Health and Sustainable Development, Federico II University, 80131 Naples, Italy
* Correspondence: gfanciu@uniss.it
† These authors contributed equally to this work.
‡ Membership of NIKE Group is provided in the Acknowledgments Section.

Simple Summary: Neuroendocrine neoplasms (NENs) comprise a heterogeneous group of tumors arising in different organs whose clinical course is variable according to histological differentiation and metastatic spread. Therapeutic options have recently expanded, but there is a need for new effective therapies, especially in less differentiated forms. Chimeric antigen receptor T cells (CAR-T) have shown efficacy in several cancers, mainly hematological, but data on NENs are scattered. We aimed to analyze the available preclinical and clinical data about CAR-T in NENs, to highlight their potential role in clinical practice. A significant therapeutic effect of CAR-T cells in NENs emerges from preclinical studies. Results from clinical trials are expected in order to define their effective role in these cancers.

Abstract: Neuroendocrine neoplasms (NENs) are a heterogeneous group of tumors with variable clinical presentation and prognosis. Surgery, when feasible, is the most effective and often curative treatment. However, NENs are frequently locally advanced or already metastatic at diagnosis. Consequently, additional local or systemic therapeutic approaches are required. Immunotherapy, based on chimeric antigen receptor T cells (CAR-T), is showing impressive results in several cancer treatments. The aim of this narrative review is to analyze the available data about the use of CAR-T in NENs, including studies in both preclinical and clinical settings. We performed an extensive search for relevant data sources, comprising full-published articles, abstracts from international meetings, and worldwide registered clinical trials. Preclinical studies performed on both cell lines and animal models indicate a significant therapeutic effect of CAR-T cells in NENs. Ongoing and future clinical trials will clarify the possible role of these drugs in patients with highly aggressive NENs.

Keywords: chimeric antigen receptor-T cells; neuroendocrine neoplasm; neuroendocrine tumor; neuroendocrine carcinoma; carcinoid tumor; somatostatin receptors

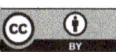

1. Introduction

Neuroendocrine neoplasms (NENs) include a heterogeneous group of tumors with variable clinical presentation and prognosis, mainly arising in the gastroenteropancreatic and pulmonary tract, with steadily increasing incidence, irrespective of site and stage [1,2]. Even though NENs usually show an indolent behavior, they are often locally advanced or already metastatic at diagnosis [1,2]. Their management is therefore challenging, and, even though the landscape of therapy has considerably expanded in the last decades [3,4], additional loco-regional or systemic approaches are required [5]. The available treatment options include somatostatin analogues (SSAs), such as octreotide and lanreotide, targeted therapies (everolimus and sunitinib), liver-directed therapies, external beam radiotherapy, peptide receptor radionuclide therapy, and chemotherapies, in variable sequences [6,7]. Prognosis is largely influenced by several factors, including patient age, tumor grade, stage, and localization [2]. Although survival rates have been improving over time, tailored therapies are needed, especially for patients with rapidly progressing diseases. The role of immunotherapy in NENs is gaining interest [8,9], and encouraging clinical results have been reported in small cell lung cancer (SCLC) [10], Merkel cell carcinoma [11], pheochromocytoma/paraganglioma [12], lung carcinoid [13], and medullary thyroid carcinoma (MTC) [14]. T cell immunotherapy using CAR-T cells is showing encouraging results in cancer treatment. CARs are recombinant receptors composed of the single-chain fragment variant (scFv) of an antibody for recognition of specific antigens, an extracellular hinge domain, a transmembrane domain, and an intracellular signal domain (Figure 1) [15]. A CAR-T cell is a T lymphocyte isolated from the patient, genetically engineered to express an antigen-specific receptor, introduced using a plasmid or viral vector, that binds directly to a cell surface antigen expressed on the cell intended to be recognized and eliminated [16]. The T cells used for CAR-T cell engineering are obtained from patient's peripheral blood cells, which are expanded ex vivo and then re-infused back in patients after lymphodepleting chemotherapy. After binding to target antigens, CAR-T cells are activated, proliferate, and exert their antitumor activity, which includes tumor lysis and induction of a secondary immune response against the tumor [17]. CAR-T cells have demonstrated remarkable success in the treatment of hematological tumors, and, to date, the European Medicines Agency (EMA) and US Food and Drug Administration (FDA) have approved six different CAR-T cell immunotherapies for these malignancies (Table 1).

Table 1. Current FDA/EMA approved CAR-T cells.

Brand Name	Generic Name	Target	Indications	FDA Approval (Year)	EMA Approval (Year)
Abecma	idecabtagene vicleucel	B-cell maturation antigen	relapsed/refractory multiple myeloma	2021	2021 (conditional)
Breyanzi	lisocabtagene maraleucel	CD19	relapsed/refractory diffuse large B-cell lymphoma, primary mediastinal large B-cell lymphoma, follicular lymphoma grade 3B, after two or more lines of systemic therapy	2021	2022 (initial orphan drug approval 2017)
Carvykti	ciltacabtagene autoleucel	CD38	Relapsed/refractory multiple myeloma	2022	2022 (orphan)
Kymriah	tisagenlecleucel	CD19	B-cell acute lymphoblastic leukemia, relapsed or refractory diffuse large B-cell lymphoma and follicular lymphoma	2017	2018 (initial orphan drug approval 2016)

Table 1. Cont.

Brand Name	Generic Name	Target	Indications	FDA Approval (Year)	EMA Approval (Year)
Tecartus	brexucabtagene autoleucel	CD19	relapsed/refractory mantle cell lymphoma	2020	2019 (conditional)
Yescarta	axicabtagene ciloleucel	CD19	diffuse large B-cell lymphoma, transformed follicular lymphoma, primary mediastinal B-cell lymphoma	2017	2018 (initial orphan drug approval 2016)

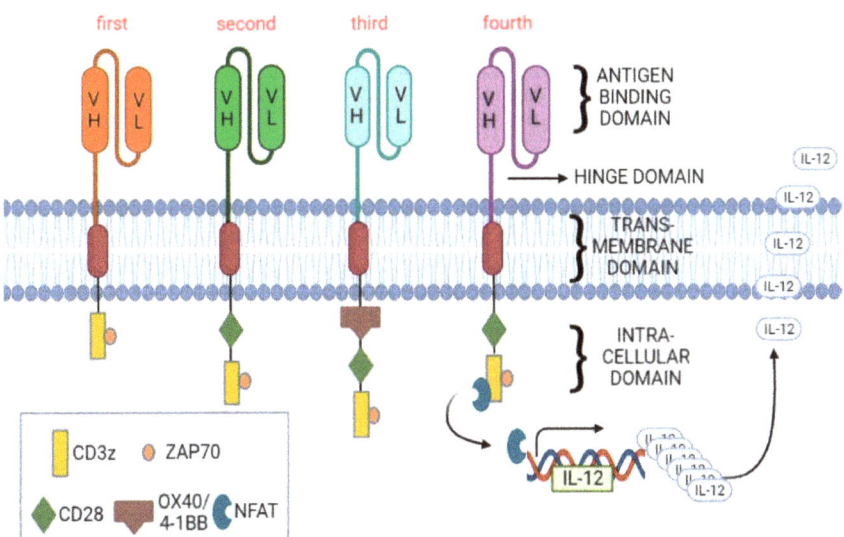

Figure 1. Diagrammatic representation of chimeric antigen receptors (CARs).

CARs are transduced on the T cell surface and interact with the selected antigens on tumor cells to induce T cell-mediated cytotoxicity. CARs are composed of a single-chain variable fragment (antigen-binding domain) composed of the variable domains, VH and VL, of the heavy and light chains of a monoclonal antibody connected via a long flexible linker to form a single-stranded fragment, which is able to recognize specific proteins on tumor cells. This portion is connected to a transmembrane domain via a hinge domain, structurally reproducing sequences of CD8α, CD28, or the Fc region of the immunoglobulins IgG1 or IgG4. The intracellular signaling domains represent the anchor of the molecule to the cell membrane and the connections with the intracellular signaling domain. This latter domain is composed of the element initiator of the T cell response, CD3-ζ, and it has been implemented over the years to enhance the cytotoxic response with the development of four different generation of CARs. While the first generation included the CD3-ζ domain only, in the subsequent ones, a costimulatory signal from CD28 (second generation) or multiple costimulatory elements besides CD28, including also 4-1BB or OX40, were introduced (third generation). Third-generation CAR-T cells showed increased differentiation towards T cell effectors, prolonged T-cell survival, and better clinical outcomes. A further development (fourth generation) of CARs was obtained by adding to the costimulatory signals the presence of transcription factors, such as NFAT, able to activate innate immune response through the production and secretion of IL-12 or other pro-inflammatory cytokines. The improved efficacy of third vs. first generation CDH17-targeting CAR-T cells was also observed in preclinical in vitro and in vivo studies against gastrointestinal NET cells (see text for detailed description).

The success and the continuous advancements achieved with CAR-T cells in hematological malignancies have encouraged their use in solid tumors, and indeed significant responses in patients with solid malignancies have been reported [18]. On this basis, we aimed to collect and discuss the available data about the CAR-T cell treatment in NENs, including both preclinical and clinical settings.

2. Search Strategy

We performed an extensive search for relevant data sources, including full-published articles in international online databases (PubMed, Web of Science, Scopus) and preliminary reports in selected international meeting abstract repositories (American Society of Clinical Oncology, ASCO; European Neuroendocrine Tumor Society, ENETS; European Society for Medical Oncology, ESMO), or short articles published as supplements of international meetings, by using the following terms: chimeric antigen receptor-T cells, CAR-T cells, receptors chimeric antigen, neuroendocrine neoplasm, neuroendocrine tumor, neuroendocrine carcinoma, carcinoid tumor, small cell lung cancer, large cell lung cancer, lung carcinoid, gastroenteropancreatic neuroendocrine tumor, gastroenteropancreatic neuroendocrine neoplasm, pheochromocytoma, paraganglioma, medullary thyroid carcinoma, pituitary tumor, somatostatin receptors. By using the same keywords adopted for reviewing published articles, we conducted an in-depth search on Registered Clinical Trials (RCTs) by using the US National Institutes of Health registry of clinical trials (http://clinicaltrials.gov) and any primary register of the World Health Organization (WHO) International Clinical Trials Registry Platform (ICTRP), http://www.who.int/ictrp/network/en/. The search was last updated on 30 June 2022.

The search revealed data on MTC, SCLC, Neuroendocrine prostate cancer (NEPC), pancreatic NENs (pNENs), and ileal and lung neuroendocrine cells.

2.1. Medullary Thyroid Carcinoma

MTC is a neuroendocrine tumor arising from calcitonin-producing parafollicular C cells of the thyroid gland, accounting for approximately 3–5% of all thyroid malignancies [19,20]. Most cases of MTC are sporadic; however, up to 25% are associated with a hereditary mutation in the REarranged during Transfection (RET) proto-oncogene [20]. Although rare, the incidence of MTC has significantly increased over the last 3 decades from 0.14 to 0.21 per 100,000 individuals, accounting for 13.4% of the total deaths attributable to thyroid cancer [21]. MTC presents with loco-regional metastasis in up to 50% of patients, distant metastasis in 10–15%, and recurrent disease develops in approximately 50% of patients [22]. The clinical course of patients with MTC is variable, ranging from mild to extremely aggressive, with a 5-year survival rate of less than 40% [23]. According to the American Thyroid Association guidelines, total thyroidectomy and dissection of cervical lymph node compartments represent the standard treatment for sporadic or hereditary MTC, but the management of advanced and progressive disease remains challenging [24]. Systemic chemotherapy has shown limited efficacy in metastatic MTC, and SSAs and everolimus have been proposed with promising results [25]. Two oral tyrosine kinase inhibitors (TKI), vandetanib and cabozantinib [26], have been approved for progressive or symptomatic MTC, showing improvement in progression-free survival (PFS) but no increase in overall survival (OV). Notably, these drugs are nonselective, and toxicity due to off-target effects is not negligible [27]. The National Comprehensive Cancer Network (NCCN) guidelines recommend that TKI therapy may not be appropriate for stable or slowly progressive, indolent disease [28]. More recently, the highly selective RET inhibitors selpercatinib (LOXO-292) and pralsetinib (BLU-667), showed efficacy in advanced MTC, but molecular testing for germline or somatic RET mutations is essential [29]. Thus, a strong need for advanced MTC effective therapies still remains. Immunotherapy represents another approach that might be better explored in the treatment of MTC. In this context, the use of chimeric antigen receptor technology could open a promising therapeutic scenario. Based on the expression of GFRα4 by MTC, Bhoj and colleagues [27] hypothesized that GFRα4 might be a putative target antigen for CAR-based T cell immunotherapy for MTC. Using phage display, they constructed P4-10bbz, a CAR that specifically targets GFRα4. This construct was cloned into a lentiviral plasmid vector, and through viral transduction GFRα4 targeting CAR-T cells were engineered. In vitro experiments showed that P4-10bbz CAR specifically responded to GFRα4. P4-10bbz CAR was expressed in a Jurkat cell line expressing an NFAT (nuclear factor of activated T-cells)-driven Green Fluorescent Protein (GFP) reporter construct. Measuring GFP expression by flow cytometry, P4-10bbz expressing Jurkat cells showed activation over basal levels when grown in wells coated with recombinant or containing soluble GFRα4 as well as when co-cultured with TT and MZ-CRC1 cells (two human MTC cell lines, which express the target antigen GFRα4). P4-10bbz CAR was also expressed in primary human T cells. When these P4-10bbz CAR-T cells were co-cultured with TT and MZ-CRC1 cells, they caused lysis of 60–70% of the cells. Increasing levels of expressed interleukin-2 (IL-2) and interferon γ (IFNγ) were detected by ELISA in the conditioned media when P4-10bbz CAR-T cells are co-cultured with GFRα4 expressing cells, further highlighting an activation of CAR-T cells. Bhoj and colleagues also demonstrated the in vivo efficacy of P4-10bbz CAR-T cells against MTC, using an MTC xenograft mouse model. The tumor mass volume, assessed by bioluminescence imaging, significantly decreased after CAR-T cell treatment. At the same time point, peripheral blood human T cells were counted by flow cytometry, showing that antitumor activity was accompanied by robust T cell expansion. In conclusion, P4-10bbz CAR-T cells effectively eradicated antigen-positive tumor cells. The response to GFRα4 is now under study in humans: NCT04877613 is an open-label phase 1 study aimed to assess the safety of different doses of GFRα4 CAR-T cells in adult patients with recurrent/metastatic MTC (progressive after at least one prior TKI-containing regimen, or in patients that were intolerant to or declined such therapy). Fludarabine and cyclophosphamide were used to induce lymphodepletion. The primary outcome is the incidence of treatment-emergent adverse events, as assessed by CTCAE v5.0. Among the secondary outcomes measures, Duration of Response, OS, and PFS are included. The study start date was 19 August 2021, with an estimated enrolment of 18 participants, and it is presently reported as "recruiting". Study completion is expected on 1 June 2039.

2.2. Small Cell Lung Carcinoma

SCLC is an aggressive, poorly differentiated, and high-grade neuroendocrine carcinoma (HG-NEC) that accounts for 15% of all lung carcinomas [30]. The incidence of SCLC has decreased in recent decades, with a prevalence of 1–5 per 10,000 people in the European community. According to the 2021 WHO classification of thoracic tumors [31], SCLC and large cell neuroendocrine carcinomas are the two lung HG-NEC subtypes sub-classified on the basis of cellular size. SCLC is the most frequent neuroendocrine lung cancer, which is commonly diagnosed as an advanced-stage disease. The gold standard treatment strategy for early-stage SCLC patients is the complete resection with mediastinal lymph node dissection [32]. However, unfortunately, the disease often rapidly recurs, with a reported rate exceeding 50%. In the setting of chemonaïve locally advanced/metastatic disease, the standard of care has been radically modified in the last decade [33]. Anti-programmed cell death-1 (anti-PD-1)/anti-programmed cell death ligand-1 (anti-PD-L1) immune checkpoint inhibitors have been incorporated into treatment algorithms for advanced SCLC [34]. This change has been made on the basis of several randomized clinical trials, demonstrating a consistent OS benefit with the early addition of immunotherapy (atezolizumab, IMPOWER 133; durvalumab, CASPIAN; pembrolizumab, Keynote-604) to platinum-based chemotherapy (cisplatin or carboplatin plus etoposide) plus chemotherapy for SCLC patients [35–37]. However, unfortunately, the overall prognosis of SCLC patients remains unfavorable, with a median OS of 10–12 months and one- and two-year OS rates of 56.2% and 21.7%, respectively [38]. Therefore, the search for more personalized, innovative, and effective therapies represents an unmet need in this context. In 2021, Taromi and colleagues analyzed the role of AC133-specific CAR-T cells for SCLC in vitro and in vivo preclinical models [39]. The AC133 epitope of CD133 has been identified as a potential target for CAR-T cells, given that the relapse of SCLC has been demonstrated to be caused by cancer stem cells (CSC) that express glycosylated AC133 form [40]. In this study, the authors carried out an assessment of the AC133-specific CAR-T cells in an orthotopic SCLC murine model as well as in SCLC cell lines. First, the authors yielded the generation of CAR-T cells using the AC133scFv derived from the anti-SC133.1mAB. Then, through cytotoxicity assays, the authors demonstrated that the CAR-T cells specifically lysed AC133-positive SCLC cells. Additionally, they demonstrated that AC133-specific CAR-T cells were able to infiltrate SCLC xenografts in vivo. Interestingly, the rates of infiltration were higher after the administration of chemotherapy to the murine models. Moreover, AC133-specific CAR-T cells determined a reduction of the tumor burden measured by magnetic resonance imaging in mice. The xenografted mice treated with AC133-specific CAR-T cells also presented a longer survival if compared to the ones who did not receive the experimental treatment. In addition, the combination of AC133-specific CAR-T cells and anti-PD-1 therapy was tested, demonstrating a synergic activity. Finally, the authors combined the AC133-specific CAR-T cells with anti-PD-1 and a third compound, a CD73 inhibitor. By using these three agents together, a further improvement in survival rates was achieved in this in vivo model of SCLC, with long-term control of the tumors. A recent study carried out by Reppel et al., evaluated the effect of disialoganglioside GD2 (GD2) CAR-T both in SCLC cells lines as well as in vivo xenograft models of primary and metastatic tumors from SCLC [41]. In fact, a hyperexpression of GD2 has been detected in SCLC cells, and it has been identified as a potentially relevant therapeutic target for immunotherapy in lung neuroendocrine cancers. GD2-CAR-T cells were obtained incorporating interleukin 15 (IL-15) in order to support CAR-T cell expansion and persistence over time. The structure of the GD2-CAR was generated using the scFv derived from the 14G2a mAb. In addition, a cassette was generated, encoding either the optimized GD2. CAR in combination with IL-15 (GD2.CAR.15) using a 2A-sequence peptide [42]. In vitro experiments demonstrated that GD2 CAR-T cells eliminated GD2 positive cells. GD2 CAR-T cells were also shown to target GD2 + SCLC in orthotopic xenograft models. Finally, through the addition of the EZH2 inhibitor tazemetostat, the authors obtained an upregulation of GD2 and an improved susceptibility to the cytotoxic effects of GD2-specific CAR-T cells. Another CAR-T cell construct developed by Crossland et al. in 2018 [43] targeted CD56, also named NCAM-1 (neuronal cell adhesion molecule 1), a glycoprotein highly expressed on the surface of malignancies with a neuronal or neuroendocrine origin, including SCLC, independently of HLA expression. CD56-CART showed significant cytolytic activity against SCLC CD56+ cell lines in vivo and in vivo. This molecule has already been the target of different antibody-based therapeutic strategies and has been proven to show antitumoral activity in previous preclinical models for different malignancies [44]. Through their work, the authors showed that CD56 CAR-T cells lyse at a high rate CD56+ SCLC and other CD56+ malignancy cell lines, with high specificity and achieving up to 64.9% of specific lysis. Moreover, they demonstrated that in xenograft mouse models infused with SCLC cell lines, CD56 expression facilitated tumor-cell killing, since mice bearing CD56+ tumors experienced a considerable reduction in tumor burden after 20 days after tumor-cell injection and an increased OS, suggesting a potential immunotherapeutic approach for CD56+ SCLC. We retrieved a single registered study (NCT03392064) on the use of CAR-T in SCLC. This is a phase 1 study aimed to evaluate the safety and tolerability of AMG 119, a CAR-T targeting delta-like protein 3 (DLL3), in SSLC patients who radiographically documented disease progression or recurrence after at least one platinum-based chemotherapy regimen. DDL3, an inhibitory Notch ligand, has been demonstrated to be highly expressed in SCLC, and it has therefore been explored as a potential therapeutic target for SCLC patients [45,46]. The primary outcomes include the incidence of dose-limiting toxicities, the incidence of treatment-emergent adverse events, and treatment-related adverse events. Among the secondary outcome measures, objective response, DOR, PFS, 1-year OS, and OS have been reported. The study started on 10 September 2018, with an estimated enrolment of 6 participants, and the estimated study completion date is 13 January 2026. Preliminary data on this study (NCT03392064) has been recently presented at the 2022 Annual Meeting of the American Society for Clinical Pharmacology and Therapeutics by Zhou and colleagues [47]. Five SCLC patients were included and all of them received AMG 119 therapy at two different doses (cohort 1: 3×10^5 CAR-T cells/kg, 3 patients; cohort 2: 1×10^6 CAR-T cells/kg, 2 patients). In both cohorts, AMG 119 determined a significant cellular expansion with long-lasting cell persistence (up to 86 days) and resulted in a well-tolerated treatment.

2.3. Neuroendocrine Prostate Carcinoma

NEPC is an aggressive variant of prostate cancer that may arise de novo or as a tumor evolution following hormonal therapies for prostate adenocarcinoma [48]. The incidence of neuroendocrine phenotypes in primary prostate cancers is approximately 1%, whereas, in lethal metastatic castrate-resistant prostate cancers, its percentage reaches 30% [49]. The prognosis of NEPC patients is poor, representing this neoplasia as the most lethal prostate cancer [50], with a median cancer-specific survival of 7 months [51]. According to NCCN guidelines, first-line therapy of NEPC consists of platinum-based combinations with taxanes or etoposide [52]. The combination of carboplatin with cabazitaxel is particularly useful for patients characterized by unfavorable genomics (i.e., loss of function mutations in PTEN, TP53, and RB1 genes); at the same time, the carboplatin–etoposide regimen is preferred for patients with pure small cell carcinomas [49]. Based on clinical and pathological features, second-line or alternative treatments could also be proposed as valuable and effective therapeutic options [53]. Moreover, in this cancer, CAR-T cell-based immunotherapy might be a promising strategy, and efforts have been made to identify NEPC-molecular targets [54,55]. The pioneering work of Lee et al. clearly demonstrated that divergent cancer differentiation states arising during prostate cancer progression are associated with changes in the expression of cell surface proteins [56]. Performing high-throughput multi-omic analyses, generated combined integrated transcriptomic and cell-surface proteomic data, and they identified carcinoembryonic antigen-related cell adhesion molecule 5 (CEACAM5) as an ideal NEPC target antigen. To test its therapeutic potential, they engineered CARs targeting CEACAM5 using lentiviral vectors and tested the efficacy and safety of these constructs in adenocarcinoma and NEPC cell lines and in patient-derived xenografts models. To quantify cytotoxicity, a co-culture assay using two engineered NEPC cell lines (MSKCC EF1—CEACAM5− or NCI-H660—CEACAM5+) transduced with CEACAM5 CAR was employed. Co-culture of CEACAM5 CAR-transduced T cells with NCI-H660 led to >80–90% cell death by 48 h, while co-culture with the MSKCC EF1 caused a minor reduction in cell viability probably due to low levels of CEACAM5 expression in the MSKCC EF1 NEPC cell line. These preliminary encouraging data led Baek and co-workers to develop a monoclonal antibody named 1G9, targeting the membrane-proximal region of CEACAM5 [57]. To assess in vitro CAR-dependent cellular cytotoxicity, anti-CEACAM5 CAR-T cells were co-cultured for 24 h with CEACAM5 + NCI–H660 and Du145-CEACAM5-NEPC cell lines. Anti-CEACAM5 CAR-T displayed high cytotoxicity in CEACAM5 + NEPC cells, and the cell killing was attributed to an increased release of IL-4, GM-CSF, and GrzB/perforin. They further evaluated the in vivo cytotoxicity in mouse xenograft models of Du145 and Du145-CAECAM5 cells. hIgG1-1G9 treatment significantly slowed tumor growth and improved mouse survival compared to control mice. Together, their results show that the newly developed anti-CEACAM5 CAR-T was able to induce in vitro and in vivo suppression of NEPC growth. Even though the results coming from this research suggest a potent antitumor effect of CEACAM5 CAR-T, studies in humans are not presently ongoing.

2.4. Pancreatic Neuroendocrine Neoplasms

In order to overcome the scarcity of available tumor-associated antigens (TAAs) that are a known target for CAR-T cell therapy in NENs, in a recent study, Feng and colleagues [58] developed an unbiased method to identify potential new TAAs that could be targeted by CAR-T cells. The authors used a phage display screening method to identify camelid animal-derived single variable domain antibodies (VHH or nanobodies) that preferentially bind to the surface of gastrointestinal (GI)-NET cells. As a result, they isolated the nanobody VHH1, which selectively binds to BON1 pancreatic neuroendocrine cells. VHH1 showed to specifically target CDH17, a cell surface adhesion protein with known overexpression in GI-NETs [59,60]. The authors demonstrated, by in vitro and in vivo experiments (using autochthonous mouse models), that VHH1-CAR-T cells (CDH17 CAR-Ts) were cytotoxic to both human and mouse tumor cells in a CDH17-dependent manner. The authors compared three CDH17 CAR-Ts approaches in three mice cohorts who were engrafted with NT-3, a pancreatic islet CDH17-expressing NET cell line, developing CDH17 + NT-3 tumors. Subsequently, after 35 days from the xenograft, CAR-T cells were infused, and the treatment was repeated after a further 5 days. The first group of mice was subjected to infusion with CDH17 CAR-Ts containing CD28 and 4-1BB costimulatory domains (VHH1-28BBz), the second group with CDH17 CAR-Ts without CD28 and 4-1BB costimulatory domains (VHH1-BBz) (Figure 1) and the third group with untransduced T Cells (CDH17-UTD). The growth curve of the tumors in each group of the mice was assessed: VHH1-28BBz CDH17 CAR-T cells induced tumor mass reduction until complete eradication of all tumors after 42 days; VHH1-BBZ showed progressive volume reduction but were not able to cause tumor elimination; conversely, CDH17-UTD therapy failed to control tumor growth. The tumors were also dissected and analyzed 10 days after the first infusion. In particular, tumoral tissues treated with VHH1-28BBz CDH17 CAR-Ts revealed the absence of neuroendocrine cells while abundant T-Cells were detected, demonstrating rapid tumor elimination.

Based on the wide and peculiar overexpression of SSTRs on neuroendocrine cancer cells [61], as well as the established efficacy in clinical practice of SSA and radiolabeled SSA in advanced NENs treatment, Mandriani and colleagues [62] developed CAR-T cells to directly target SSTRs. The innovative CAR-T construct included two molecules of the SSA octreotide, which binds with high affinity to SSTR2 and SSTR5, and the costimulatory molecule CD28. The CAR-Ts were cloned in a retroviral vector and subsequently transduced in CD8+ cells. CAR-T cells were then co-incubated with different human NEN cell lines from pNEN, namely BON1, QGP1, and CM, that were previously screened for SSTR 1–5 overexpression. In vitro cytotoxicity was assessed by bioluminescence after 72 h of co-culture, showing tumor cell death in 58% ($\pm$8%), 53% ($\pm$1%), and 42% ($\pm$3%). In the same study, the authors evaluated the anti-SSRT CAR-T therapy effects in mice, subcutaneously engrafted with two different SSTR + NET cell lines (BON1 and CM). When NET xenografts reached 1 mm 3, mice were randomized to receive phosphate-buffered saline (PBS), UTD T cells, or anti-SSTR CAR-T cells by tail vein injection. In vivo tumor growth was assessed by bioluminescence. Mice treated with anti-SSTR CAR-T cells showed a significant reduction in tumor growth as compared with the animals treated with UTD T cells or PBS; the difference in tumor growth reached statistical significance ($p < 0.05$) after 14 and 21 days for CM and BON1 tumors, respectively. No evident adverse effects to the animals were detected up to 4 weeks after treatment

2.5. Ileal and Lung Neuroendocrine Cells

Finally, the study above reported (61) that CAR-T cells were co-incubated with human NEN cell lines from intestinal NET (CNDT2.5) and lung carcinoid (H727). In vitro cytotoxicity showed tumor cell death in 37% ($\pm$7%) and 31% ($\pm$14%), respectively. No in vivo data are reported.

Figure 2 summarizes the CAR-T cells against NEN antigens (GFRα4, CD133, GD2, CD56, CEACAM5, CDH17, and SSTR) developed in the last few years.

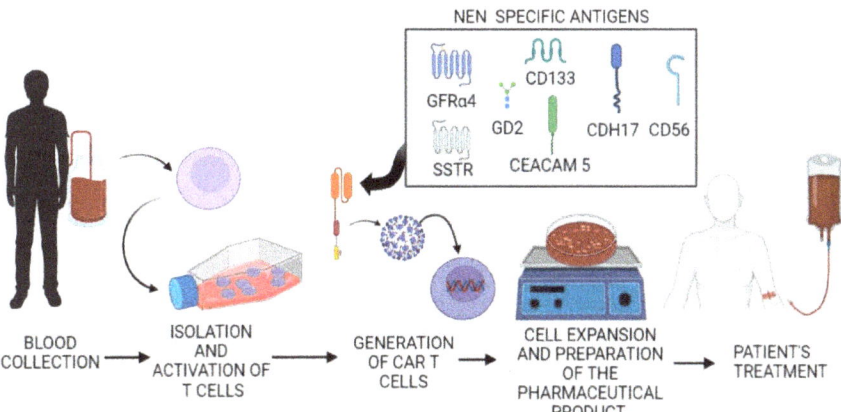

Figure 2. The process of developing CAR-T cells as a therapeutic approach for NEN.

T cells are isolated from a patient's blood (or from a donor), are expanded, and then activated in vitro. The culture is then genetically engineered to express the CAR constructs (in the square are reported target antigens used in the preparations directed against NEN, as discussed in the text). CAR-T cells undergo to further in vitro expansion and are prepared as a pharmacological product that will be administered to the patient.

2.6. Potential Future Applications

Potentially interesting data may also arise from studies not specifically designed for NENs. For example, 3 phase I and Ib clinical trials developed by Katz and colleagues [63–65] evaluated the use of regional administration of anti-CEA CAR-T cell therapy targeting CEA+ liver metastasis from digestive tract adenocarcinomas through intra-hepatic artery infusion, showing clinical efficacy and safety.

Interestingly, CEA is known to be overexpressed in MTC and other different types of NENs [66,67]. Clinically, excellent targeting of MTC has been found with radiolabeled anti-CEA antibodies, and antitumor effects have been achieved with ^{131}I-labelled anti-CEA antibodies, suggesting a high potential of pretargeting for diagnostic and theranostic applications in MTC patients [68–72]. Thus, anti-CEA CAR-T cell therapy might be potentially useful in refractory MTC and/or other CEA+ NENs.

3. Conclusions

In the last few years, preclinical studies performed on NEN cell lines and NEN animal models suggested the potential relevance of CAR-T cells for NEN treatment. Ongoing and future clinical trials will clarify their actual efficacy in these tumors. Given the limitations of safety [73,74] and costs (possibly reaching and/or exceeding $400,000) [75], the assessment of the health outcomes versus alternative therapies will represent a crucial point. The chance of such an individualized approach should then be preferred, rather than as a general approach, only in selected patients with highly aggressive NENs, lacking other therapeutic options, as already occurs in hematological malignancies and other solid tumors.

Author Contributions: G.F., R.M., A.L.S., F.C., T.F., N.M., A.P. and V.D.V. were responsible for the design, the methodology, the draft preparation, the reviewing, and editing. A.C. and A.F. were responsible for the supervision. All authors have read and agreed to the published version of the manuscript.

Funding: This work was supported by the Italian Ministry of Education, University and Research (MIUR): PRIN 2017Z3N3YC.

Acknowledgments: This review is part of the "Neuroendocrine Tumors Innovation Knowledge and Education" project led by Annamaria Colao and Antongiulio Faggiano, which aims at increasing the knowledge on neuroendocrine tumors. The authors would like to acknowledge all the Collaborators of this project: Manuela Albertelli, Barbara Altieri, Luigi Barrea, Nazarena Betella, Severo Campione, Giuseppe Cannavale, Roberta Centello, Alessia Cozzolino, Paola Crivelli, Federica de Cicco, Andrea Dicitore, Sara Di Meglio, Sergio Di Molfetta, Andrea Dotto, Tiziana Feola, Francesco Ferraù, Emanuele Filice, Marco Gallo, Elisa Giannetta, Federica Grillo, Erika Grossrubatcher, Elia Guadagno, Andrea Isidori, Valentina Guarnotta, Elisabetta Lavezzi, Fabio Lo Calzo, Pasqualino Malandrino, Chiara Martini, Andrea Lania, Rossella Mazzilli, Erika Messina, Roberto Minotta, Giovanna Muscogiuri, Soraya Olana, Genoveffa Pizza, Gabriella Pugliese, Giulia Puliani, Alberto Ragni, Manila Rubino, Rosaria Maddalena Ruggeri, Franz Sesti, Maria Grazia Tarsitano, Alessandro Veresani, Giovanni Vitale, Virginia Zamponi, Isabella Zanata, and Maria Chiara Zatelli.

Conflicts of Interest: The authors declare no conflict of interest. The funders had no role in the design of the study; in the collection, analyses, or interpretation of data; in the writing of the manuscript, or in the decision to publish the results.

References

1. Faggiano, A.; Ferolla, P.; Grimaldi, F.; Campana, D.; Manzoni, M.; Davi, M.V.; Bianchi, A.; Valcavi, R.; Papini, E.; Giuffrida, D.; et al. Natural history of gastro-entero-pancreatic and thoracic neuroendocrine tumors. Data from a large prospective and retrospective Italian epidemiological study: The NET management study. *J. Endocrinol. Investig.* **2012**, *35*, 817–823. [CrossRef]
2. Dasari, A.; Shen, C.; Halperin, D.; Zhao, B.; Zhou, S.; Xu, Y.; Shih, T.; Yao, J.C. Trends in the Incidence, Prevalence, and Survival Outcomes in Patients With Neuroendocrine Tumors in the United States. *JAMA Oncol.* **2017**, *3*, 1335–1342. [CrossRef] [PubMed]
3. Faggiano, A.; Lo Calzo, F.; Pizza, G.; Modica, R.; Colao, A. The safety of available treatments options for neuroendocrine tumors. *Expert Opin. Drug Saf.* **2017**, *16*, 1149–1161. [CrossRef]
4. Das, S.; Dasari, A. Novel therapeutics for patients with well-differentiated gastroenteropancreatic neuroendocrine tumors. *Ther. Adv. Med. Oncol.* **2021**, *13*, 17588359211018047. [CrossRef] [PubMed]
5. Pavel, M.; O'Toole, D.; Costa, F.; Capdevila, J.; Gross, D.; Kianmanesh, R.; Krenning, E.; Knigge, U.; Salazar, R.; Pape, U.F.; et al. ENETS Consensus Guidelines Update for the Management of Distant Metastatic Disease of Intestinal, Pancreatic, Bronchial Neuroendocrine Neoplasms (NEN) and NEN of Unknown Primary Site. *Neuroendocrinology* **2016**, *103*, 172–185. [CrossRef]
6. Faggiano, A.; Di Maio, S.; Mocerino, C.; Ottaviano, M.; De Divitiis, C.; Guarnotta, V.; Dolce, P.; Modica, R.; Puliafito, I.; Tozzi, L.; et al. Therapeutic sequences in patients with grade 1–2 neuroendocrine tumors (NET): An observational multicenter study from the ELIOS group. *Endocrine* **2019**, *66*, 417–424. [CrossRef]
7. Lamberti, G.; Faggiano, A.; Brighi, N.; Tafuto, S.; Ibrahim, T.; Brizzi, M.P.; Pusceddu, S.; Albertelli, M.; Massironi, S.; Panzuto, F.; et al. Nonconventional Doses of Somatostatin Analogs in Patients With Progressing Well-Differentiated Neuroendocrine Tumor. *J. Clin. Endocrinol. Metab.* **2020**, *105*, 194–200. [CrossRef]
8. Al-Toubah, T.; Cives, M.; Strosberg, J. Novel immunotherapy strategies for treatment of neuroendocrine neoplasms. *Transl. Gastroenterol. Hepatol.* **2020**, *5*, 54. [CrossRef] [PubMed]
9. Albertelli, M.; Dotto, A.; Nista, F.; Veresani, A.; Patti, L.; Gay, S.; Sciallero, S.; Boschetti, M.; Ferone, D. Present and future of immunotherapy in Neuroendocrine Tumors. *Rev. Endocr. Metab. Disord.* **2021**, *22*, 615–636. [CrossRef]
10. Fazio, N.; Abdel-Rahman, O. Immunotherapy in Neuroendocrine Neoplasms: Where Are We Now? *Curr. Treat. Options Oncol.* **2021**, *22*, 19. [CrossRef]
11. Gallo, M.; Guarnotta, V.; De Cicco, F.; Rubino, M.; Faggiano, A.; Colao, A.; Group, N. Immune checkpoint blockade for Merkel cell carcinoma: Actual findings and unanswered questions. *J. Cancer Res. Clin. Oncol.* **2019**, *145*, 429–443. [CrossRef] [PubMed]
12. Fanciulli, G.; Di Molfetta, S.; Dotto, A.; Florio, T.; Feola, T.; Rubino, M.; de Cicco, F.; Colao, A.; Faggiano, A.; Nike, G. Emerging Therapies in Pheochromocytoma and Paraganglioma: Immune Checkpoint Inhibitors in the Starting Blocks. *J. Clin. Med.* **2020**, *10*, 88. [CrossRef] [PubMed]
13. Di Molfetta, S.; Feola, T.; Fanciulli, G.; Florio, T.; Colao, A.; Faggiano, A.; Nike, G. Immune Checkpoint Blockade in Lung Carcinoids with Aggressive Behaviour: One More Arrow in Our Quiver? *J. Clin. Med.* **2022**, *11*, 1019. [CrossRef] [PubMed]
14. Di Molfetta, S.; Dotto, A.; Fanciulli, G.; Florio, T.; Feola, T.; Colao, A.; Faggiano, A. Immune Checkpoint Inhibitors: New Weapons Against Medullary Thyroid Cancer? *Front. Endocrinol.* **2021**, *12*, 667784. [CrossRef] [PubMed]
15. Gauthier, J.; Yakoub-Agha, I. Chimeric antigen-receptor T-cell therapy for hematological malignancies and solid tumors: Clinical data to date, current limitations and perspectives. *Curr. Res. Transl. Med.* **2017**, *65*, 93–102. [CrossRef]
16. Sterner, R.C.; Sterner, R.M. CAR-T cell therapy: Current limitations and potential strategies. *Blood Cancer J.* **2021**, *11*, 69. [CrossRef]
17. Sadelain, M.; Brentjens, R.; Riviere, I. The basic principles of chimeric antigen receptor design. *Cancer Discov.* **2013**, *3*, 388–398. [CrossRef]
18. Ma, S.; Li, X.; Wang, X.; Cheng, L.; Li, Z.; Zhang, C.; Ye, Z.; Qian, Q. Current Progress in CAR-T Cell Therapy for Solid Tumors. *Int. J. Biol. Sci.* **2019**, *15*, 2548–2560. [CrossRef]

19. Tuttle, R.M.; Ball, D.W.; Byrd, D.; Daniels, G.H.; Dilawari, R.A.; Doherty, G.M.; Duh, Q.Y.; Ehya, H.; Farrar, W.B.; Haddad, R.I.; et al. Medullary carcinoma. *J. Natl. Compr. Cancer Netw.* 2010, *8*, 512–530. [CrossRef]
20. Viola, D.; Elisei, R. Management of Medullary Thyroid Cancer. *Endocrinol. Metab. Clin. N. Am.* 2019, *48*, 285–301. [CrossRef]
21. Randle, R.W.; Balentine, C.J.; Leverson, G.E.; Havlena, J.A.; Sippel, R.S.; Schneider, D.F.; Pitt, S.C. Trends in the presentation, treatment, and survival of patients with medullary thyroid cancer over the past 30 years. *Surgery* 2017, *161*, 137–146. [CrossRef] [PubMed]
22. Sippel, R.S.; Kunnimalaiyaan, M.; Chen, H. Current management of medullary thyroid cancer. *Oncologist* 2008, *13*, 539–547. [CrossRef] [PubMed]
23. Roy, M.; Chen, H.; Sippel, R.S. Current understanding and management of medullary thyroid cancer. *Oncologist* 2013, *18*, 1093–1100. [CrossRef]
24. Wells, S.A., Jr.; Asa, S.L.; Dralle, H.; Elisei, R.; Evans, D.B.; Gagel, R.F.; Lee, N.; Machens, A.; Moley, J.F.; Pacini, F.; et al. Revised American Thyroid Association guidelines for the management of medullary thyroid carcinoma. *Thyroid* 2015, *25*, 567–610. [CrossRef]
25. Faggiano, A.; Modica, R.; Severino, R.; Camera, L.; Fonti, R.; Del Prete, M.; Chiofalo, M.G.; Aria, M.; Ferolla, P.; Vitale, G.; et al. The antiproliferative effect of pasireotide LAR alone and in combination with everolimus in patients with medullary thyroid cancer: A single-center, open-label, phase II, proof-of-concept study. *Endocrine* 2018, *62*, 46–56. [CrossRef] [PubMed]
26. Grillo, F.; Florio, T.; Ferrau, F.; Kara, E.; Fanciulli, G.; Faggiano, A.; Colao, A.; Group, N. Emerging multitarget tyrosine kinase inhibitors in the treatment of neuroendocrine neoplasms. *Endocr. Relat. Cancer* 2018, *25*, R453–R466. [CrossRef] [PubMed]
27. Okafor, C.; Hogan, J.; Raygada, M.; Thomas, B.J.; Akshintala, S.; Glod, J.W.; Del Rivero, J. Update on Targeted Therapy in Medullary Thyroid Cancer. *Front. Endocrinol.* 2021, *12*, 708949. [CrossRef] [PubMed]
28. Haddad, R.I.; Bischoff, L.; Ball, D.; Bernet, V.; Blomain, E.; Busaidy, N.L.; Campbell, M.; Dickson, P.; Duh, Q.Y.; Ehya, H.; et al. NCCN clinical practice guidelines in oncology: Thyroid carcinoma., V 2.2022 ed. *J. Natl. Compr. Cancer Netw.* 2022, *20*, 925–951. [CrossRef]
29. Kim, M.; Kim, B.H. Current Guidelines for Management of Medullary Thyroid Carcinoma. *Endocrinol. Metab.* 2021, *36*, 514–524. [CrossRef]
30. Rudin, C.M.; Brambilla, E.; Faivre-Finn, C.; Sage, J. Small-cell lung cancer. *Nat. Rev. Dis. Primers* 2021, *7*, 3. [CrossRef]
31. WHO. *WHO Classification of Tumors 2021: Thoracic Tumors*; WHO: Geneva, Switzerland, 2021.
32. Dingemans, A.C.; Fruh, M.; Ardizzoni, A.; Besse, B.; Faivre-Finn, C.; Hendriks, L.E.; Lantuejoul, S.; Peters, S.; Reguart, N.; Rudin, C.M.; et al. Small-cell lung cancer: ESMO Clinical Practice Guidelines for diagnosis, treatment and follow-up(). *Ann. Oncol.* 2021, *32*, 839–853. [CrossRef] [PubMed]
33. Arriola, E.; Gonzalez-Cao, M.; Domine, M.; De Castro, J.; Cobo, M.; Bernabe, R.; Navarro, A.; Sullivan, I.; Trigo, J.M.; Mosquera, J.; et al. Addition of Immune Checkpoint Inhibitors to Chemotherapy vs Chemotherapy Alone as First-Line Treatment in Extensive-Stage Small-Cell Lung Carcinoma: A Systematic Review and Meta-Analysis. *Oncol. Ther.* 2022, *10*, 167–184. [CrossRef] [PubMed]
34. Ganti, A.K.P.; Loo, B.W.; Bassetti, M.; Blakely, C.; Chiang, A.; D'Amico, T.A.; D'Avella, C.; Dowlati, A.; Downey, R.J.; Edelman, M.; et al. Small Cell Lung Cancer, Version 2.2022, NCCN Clinical Practice Guidelines in Oncology. *J. Natl. Compr. Cancer Netw.* 2021, *19*, 1441–1464. [CrossRef]
35. Horn, L.; Mansfield, A.S.; Szczesna, A.; Havel, L.; Krzakowski, M.; Hochmair, M.J.; Huemer, F.; Losonczy, G.; Johnson, M.L.; Nishio, M.; et al. First-Line Atezolizumab plus Chemotherapy in Extensive-Stage Small-Cell Lung Cancer. *N. Engl. J. Med.* 2018, *379*, 2220–2229. [CrossRef] [PubMed]
36. Paz-Ares, L.; Dvorkin, M.; Chen, Y.; Reinmuth, N.; Hotta, K.; Trukhin, D.; Statsenko, G.; Hochmair, M.J.; Ozguroglu, M.; Ji, J.H.; et al. Durvalumab plus platinum-etoposide versus platinum-etoposide in first-line treatment of extensive-stage small-cell lung cancer (CASPIAN): A randomised, controlled, open-label, phase 3 trial. *Lancet* 2019, *394*, 1929–1939. [CrossRef]
37. Rudin, C.M.; Awad, M.M.; Navarro, A.; Gottfried, M.; Peters, S.; Csoszi, T.; Cheema, P.K.; Rodriguez-Abreu, D.; Wollner, M.; Yang, J.C.; et al. Pembrolizumab or Placebo Plus Etoposide and Platinum as First-Line Therapy for Extensive-Stage Small-Cell Lung Cancer: Randomized, Double-Blind, Phase III KEYNOTE-604 Study. *J. Clin. Oncol.* 2020, *38*, 2369–2379. [CrossRef]
38. Huang, L.L.; Hu, X.S.; Wang, Y.; Li, J.L.; Wang, H.Y.; Liu, P.; Xu, J.P.; He, X.H.; Hao, X.Z.; Jiang, P.D.; et al. Survival and pretreatment prognostic factors for extensive-stage small cell lung cancer: A comprehensive analysis of 358 patients. *Thorac. Cancer* 2021, *12*, 1943–1951. [CrossRef]
39. Taromi, S.; Firat, E.; Simonis, A.; Braun, L.M.; Apostolova, P.; Elze, M.; Passlick, B.; Schumacher, A.; Lagies, S.; Frey, A.; et al. RETRACTED: Enhanced AC133-specific CAR T cell therapy induces durable remissions in mice with metastatic small cell lung cancer. *Cancer Lett.* 2021, *520*, 385–399. [CrossRef]
40. Sarvi, S.; Mackinnon, A.C.; Avlonitis, N.; Bradley, M.; Rintoul, R.C.; Rassl, D.M.; Wang, W.; Forbes, S.J.; Gregory, C.D.; Sethi, T. CD133+ cancer stem-like cells in small cell lung cancer are highly tumorigenic and chemoresistant but sensitive to a novel neuropeptide antagonist. *Cancer Res.* 2014, *74*, 1554–1565. [CrossRef]
41. Reppel, L.; Tsahouridis, O.; Akulian, J.; Davis, I.J.; Lee, H.; Fuca, G.; Weiss, J.; Dotti, G.; Pecot, C.V.; Savoldo, B. Targeting disialoganglioside GD2 with chimeric antigen receptor-redirected T cells in lung cancer. *J. Immunother. Cancer* 2022, *10*, e003897. [CrossRef]

42. Chen, Y.; Sun, C.; Landoni, E.; Metelitsa, L.; Dotti, G.; Savoldo, B. Eradication of Neuroblastoma by T Cells Redirected with an Optimized GD2-Specific Chimeric Antigen Receptor and Interleukin-15. *Clin. Cancer Res.* **2019**, *25*, 2915–2924. [CrossRef] [PubMed]
43. Crossland, D.L.; Denning, W.L.; Ang, S.; Olivares, S.; Mi, T.; Switzer, K.; Singh, H.; Huls, H.; Gold, K.S.; Glisson, B.S.; et al. Antitumor activity of CD56-chimeric antigen receptor T cells in neuroblastoma and SCLC models. *Oncogene* **2018**, *37*, 3686–3697. [CrossRef] [PubMed]
44. Shah, M.H.; Lorigan, P.; O'Brien, M.E.; Fossella, F.V.; Moore, K.N.; Bhatia, S.; Kirby, M.; Woll, P.J. Phase I study of IMGN901, a CD56-targeting antibody-drug conjugate, in patients with CD56-positive solid tumors. *Investig. New Drugs* **2016**, *34*, 290–299. [CrossRef] [PubMed]
45. Leonetti, A.; Facchinetti, F.; Minari, R.; Cortellini, A.; Rolfo, C.D.; Giovannetti, E.; Tiseo, M. Notch pathway in small-cell lung cancer: From preclinical evidence to therapeutic challenges. *Cell Oncol.* **2019**, *42*, 261–273. [CrossRef]
46. Owen, D.H.; Giffin, M.J.; Bailis, J.M.; Smit, M.D.; Carbone, D.P.; He, K. DLL3: An emerging target in small cell lung cancer. *J. Hematol. Oncol.* **2019**, *12*, 61. [CrossRef]
47. Zhou, D.; Byers, L.; Sable, B.; Smit, M.; Sadraei, N.H.; Dutta, S.; Upreti, V. Clinical pharmacology characterization of AMG 119, a chimeric antigen receptor T (CAR-T) cell therapy targeting Delta-Like Ligand 3 (DLL3), in patients with relapsed patients with relapsed/refractory Small Cell Lung Cancer. In *Clinical Pharmacology & Therapeutics*; Wiley: New York, NY, USA, 2022; Volume 111.
48. Conteduca, V.; Oromendia, C.; Eng, K.W.; Bareja, R.; Sigouros, M.; Molina, A.; Faltas, B.M.; Sboner, A.; Mosquera, J.M.; Elemento, O.; et al. Clinical features of neuroendocrine prostate cancer. *Eur. J. Cancer* **2019**, *121*, 7–18. [CrossRef]
49. Epstein, J.I.; Amin, M.B.; Beltran, H.; Lotan, T.L.; Mosquera, J.M.; Reuter, V.E.; Robinson, B.D.; Troncoso, P.; Rubin, M.A. Proposed morphologic classification of prostate cancer with neuroendocrine differentiation. *Am. J. Surg. Pathol.* **2014**, *38*, 756–767. [CrossRef]
50. Kranitz, N.; Szepesvary, Z.; Kocsis, K.; Kullmann, T. Neuroendocrine Cancer of the Prostate. *Pathol. Oncol. Res.* **2020**, *26*, 1447–1450. [CrossRef]
51. Alanee, S.; Moore, A.; Nutt, M.; Holland, B.; Dynda, D.; El-Zawahry, A.; McVary, K.T. Contemporary Incidence and Mortality Rates of Neuroendocrine Prostate Cancer. *Anticancer Res.* **2015**, *35*, 4145–4150.
52. Bhagirath, D.; Liston, M.; Akoto, T.; Lui, B.; Bensing, B.A.; Sharma, A.; Saini, S. Novel, non-invasive markers for detecting therapy induced neuroendocrine differentiation in castration-resistant prostate cancer patients. *Sci. Rep.* **2021**, *11*, 8279. [CrossRef]
53. Beltran, H.; Demichelis, F. Therapy considerations in neuroendocrine prostate cancer: What next? *Endocr. Relat. Cancer* **2021**, *28*, T67–T78. [CrossRef] [PubMed]
54. Beltran, H.; Prandi, D.; Mosquera, J.M.; Benelli, M.; Puca, L.; Cyrta, J.; Marotz, C.; Giannopoulou, E.; Chakravarthi, B.V.; Varambally, S.; et al. Divergent clonal evolution of castration-resistant neuroendocrine prostate cancer. *Nat. Med.* **2016**, *22*, 298–305. [CrossRef] [PubMed]
55. Wang, Y.; Wang, Y.; Ci, X.; Choi, S.Y.C.; Crea, F.; Lin, D.; Wang, Y. Molecular events in neuroendocrine prostate cancer development. *Nat. Rev. Urol.* **2021**, *18*, 581–596. [CrossRef]
56. Lee, J.K.; Bangayan, N.J.; Chai, T.; Smith, B.A.; Pariva, T.E.; Yun, S.; Vashisht, A.; Zhang, Q.; Park, J.W.; Corey, E.; et al. Systemic surfaceome profiling identifies target antigens for immune-based therapy in subtypes of advanced prostate cancer. *Proc. Natl. Acad. Sci. USA* **2018**, *115*, E4473–E4482. [CrossRef] [PubMed]
57. Baek, D.S.; Kim, Y.J.; Vergara, S.; Conard, A.; Adams, C.; Calero, G.; Ishima, R.; Mellors, J.W.; Dimitrov, D.S. A highly-specific fully-human antibody and CAR-T cells targeting CD66e/CEACAM5 are cytotoxic for CD66e-expressing cancer cells in vitro and in vivo. *Cancer Lett.* **2022**, *525*, 97–107. [CrossRef] [PubMed]
58. Feng, Z.; He, X.; Zhang, X.; Wu, Y.; Xing, B.; Knowles, A.; Shan, Q.; Miller, S.; Hojnacki, T.; Ma, J.; et al. Potent suppression of neuroendocrine tumors and gastrointestinal cancers by CDH17CAR T cells without toxicity to normal tissues. *Nat. Cancer* **2022**, *3*, 581–594. [CrossRef] [PubMed]
59. Su, M.C.; Yuan, R.H.; Lin, C.Y.; Jeng, Y.M. Cadherin-17 is a useful diagnostic marker for adenocarcinomas of the digestive system. *Mod. Pathol.* **2008**, *21*, 1379–1386. [CrossRef]
60. Snow, A.N.; Mangray, S.; Lu, S.; Clubwala, R.; Li, J.; Resnick, M.B.; Yakirevich, E. Expression of cadherin 17 in well-differentiated neuroendocrine tumours. *Histopathology* **2015**, *66*, 1010–1021. [CrossRef]
61. Barbieri, F.; Albertelli, M.; Grillo, F.; Mohamed, A.; Saveanu, A.; Barlier, A.; Ferone, D.; Florio, T. Neuroendocrine tumors: Insights into innovative therapeutic options and rational development of targeted therapies. *Drug Discov. Today* **2014**, *19*, 458–468. [CrossRef]
62. Mandriani, B.; Pelle, E.; Mannavola, F.; Palazzo, A.; Marsano, R.M.; Ingravallo, G.; Cazzato, G.; Ramello, M.C.; Porta, C.; Strosberg, J.; et al. Development of anti-somatostatin receptors CAR T cells for treatment of neuroendocrine tumors. *J. Immunother. Cancer* **2022**, *10*, e004854. [CrossRef]
63. Katz, S.C.; Burga, R.A.; McCormack, E.; Wang, L.J.; Mooring, W.; Point, G.R.; Khare, P.D.; Thorn, M.; Ma, Q.; Stainken, B.F.; et al. Phase I Hepatic Immunotherapy for Metastases Study of Intra-Arterial Chimeric Antigen Receptor-Modified T-cell Therapy for CEA+ Liver Metastases. *Clin. Cancer Res.* **2015**, *21*, 3149–3159. [CrossRef] [PubMed]

64. Katz, S.C.; Hardaway, J.; Prince, E.; Guha, P.; Cunetta, M.; Moody, A.; Wang, L.J.; Armenio, V.; Espat, N.J.; Junghans, R.P. HITM-SIR: Phase Ib trial of intraarterial chimeric antigen receptor T-cell therapy and selective internal radiation therapy for CEA(+) liver metastases. *Cancer Gene Ther.* **2020**, *27*, 341–355. [CrossRef] [PubMed]
65. Katz, S.C.; Moody, A.E; Guha, P.; Hardaway, J.C.; Prince, E.; LaPorte, J.; Stancu, M.; Slansky, J.E.; Jordan, K.R.; Schulick, R.D.; et al. HITM-SURE: Hepatic immunotherapy for metastases phase Ib anti-CEA CAR-T study utilizing pressure enabled drug delivery. *J. Immunother. Cancer* **2020**, *8*, e001097. [CrossRef]
66. Gold, P.; Freedman, S.O. Specific carcinoembryonic antigens of the human digestive system. *J. Exp. Med.* **1965**, *122*, 467–481. [CrossRef] [PubMed]
67. Ishikawa, N.; Hamada, S. Association of medullary carcinoma of the thyroid with carcinoembryonic antigen. *Br. J. Cancer* **1976**, *34*, 111–115. [CrossRef] [PubMed]
68. Hamada, S.; Hamada, S. Localization of carcinoembryonic antigen in medullary thyroid carcinoma by immunofluorescent techniques. *Br. J. Cancer* **1977**, *36*, 572–576. [CrossRef] [PubMed]
69. Edington, H.D.; Watson, C.G.; Levine, G.; Tauxe, W.N.; Yousem, S.A.; Unger, M.; Kowal, C.D. Radioimmunoimaging of metastatic medullary carcinoma of the thyroid gland using an indium-111-labeled monoclonal antibody to CEA. *Surgery* **1988**, *104*, 1004–1010.
70. De Labriolle-Vaylet, C.; Cattan, P.; Sarfati, E.; Wioland, M.; Billotey, C.; Brocheriou, C.; Rouvier, E.; de Roquancourt, A.; Rostene, W.; Askienazy, S.; et al. Successful surgical removal of occult metastases of medullary thyroid carcinoma recurrences with the help of immunoscintigraphy and radioimmunoguided surgery. *Clin. Cancer Res.* **2000**, *6*, 363–371.
71. Bodet-Milin, C.; Faivre-Chauvet, A.; Carlier, T.; Rauscher, A.; Bourgeois, M.; Cerato, E.; Rohmer, V.; Couturier, O.; Drui, D.; Goldenberg, D.M.; et al. Immuno-PET Using Anticarcinoembryonic Antigen Bispecific Antibody and 68Ga-Labeled Peptide in Metastatic Medullary Thyroid Carcinoma: Clinical Optimization of the Pretargeting Parameters in a First-in-Human Trial. *J. Nucl. Med.* **2016**, *57*, 1505–1511. [CrossRef]
72. Bodet-Milin, C.; Bailly, C.; Touchefeu, Y.; Frampas, E.; Bourgeois, M.; Rauscher, A.; Lacoeuille, F.; Drui, D.; Arlicot, N.; Goldenberg, D.M.; et al. Clinical Results in Medullary Thyroid Carcinoma Suggest High Potential of Pretargeted Immuno-PET for Tumor Imaging and Theranostic Approaches. *Front. Med.* **2019**, *6*, 124. [CrossRef]
73. Zhang, Q.; Ping, J.; Huang, Z.; Zhang, X.; Zhou, J.; Wang, G.; Liu, S.; Ma, J. CAR-T Cell Therapy in Cancer: Tribulations and Road Ahead. *J. Immunol. Res.* **2020**, *2020*, 1924379. [CrossRef] [PubMed]
74. Marofi, F.; Motavalli, R.; Safonov, V.A.; Thangavelu, L.; Yumashev, A.V.; Alexander, M.; Shomali, N.; Chartrand, M.S.; Pathak, Y.; Jarahian, M.; et al. CAR T cells in solid tumors: Challenges and opportunities. *Stem Cell Res. Ther.* **2021**, *12*, 81. [CrossRef] [PubMed]
75. Lin, J.K.; Muffly, L.S.; Spinner, M.A.; Barnes, J.I.; Owens, D.K.; Goldhaber-Fiebert, J.D. Cost Effectiveness of Chimeric Antigen Receptor T-Cell Therapy in Multiply Relapsed or Refractory Adult Large B-Cell Lymphoma. *J. Clin. Oncol.* **2019**, *37*, 2105–2119. [CrossRef] [PubMed]

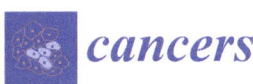

Article

A Phase 2 Trial of Ibrutinib and Nivolumab in Patients with Relapsed or Refractory Classical Hodgkin's Lymphoma

Walter Hanel [1,†], Polina Shindiapina [1,†], David A. Bond [1], Yazeed Sawalha [1], Narendranath Epperla [1], Timothy Voorhees [1], Rina Li Welkie [1], Ying Huang [1], Gregory K. Behbehani [1], Xiaoli Zhang [2], Eric McLaughlin [2], Wing K. Chan [1], Jonathan E. Brammer [1], Samantha Jaglowski [1], John C. Reneau [1], Beth A. Christian [1], Basem M. William [3], Jonathon B. Cohen [4], Robert A. Baiocchi [1], Kami Maddocks [1], Kristie A. Blum [4,*,‡] and Lapo Alinari [1,*,‡]

1. Division of Hematology, Department of Medicine, The Ohio State University, 460 W 10th Ave., Columbus, OH 43210, USA
2. Center for Biostatistics, Department of Biomedical Informatics, The Ohio State University, Columbus, OH 43210, USA
3. Blood and Marrow Transplant and Cell Therapy Program, OhioHealth, 500 Thomas Ln #A3, Columbus, OH 43214, USA
4. Department of Hematology and Medical Oncology, Winship Cancer Institute, Emory University, 1365 Clifton Road NE, B4013, Atlanta, GA 30322, USA
* Correspondence: kristie.blum@emoryhealthcare.org (K.A.B.); lapo.alinari@osumc.edu (L.A.); Tel.: +1-404-778-5933 (K.A.B.); +1-614-293-5594 (L.A.)
† These authors contributed equally to this work.
‡ These authors contributed equally to this work.

Citation: Hanel, W.; Shindiapina, P.; Bond, D.A.; Sawalha, Y.; Epperla, N.; Voorhees, T.; Welkie, R.L.; Huang, Y.; Behbehani, G.K.; Zhang, X.; et al. A Phase 2 Trial of Ibrutinib and Nivolumab in Patients with Relapsed or Refractory Classical Hodgkin's Lymphoma. *Cancers* 2023, 15, 1437. https://doi.org/10.3390/cancers15051437

Academic Editor: David Wong

Received: 28 December 2022
Revised: 15 February 2023
Accepted: 22 February 2023
Published: 24 February 2023

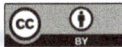

Copyright: © 2023 by the authors. Licensee MDPI, Basel, Switzerland. This article is an open access article distributed under the terms and conditions of the Creative Commons Attribution (CC BY) license (https:// creativecommons.org/licenses/by/ 4.0/).

Simple Summary: Relapsed or refractory classical Hodgkin lymphoma remains a difficult treatment challenge. Despite responses with the checkpoint inhibitors nivolumab and pembrolizumab, patients eventually progress. Combining other treatments with checkpoint inhibitors may provide more frequent and durable responses in this setting. We conducted a phase II study in relapsed or refractory Hodgkin lymphoma combining nivolumab with the Bruton's tyrosine kinase inhibitor ibrutinib. Although we did not find an increase in the response rate of this combination compared to that previously reported, responses tended to be durable even in patients who progressed on nivolumab therapy prior to enrollment. Larger studies combining Bruton's tyrosine kinase inhibitors with checkpoint blockade are warranted, especially in patients who had progressed previously on checkpoint inhibitor therapy.

Abstract: Background: Relapsed or refractory classical Hodgkin lymphoma (cHL) remains a difficult treatment challenge. Although checkpoint inhibitors (CPI) have provided clinical benefit for these patients, responses are generally not durable, and progression eventually occurs. Discovering combination therapies which maximize the immune response of CPI therapy may overcome this limitation. We hypothesized that adding ibrutinib to nivolumab will lead to deeper and more durable responses in cHL by promoting a more favorable immune microenvironment leading to enhanced T-cell-mediated anti-lymphoma responses. Methods: We conducted a single arm, phase II clinical trial testing the efficacy of nivolumab in combination with ibrutinib in patients ≥18 years of age with histologically confirmed cHL who had received at least one prior line of therapy. Prior treatment with CPIs was allowed. Ibrutinib was administered at 560 mg daily until progression in combination with nivolumab 3 mg/kg IV every 3 weeks for up to 16 cycles. The primary objective was complete response rate (CRR) assessed per Lugano criteria. Secondary objectives included overall response rate (ORR), safety, progression free survival (PFS), and duration of response (DoR). Results: A total of 17 patients from two academic centers were enrolled. The median age of all patients was 40 (range 20–84). The median number of prior lines of treatment was five (range 1–8), including 10 patients (58.8%) who had progressed on prior nivolumab therapy. Most treatment related events were mild (<Grade 3) and expected from the individual side effect profiles of ibrutinib and nivolumab. In the intent to treat population (*n* = 17), the ORR and CRR were 51.9% (9/17) and 29.4% (5/17), which

did not meet the prespecified efficacy endpoint of a CRR of 50%. In patients who received prior nivolumab therapy (n = 10), the ORR and CRR were 50.0% (5/10) and 20.0% (2/10), respectively. At a median follow up of 8.9 months, the median PFS was 17.3 months, and the median DOR was 20.2 months. There was no statistically significant difference in median PFS between patients who received previous nivolumab therapy versus patients who were nivolumab naïve (13.2 months vs. 22.0 months, $p = 0.164$). Conclusions: Combined nivolumab and ibrutinib led to a CRR of 29.4% in R/R cHL. Although this study did not meet its primary efficacy endpoint of a CRR of 50%, likely due to enrollment of heavily pretreated patients including over half of who had progressed on prior nivolumab treatment, responses that were achieved with combination ibrutinib and nivolumab therapy tended to be durable even in the case of prior progression on nivolumab therapy. Larger studies investigating the efficacy of dual BTK inhibitor/immune checkpoint blockade, particularly in patients who had previously progressed on checkpoint blockade therapy, are warranted.

Keywords: Hodgkin's lymphoma; nivolumab; ibrutinib

1. Introduction

Although classical Hodgkin's lymphoma (cHL) is a generally curable disease with combination chemotherapy, treatment of patients who relapse after chemotherapy remains a difficult challenge [1,2]. Autologous stem cell transplant (auto-HCT) continues to be the standard of care for patients with chemo-sensitive relapse and who are able to tolerate further treatment [3]. For patients who relapse after auto-HCT or who are unable to tolerate auto-HCT, targeted treatment options including anti-CD30 therapy with brentuximab or checkpoint inhibitors (CPI) with either nivolumab or pembrolizumab have improved patient outcomes [4–8].

Nivolumab is a monoclonal antibody that inhibits programmed death receptor 1 (PD1), a negative regulatory receptor of T-cells, leading to more effective immune-mediated antitumor responses in many tumor types including cHL [5–7]. Patients treated with nivolumab after relapsing after an auto-HCT on the Checkmate-205 study had an overall response rate (ORR) and complete response rate (CRR) of 69% and 16%, respectively, with a median progression free survival (PFS) of 14.7 months while treatment with pembrolizumab on the KEYNOTE-087 study showed an ORR and CRR of 71.9% and 27.6% with a PFS of 13.7 months [5–7]. More recently, data from the KEYNOTE-204 trial randomizing patients either postauto HCT or who were ineligible for auto-HCT to either pembrolizumab or brentuximab showed superiority for pembrolizumab with an ORR, CRR, and median PFS of 65.6%, 25%, and 13.2 months [8]. Despite the progress that has been made with CPI monotherapy in the relapsed setting, patients will eventually progress on therapy with no effective available treatment options after failure of both CPI and anti-CD30 therapy aside from allogeneic-HCT (allo-HCT), which is feasible in only selected patients. Thus, new approaches to maximize responses to CPI therapy may significantly increase the depth and durability of responses and further improve patient outcomes.

Bruton tyrosine kinase inhibitor (BTKi) therapy has revolutionized the treatment of chronic lymphocytic leukemia (CLL) and has also been found to be effective in certain types of B-cell non-Hodgkin's Lymphoma (NHL) [9]. Aside from direct cytotoxic effects, BTKi therapy has been shown to have immune modulatory properties [10]. Patients with CLL treated with ibrutinib after 8 weeks have increased CD8 cells with increased effector T cells to Treg ratios [11]. Longer-term treatment of ibrutinib may reverse T-cell exhaustion by reducing PD-1 expression on chronically activated CD8 T-cells and reconstitution of T cell cytokine production [12,13]. In addition, ibrutinib is known to potentiate Th1-mediated immune responses through inhibition of interleukin-2–inducible kinase (ITK) [14]. However, ibrutinib can also suppress NK-cell-mediated cytotoxicity and suppresses TLR-induced phagocytosis of tumor cells by monocytes [15–17], indicating potentially mixed effects on different immune subtypes. Immunohistochemistry for BTK has shown staining in the immune cells within the cHL microenvironment without staining the Reed Sternberg (RS) cells themselves [18], suggesting that BTKi therapy in cHL may play a role in modulation of the immune microenvironment rather than being directly cytotoxic to RS cells themselves. On the other hand, the src family kinases Lyn, Fyn, and Syk, which are expressed in RS cells and are known to be inhibited as an off-target effect by ibrutinib, lead to potential direct RS cytotoxicity in addition to the immunomodulatory effects discussed above [19].

Initial case reports of two patients with heavily pretreated cHL in the post allo-HCT period treated with ibrutinib showed a near CR in one patient who eventually progressed at 4 months and an ongoing CR in another patient out to 6 months [20]. In a case series of seven heavily pretreated cHL patients including three patients who relapsed after allo-HCT treated with single-agent ibrutinib, four patients responded, three of which had CRs and two of which were still ongoing at 3 and 15 months [21]. A phase II trial (NCT02824029) evaluating ibrutinib monotherapy in R/R cHL is currently ongoing.

Based on the possible T-cell and tumor microenvironment effects of ibrutinib as well as the monotherapy activity of patients with relapsed cHL, we investigated whether combination therapy with ibrutinib and nivolumab would lead to deeper and more durable responses in R/R Hodgkin's lymphoma.

2. Materials and Methods
2.1. Study Design and Patients

This was a single arm phase II trial of nivolumab plus ibrutinib (NCT02940301) conducted across two centers (The James Comprehensive Cancer Center and Emory University Hospital). Patients 18 years of age or older with cHL who received at least one prior treatment were enrolled. Patients were allowed to have received prior CPI, but patients could not have received prior ibrutinib. Prior auto-HCT was not required but permitted, while prior allogeneic-HCT was excluded. Patients were allowed to come off early to undergo either auto-HCT or allo-HCT at the discretion of the treating physician.

2.2. Treatments

Nivolumab (3 mg/kg) was given on day 1 of a 21-day cycle while Ibrutinib (560 mg) was given continuously on days 1–21. Nivolumab was continued until disease progression for a maximum of 16 cycles. Ibrutinib was continued until disease progression. All patients were started at dose level (DL) 0 (nivolumab 3 mg/kg, ibrutinib 560 mg), and dose reductions for toxicity were performed according to the following dose levels: DL-1, nivolumab 2 mg/kg, ibrutinib 420 mg; DL-2, nivolumab 1 mg/kg, ibrutinib 280 mg).

2.3. End Points and Assessments

The primary endpoint of this study was complete response rate (CRR) as assessed with CT or CT-PET per Lugano criteria [22]. Imaging was performed prior to cycles 4, 7, 10, and 16 and every 8 cycles thereafter. Secondary endpoints include overall response rate (ORR), progression free survival (PFS), duration of response (DOR), and toxicity. Patients who withdrew early due to toxicity or disease progression prior to disease response assessment were included in the denominator when calculating the CRR and ORR as part of the intent to treat population. Patients coming off trial early to undergo an HCT were censored at the time of transplant. The data cutoff for this study was 5/1/2022.

2.4. Immune Phenotyping by CyTOF

Blood was collected from the study subjects on Cycle 1 Day 1 prior to administration of the first dose of treatment, and on Cycle 4 Day 1. Whole blood was fixed using proteomic stabilization buffer (Smart Tube PROT-1). Fixed blood was stored at −80 °C. Prior to staining, fixed blood was defrosted. Red blood cells were lysed in water. PBMCs were recovered and washed in phosphate buffer saline, followed by cell staining buffer (CSB; Fluidigm 201068). Two million fixed PBMCs were used per staining reaction. Surface and intracellular antigen staining was performed using standard techniques. Briefly, Fc-blocked cells were resuspended in 50 µL of cell staining buffer. An amount of 50 µL of the surface marker antibody cocktail was added to each tube (final volume 100 µL). Samples were shaken for 50 min at room temperature. After surface staining, cells were washed with CSB, fixed in 1.5% paraformaldehyde, and permeabilized with $-20\ °C$ methanol for 15 min. Subsequently, cells were washed in PBS and CSB and stained with intracellular antibodies at room temperature with shaking, in a final volume of 100 µL. Following additional wash steps, cells were fixed in PBS containing 1.5% paraformaldehyde and a 1:5000 dilution of the iridium intercalator pentamethylcyclopentadienyl-Ir(III)-dipyridophenazine (Fluidigm, San Francisco, CA, USA) for 12–26 h. Excess intercalator was washed away prior to data collection. Data was collected using a Helios™ mass cytometer (Fluidigm) at a rate of 200–400 events per second. Events in the amounts of 600,000–1,000,000 per sample were collected. Data visualization and data analysis were performed on the cloud-based platform Cytobank (Cytobank, Inc., Brea, CA, USA). Cell populations of interest were identified using manual gating. For a more detailed description of cyTOF methods, see the supplemental section.

Antibody clones and vendors, as well as metal conjugates, are listed in Table S7. Metal-labeled antibodies were purchased from Fluidigm. Antibodies purchased from other vendors were conjugated to metals purchased from Fluidigm according to the manufacturer's instructions using the multimetal labeling kit (Fluidigm 201300).

2.5. Statistics

To determine target enrollment, Simon's two-stage design was used to test the null hypothesis that the true CR rate is <20% versus the alternative hypothesis that the true CR rate is >50%. With Type I and II errors constrained to 0.10, ten patients were initially enrolled. Of these patients, 3 patients achieved a CR (30%), warranting expansion of the total enrollment to 17 patients. PFS and DOR data were analyzed by Kaplan–Meier method with significance determined by log rank analysis.

For cyTOF analyses, comparisons were performed using unpaired t-test to detect significant differences in immune cell population prevalence between responders and nonresponders, followed by false discovery rate adjustment. Data analysis was performed using a combination of manual gating using Cytobank software. Principal component analysis was performed to assess clustering of responding patients compared to nonresponding patients. The first and second components were plotted for the various immune expression populations at Cycle 1, and T cell profiles at Cycle 1, Cycle 4, and Cycles 12–16. Individual expression levels were compared by response using Wilcoxon rank-sum tests. Results of two-sample t-tests are also presented given the low power of Wilcoxon tests with small sample sizes. Due to the exploratory nature of these analyses, p-values were not adjusted for multiple comparisons. Statistical analyses were performed using SAS version 9.4 (SAS Institute Inc., Cary, NC, USA).

3. Results

3.1. Patient Baseline Characteristics

A total of 17 patients were enrolled between the dates of 3/2017 and 3/2021 (Table 1). The median age was 40, with 5 patients >60 years of age. Patients received a median of 5 prior therapies (range 1–8), including brentuximab in 76.5% and nivolumab in 58.8%. Eight of ten patients previously treated with nivolumab progressed while receiving nivolumab. Of the remaining 2 patients, one patient had stable disease while on therapy, and the other patient completed 12 cycles of maintenance post auto-HCT. The median time from the last CPI was 4.9 months. Eight patients (47.1%) underwent a prior auto-HCT.

Table 1. Patient Characteristics.

Demographics	N = 17
Age, years, median (range)	40 (20–84)
Sex, no (%)	
Male	8 (47.1%)
Female	9 (52.9%)
Race, no (%)	
White	16 (94.1%)
Black or African American	1 (5.9%)
Diagnosis	
Classical Hodgkin's lymphoma	17 (100%)
Prior lines of treatment, median (range)	5 (1–8)
Prior combination chemotherapy N (%)	15 (88.2%)
ABVD	12 (70.6%)
AVD + BV	1 (5.9%)
AVD	1 (5.9%)
other	1 (5.9%)
Prior autologous stem cell transplant, N (%)	8 (47.1%)
Prior brentuximab, N (%)	13 (76.5%)
Prior nivolumab, N (%)	10 (58.8%)

Abbreviations: ABVD = Adriamycin, bleomycin, vinblastine, dacarbazine; AVD = Adriamycin, vinblastine, Dacarbazine; BV = brentuximab.

3.2. Efficacy

The ORR and CRR of all patients in the intent to treat population ($n = 17$) was 52.9% (95% CI, 31.0–73.8%) and 29.4% (95% CI, 12.9–53.4%), respectively (Table 2). Seven patients achieved their best response on first disease assessment (prior to Cycle 4) while two achieved a deeper response with further therapy: One patient converted from a PR to a CR at the second response assessment while the other patient converted from SD to a PR. With a median follow up of 8.9 months, the median PFS was 17.3 months with a median DOR of 20.2 months (Figure 1).

When stratifying patients according to previous nivolumab, the ORR and CRR for nivolumab naïve patients ($n = 7$) was 57.1% (95% CI, 25.0–84.2%) and 42.8% (95% CI, 15.7–75.0%). In patients treated with prior nivolumab ($n = 10$), the ORR and CRR were 50% (95% CI, 23.7–76.3%) and 20% (95% CI, 0–44.8%). The majority of patients receiving prior CPI therapy had progressed while on therapy ($n = 8$ of 10). Five of these patients with prior progression responded to the combination of nivolumab and ibrutinib, and two of these five achieved a CR. There was no significant difference in the median PFS (22.0 months vs. 13.3 months) between patients with prior nivolumab and patients who were nivolumab naïve ($p = 0.164$) (Figure 2).

Four patients came off trial to receive HCTs ($n = 2$ auto, $n = 2$ allo). Of the patients that underwent auto-HCT, the first patient had stable disease at the time of coming off trial. This patient underwent ICE chemotherapy followed by auto-HCT and converted into CR post-HCT. This patient remained in CR at the time of data cutoff. The second patient achieved a CR on trial and proceeded directly to auto-HCT without chemotherapy and remained in CR at the time of data cutoff. Of the patients that underwent allo-HCT, the first patient had a CR at the time of transplant and had no evidence of acute graft versus host disease (GVHD) in the post-transplant period but did eventually relapse one year after transplant and went on an alternate therapy. Their last nivolumab infusion was 57 days prior to their allo-HCT. The second patient had a partial response at the time of HCT and developed severe acute GVHD involving the skin, liver, and colon in the post-HCT period, which persisted as chronic GVHD. This patient received their allo-HCT 42 days after receiving their last nivolumab infusion. The patient was disease-free post allo-HCT but eventually died due to complications of chronic GVHD. A swimmer's plot summarizing the outcome of each individual patient enrolled is shown in Figure 3.

Table 2. Response and Outcomes.

Best Response	N = 17
Overall response (95% CI)	52.9 (31.0–73.8)
Complete response (95% CI)	29.4 (12.9–53.4)
Partial response (95% CI)	23.5 (9.0–47.7)
Stable disease (95% CI)	23.5 (9.0–47.5)
Progressive disease (95% CI)	5.9 (0–28.9)
Not evaluable due to toxicity (95% CI)	11.7 (2.0–35.6)
Off-treatment Reason	N = 16
Disease progression (percent)	7 (43.8%)
Adverse event (percent)	4 (25.0%)
Auto-HCT transplant (percent)	2 (12.5%)
Allo-HCT transplant (percent)	2 (12.5%)
Patient withdrawal	1 (6.3%)
Progression-free survival	
Number of events	7
Number censored	10
Median	17.3
Median follow-up (months)	8.9
Duration of response	
Number of events	3
Number censored	7
Median	20.2
Median follow-up (months)	6.1

Abbreviations: HCT, hematopoietic stem cell transplant; CI, confidence interval.

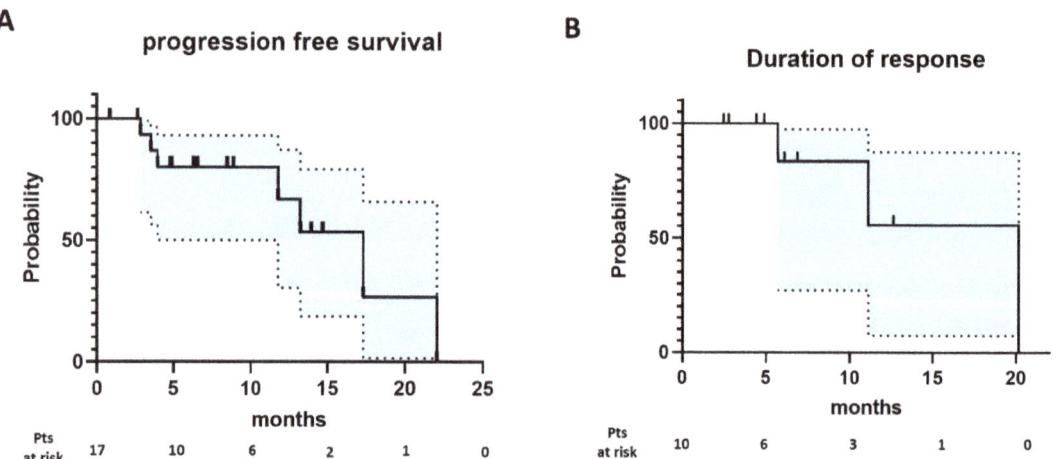

Figure 1. Kaplan–Meier curve for progression-free survival (**A**, $n = 17$) and duration of response (**B**, $n = 10$) are shown.

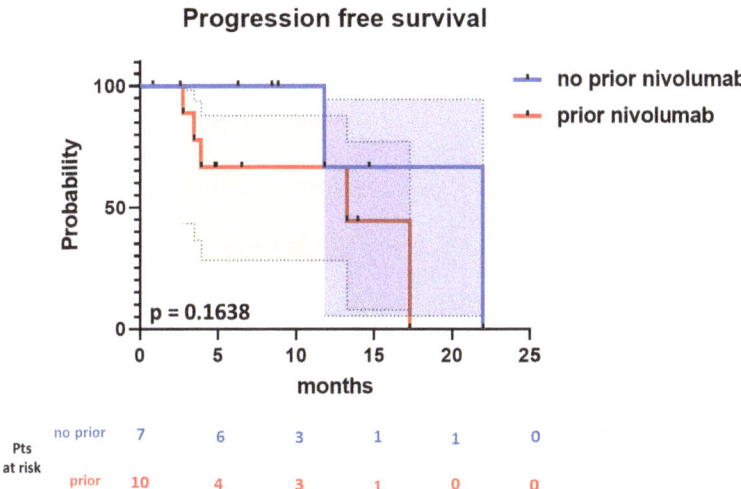

Figure 2. Progression-free survival stratified into nivolumab naïve patients (blue line) and patients with prior nivolumab (red line).

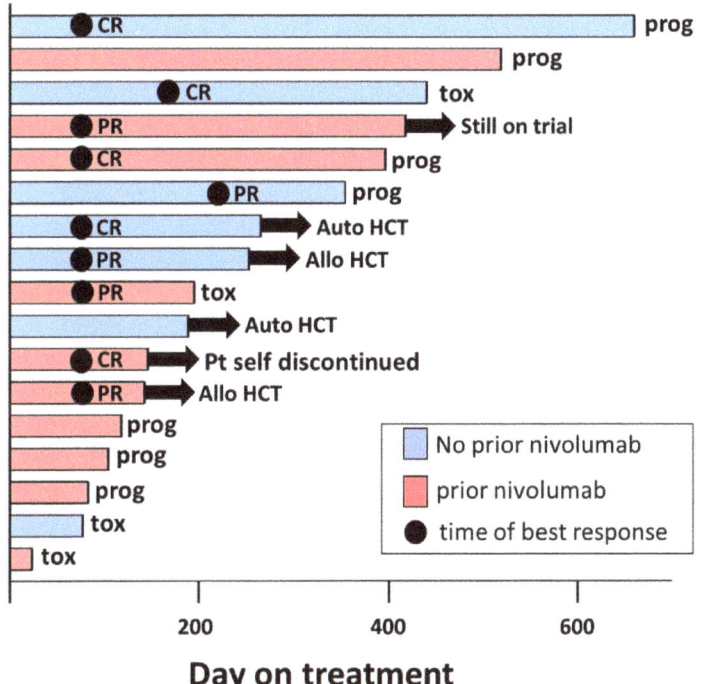

Figure 3. Swimmer's plot of all patients enrolled in trial.

3.3. Safety

Most treatment-related events were mild (<Grade 3) and expected from the individual side effect profiles of ibrutinib and nivolumab (Table 3). Four patients did have to discontinue treatment due to treatment-related side effects. One of these patients had persistent grade 2 LFT elevation despite holding therapy, another patient had a grade 3 rash, and the third patient had grade 3 hematuria. Biopsies were not acquired to further clarify if the

etiology of these side effects was in fact immune related. Due to the overlapping side effect profiles of the individual drugs, specific relation to either ibrutinib or nivolumab could not be definitively concluded in these cases. The last patient came off trial after having sepsis with an associated pericardial effusion. In each of these cases, the side effect did resolve with treatment discontinuation. None of the patients enrolled on trial required treatment with high-dose steroids for side effect resolution.

Table 3. Treatment-related Adverse Events in $\geq$ 10% of pts.

	Any Grade	Grade $\geq$ 3
Anemia	6 (35)	0 (0)
Lymphopenia	6 (35)	2 (12)
Fatigue	5 (29)	0 (0)
Thrombocytopenia	5 (29)	0 (0)
Myalgia	5 (29)	0 (0)
Rash	4 (24)	3 (18)
Hypertension	4 (24)	0 (0)
Blood and lymphatic system disorders	3 (18)	0 (0)
Gastroesophageal reflux	3 (18)	0 (0)
Fever	3 (18)	0 (0)
Dysgeusia	3 (18)	0 (0)
Diarrhea	2 (12)	0 (0)
Dyspepsia	2 (12)	0 (0)
Dysphagia	2 (12)	0 (0)
Nausea	2 (12)	0 (0)
Emesis	2 (12)	0 (0)
Urinary tract infection	2 (12)	1 (6)
Ecchymosis	2 (12)	0 (0)
AST increased	2 (12)	0 (0)
Neutropenia	2 (12)	0 (0)
Weight gain	2 (12)	0 (0)
Leukopenia	2 (12)	0 (0)
Hematuria	2 (12)	1 (6)
Pruritis	2 (12)	0 (0)
Skin and subcutaneous disorders	2 (12)	1 (6)

3.4. Exploratory Immune Phenotyping

Immune phenotyping of T cell populations in fixed whole blood from available samples (nine responders and five nonresponders) was performed with mass cytometry. Twenty CD4+ and 20 CD8+ T cell subsets, including cells expressing cytotoxic molecules (granzyme B and perforin), transcription factors (T-bet, GATA3, and FoxP3), naïve and memory markers (CD45RA, CD45RO, and CD62L), markers of activation (HLA-DR and CD28), degranulation (NKG2D), immunomodulatory/apoptosis inducer (CD95, also known as Fas), exhaustion (LAG3 and Tim-3) and anergy (CD57), and checkpoint molecules (PD-1, CTLA4, PD-L1, and PD-L2) were evaluated.

Due to the interference of nivolumab treatment with effective binding of the PD-1 targeting antibody clone EH12.2H7 that was used in this study, which has been described elsewhere [23], we were not able to investigate the true proportion of circulating PD-1+

T cells in subjects after initiation of nivolumab treatment. Furthermore, many of the subjects were exposed to nivolumab before enrollment on this trial, which, in some cases, affected our ability to detect PD-1 expression. We selected a group of subjects that had not received nivolumab within 200 days of beginning the trial for analysis of PD-1 expression on Cycle 1, Day 1 (Table S1), and PD-1 was detected on the surface of multiple circulating T cell subsets (Table S1). We observed no significant differences in the expression of PD-1 in various T cell populations between responders and nonresponders in this subset of patients (Tables S1–S3, Figure S1). Further investigation of subpopulations of CD4+/PD-1+ and CD8+/PD-1+ T cells also showed no significant differences (Tables S2 and S3, Figure S1). Exploratory analysis across all markers revealed that nonresponders had a higher median percentage of CTLA4 (exhaustion marker) expression in CD4+/PD-1+ T cells although these results were not statistically significant after adjustment for multiple comparisons (Table S4, Figure S2).

Exploratory analysis of the prevalence of various circulating T cell subsets between responders and nonresponders before and after initiation of treatment that included all subjects revealed no differences on Cycle 1, Day 1 and Cycle 4, Day 1, between responders and nonresponders, after adjusting for multiple comparisons (Tables S4–S6). Given the known Th1 expansion induced by ibrutinib, we performed a focused analysis of the baseline and the Cycle 4, Day 1 populations of Th1 (CD4+Tbet+) and Th2 (CD4+GATA3+) subsets between responders and nonresponders (Figure S3). We found a higher baseline percentage of Th1 cells in responders that did slightly increase at Cycle 4, while nonresponders had lower levels of baseline Th1 cells that slightly decreased with treatment (Figure S3, left). Conversely, Th2 cells decreased in responders while increasing in nonresponders (Figure S3, right). However, both the average baseline levels of both T-cell subsets as well as the changes from Cycle 1 to Cycle 4 were not statistically significant between responders and nonresponders.

4. Discussion

In these heavily pretreated patients with a median number of prior lines of treatment of five, including 76.5% who received prior brentuximab, they achieved an ORR and CRR of 52.9% and 29.4%, respectively, which did not meet the prespecified efficacy endpoint of a CRR of 50%. The median PFS of all patients was 17.3 months. Therapy was generally well tolerated and toxicities that were encountered were anticipated based on the individual side effect profiles of ibrutinib and nivolumab. There was no appreciable increase in immune-related adverse events compared to what would be anticipated with nivolumab monotherapy, with no patients requiring treatment with high-dose steroids.

There is significant interest in improving upon the response rate and duration of response of CPI therapy in patients with relapsed cHL who either fail auto-HCT or are unable to tolerate auto-HCT. Several trials have been conducted to date exploring combination therapies with nivolumab to achieve improved responses both in the second line setting and in the multiply relapsed setting, including brentuximab, ICE chemotherapy, ipiliumumab, and brentuximab/ipililumamb [24–27]. In this phase II study, we investigated if ibrutinib, with its known immunomodulatory activity, could improve upon the responses of nivolumab therapy in patients with relapsed cHL. This combination has also been investigated in other B-cell malignancies including relapsed/refractory CLL with or without Richter's transformation and other B-cell NHLs with activity similar to single-agent ibrutinib in the B-cell NHL cohort. However, the combination of ibrutinib and nivolumab resulted in a promising ORR of 65% with two CRs and 11 PRs in the Richter's transformation cohort [28]. All patients in this study were ibrutinib- and CPI-naïve. A more recent phase II study of patients with Richter's transformation enrolled patients with and without prior exposure to a Btk inhibitor with lower responses (64% vs. 23%) between Btk-naïve vs. Btk-exposed patients [29]. Our study was distinct in allowing patients with prior CPI therapy to be enrolled, which allowed us to also study whether the addition of ibrutinib could lead to durable responses in patients who have previously progressed on CPI.

When stratifying patients further by prior CPI use, we found an ORR and CRR for CPI-naïve patients ($n = 7$) of 57.1% and 42.8%, respectively, and 50% and 20% for patients who received previous CPI ($n = 10$). There is published retrospective data demonstrating the efficacy of CPI retreatment in relapsed/refractory cHL patients [30,31]. In the first study, seven patients who initially received either a CR or PR to nivolumab went on to achieve an ORR and CRR of 100% and 57.1%, respectively [27]. In the second study, a series of 23 patients who achieved a CRR to prior nivolumab therapy went on to achieve an ORR and CRR of 67% and 33.3%, respectively [28]. However, as patients in these studies had discontinued anti-PD1 therapy because of durable responses while on therapy, data on responses in the setting of CPI reintroduction in patients who had previously progressed on therapy is lacking. Our results do suggest that combination therapy with nivolumab and ibrutinib may possibly resensitize patients to checkpoint blockade, but given the fact that ibrutinib can have single-agent activity in relapsed and refractory cHL, a randomized study in patients who progressed on prior CPI comparing ibrutinib monotherapy with ibrutinib with CPI would be needed to firmly establish this possibility.

The most abundant cells in the surrounding inflammatory cHL infiltrate consist of CD4+ T-cells with a T helper 2 (Th2) and T regulatory (Treg) phenotype, which provide continuous CD40L and cytokine stimulation for RS cell survival and proliferation [32]. This interaction between Th2, Treg, and RS cells also facilitate immunologic escape of the RS cells by inhibiting cytotoxic T-lymphocytes and disrupting the Th1/Th2 balance. Ibrutinib can inhibit ITK, which is necessary for Th2 signaling and proliferation while Th1 cells do not appear to be affected likely due to the compensatory resting lymphocyte kinase (RLK), which is specific to the Th1 lineage [33]. Thus, blockade of ITK may induce a shift from Th2-mediated immunity to a Th1 response thus triggering a shift to a cytotoxic T-cell and effector-cell-mediated cHL cell killing and preventing immunologic escape in this disease. This effect may be further enhanced by the known Th1 enhancement with PD1 blockade. Our data did show an increase in the Th1 cell population in responders without concomitant increase in Th2 cells after introduction treatment of both ibrutinib and nivolumab, potentially suggesting that this mechanism of ibrutinib-induced immune enhancement may not be present in nonresponders and may in part explain their poor responses. Larger patient numbers would be needed to establish this possibility and its utility as a biomarker of ongoing response. It is important to note that an enhanced Th1 response to PD1 inhibitors has been associated with life-threatening immune-related adverse events at least in case reports. However, we did not encounter these potentially fatal immune-related side effects in this trial [31].

Deep immune profiling of the circulating T cell repertoire in responders and nonresponders (not exposed to nivolumab in the 200 days preceding trial enrollment) showed expression of PD-1 on functionally diverse circulating T cell subsets, including cytotoxic and helper T cells, and naïve and memory, activated, and degranulating T cells, as well as those expressing markers of exhaustion and anergy, and checkpoint molecules. Comparison between responders and nonresponders did not show significant differences in circulating T cell populations. It may be possible that differences in the tumor microenvironment that are not reflected in the circulating T cell repertoire may account for differential responses to therapy, or a higher number of subjects may be needed to discern significant differences.

There are several limitations to this study. As it is a single-arm study, it is not possible to evaluate whether combination treatment with nivolumab and ibrutinib is superior to nivolumab alone. Furthermore, the patient population with respect to their prior treatments, most notably the use of prior nivolumab, was heterogenous, thus limiting our ability to make individual conclusions on a specific subset of patients given the smaller numbers in these subsets (e.g., nivolumab-naïve vs. nivolumab-experienced). Finally, as patients were allowed to proceed to either autologous or allogeneic transplant on this trial, censoring at the time of transplant further limited the determination of durability of responses of the ibrutinib and nivolumab combination.

5. Conclusions

Combination treatment with nivolumab and ibrutinib therapy was generally tolerated and achieved responses in heavily pretreated patients with cHL including in some patients who had received prior CPI therapy. Larger studies of the use of this combination in cHL in both CPI-naïve patients and patients previously treated with CPI are warranted.

Supplementary Materials: The following supporting information can be downloaded at: https://www.mdpi.com/article/10.3390/cancers15051437/s1, Table S1. Comparison of the median percentage of PD-1+ cells in T cell subsets of the subjects that were not exposed to nivolumab for at least 200 days before enrollment on the trial, Cycle 1, Day 1. Table S2. Comparison of the median percentages of cells expressing the designated immune markers among CD8+/PD-1+ T cells in the subjects that were not exposed to nivolumab for at least 200 days before enrollment on the trial, Cycle 1, Day 1. Table S3. Comparison of the median percentages of cells expressing the designated immune markers among CD4+/PD-1+ T cells in the subjects that were not exposed to nivolumab for at least 200 days before enrollment on the trial, Cycle 1, Day 1. Table S4. Comparison of the median percentages of T cells expressing the designated immune markers between all responders and all non-responders, Cycle 1, Day 1. Table S5. Comparison of the median percentages of T cells expressing the designated immune markers between all responders and all non-responders, Cycle 4, Day 1. Table S6. Comparison of the median percentages of T cells expressing the designated immune markers between all responders and all non-responders, Cycle 4, Day 1. Table S7. Antibodies used for mass cytometry. Figure S1. Quantification of the average PD1 positive cells between responders ($n = 7$) and non-responders ($n = 3$) at baseline in all T-cells (left), CD8+ T-cells (middle) and CD4+ T-cells (right). Each dot represents an individual patient. Figure S2. Representative percentage of CD4+/PD-1+ cells on C1D1 (left) and analysis of CTLA-4 expression in CD4+/PD-1+ T cells (right) showed a trend towards higher percentage of CTLA4+ in non-responders. p-value 0.068 (Wilcoxon) and 0.09 (t-test). Center lines show the medians; box limits indicate the 25th and 75th percentiles; whiskers extend 1.5 times the interquartile range from the 25th and 75th percentiles, outliers are represented by dots. $n = 7$ (responders) and 3 (non-responders). Figure S3. Quantification of the average Th1 (left, CD4+Tbet+) and Th2 (CD4+GATA3+) cells at the indicated time points in responders (blue, $n = 9$) and non-responders (red, $n = 4$). Each dot represents an individual patient.

Author Contributions: L.A. and K.A.B. conceived and led the project and analyzed the data. W.H. collected the data, analyzed the data, and wrote the manuscript. P.S. performed experiments and analyzed the data. D.A.B., Y.S., N.E., T.V., J.E.B., S.J., J.C.R., B.A.C., B.M.W., J.B.C., R.A.B., K.M. and K.A.B. enrolled patients in the clinical trial. R.L.W., Y.H., X.Z., and E.M. contributed to the trial design and performed the statistical analysis. G.K.B. and W.K.C. contributed to the analysis and scientific discussion. All authors reviewed, edited, and approved the final version of the manuscript. All authors have read and agreed to the published version of the manuscript.

Funding: American Society of Clinical Oncology Young Investigator Award (L.A., T.V.).

Institutional Review Board Statement: The study was conducted in accordance with the Declaration of Helsinki and was approved by the Institutional Review Board (or Ethics Committee) of Ohio State University (protocol code 2016C0122, date of approval 26 October 2016).

Informed Consent Statement: Informed consent was obtained from all subjects involved in this study.

Data Availability Statement: For all original data, please contact L.A. (lapo.alinari@osumc.edu).

Acknowledgments: We acknowledge the members of the study team at Ohio State University and Emory for their dedication to this study. We thank the clinical teams who provided care for the study patients as well as the participating patients and those who support them.

Conflicts of Interest: The following author has disclosed conflicts of interest: B.W.: Consultancy, Guidepoint Global; Advisory Board, MorphoSys. All other authors declare no relevant conflicts of interest. The funders (Pharmacyclics) reviewed the final draft of the manuscript but had no role in the design of the study; in the collection, analyses, or interpretation of data; in the writing of the manuscript; or in the decision to publish the results.

References

1. Epperla, N.; Hamadani, M. Double-refractory Hodgkin lymphoma: Tackling relapse after brentuximab vedotin and checkpoint inhibitors. *Hematology* **2021**, *2021*, 247–253. [CrossRef]
2. Moskowitz, A.J.; Herrera, A.F.; Beaven, A.W. Relapsed and Refractory Classical Hodgkin Lymphoma: Keeping Pace With Novel Agents and New Options for Salvage Therapy. *Am. Soc. Clin. Oncol. Educ. Book* **2019**, *39*, 477–486. [CrossRef] [PubMed]
3. Broccoli, A.; Zinzani, P.L. The role of transplantation in Hodgkin lymphoma. *Br. J. Haematol.* **2019**, *184*, 93–104. [CrossRef] [PubMed]
4. Chen, R.; Gopal, A.K.; Smith, S.E.; Ansell, S.M.; Rosenblatt, J.D.; Savage, K.J.; Connors, J.M.; Engert, A.; Larsen, E.K.; Huebner, D.; et al. Five-year survival and durability results of brentuximab vedotin in patients with relapsed or refractory Hodgkin lymphoma. *Blood* **2016**, *128*, 1562–1566. [CrossRef] [PubMed]
5. Chen, R.; Zinzani, P.L.; Fanale, M.A.; Armand, P.; Johnson, N.A.; Brice, P.; Radford, J.; Ribrag, V.; Molin, D.; Vassilakopoulos, T.P.; et al. Phase II Study of the Efficacy and Safety of Pembrolizumab for Relapsed/Refractory Classic Hodgkin Lymphoma. *J. Clin. Oncol.* **2017**, *35*, 2125–2132. [CrossRef] [PubMed]
6. Chen, R.; Zinzani, P.L.; Lee, H.J.; Armand, P.; Johnson, N.A.; Brice, P.; Radford, J.; Ribrag, V.; Molin, D.; Vassilakopoulos, T.P.; et al. Pembrolizumab in relapsed or refractory Hodgkin lymphoma: 2-year follow-up of KEYNOTE-087. *Blood* **2019**, *134*, 1144–1153. [CrossRef]
7. Armand, P.; Engert, A.; Younes, A.; Fanale, M.; Santoro, A.; Zinzani, P.L.; Timmerman, J.M.; Collins, G.P.; Ramchandren, R.; Cohen, J.B.; et al. Nivolumab for Relapsed/Refractory Classic Hodgkin Lymphoma after Failure of Autologous Hematopoietic Cell Transplantation: Extended Follow-Up of the Multicohort Single-Arm Phase II CheckMate 205 Trial. *J. Clin. Oncol.* **2018**, *36*, 1428–1439. [CrossRef]
8. Kuruvilla, J.; Ramchandren, R.; Santoro, A.; Paszkiewicz-Kozik, E.; Gasiorowski, R.; Johnson, N.A.; Fogliatto, L.M.; Goncalves, I.; de Oliveira, J.S.R.; Buccheri, V.; et al. Pembrolizumab versus brentuximab vedotin in relapsed or refractory classical Hodgkin lymphoma (KEYNOTE-204): An interim analysis of a multicentre, randomised, open-label, phase 3 study. *Lancet Oncol.* **2021**, *22*, 512–524. [CrossRef]
9. Alinari, L.; Quinion, C.; Blum, K.A. Bruton's tyrosine kinase inhibitors in B-cell non-Hodgkin's lymphomas. *Clin. Pharmacol. Ther.* **2015**, *97*, 469–477. [CrossRef]
10. Zhu, S.; Gokhale, S.; Jung, J.; Spirollari, E.; Tsai, J.; Arceo, J.; Wu, B.W.; Victor, E.; Xie, P. Multifaceted Immunomodulatory Effects of the BTK Inhibitors Ibrutinib and Acalabrutinib on Different Immune Cell Subsets—Beyond B Lymphocytes. *Front. Cell Dev. Biol.* **2021**, *9*, 727531. [CrossRef]
11. Long, M.; Beckwith, K.; Do, P.; Mundy, B.L.; Gordon, A.; Lehman, A.M.; Maddocks, K.J.; Cheney, C.; Jones, J.A.; Flynn, J.M.; et al. Ibrutinib treatment improves T cell number and function in CLL patients. *J. Clin. Investig.* **2017**, *127*, 3052–3064. [CrossRef] [PubMed]
12. Parry, H.M.; Mirajkar, N.; Cutmore, N.; Zuo, J.; Long, H.; Kwok, M.; Oldrieve, C.; Hudson, C.; Stankovic, T.; Paneesha, S.; et al. Long-Term Ibrutinib Therapy Reverses CD8(+) T Cell Exhaustion in B Cell Chronic Lymphocytic Leukaemia. *Front. Immunol.* **2019**, *10*, 2832. [CrossRef] [PubMed]
13. Davis, J.E.; Handunnetti, S.M.; Ludford-Menting, M.; Sharpe, C.; Blombery, P.; Anderson, M.A.; Roberts, A.W.; Seymour, J.F.; Tam, C.S.; Ritchie, D.S.; et al. Immune recovery in patients with mantle cell lymphoma receiving long-term ibrutinib and venetoclax combination therapy. *Blood Adv.* **2020**, *4*, 4849–4859. [CrossRef]
14. Dubovsky, J.A.; Beckwith, K.A.; Natarajan, G.; Woyach, J.A.; Jaglowski, S.; Zhong, Y.; Hessler, J.D.; Liu, T.M.; Chang, B.Y.; Larkin, K.M.; et al. Ibrutinib is an irreversible molecular inhibitor of ITK driving a Th1-selective pressure in T lymphocytes. *Blood* **2013**, *122*, 2539–2549. [CrossRef]
15. Hassenruck, F.; Knodgen, E.; Gockeritz, E.; Midda, S.H.; Vondey, V.; Neumann, L.; Herter, S.; Klein, C.; Hallek, M.; Krause, G. Sensitive Detection of the Natural Killer Cell-Mediated Cytotoxicity of Anti-CD20 Antibodies and Its Impairment by B-Cell Receptor Pathway Inhibitors. *BioMed Res. Int.* **2018**, *2018*, 1023490. [CrossRef] [PubMed]
16. Da Roit, F.; Engelberts, P.J.; Taylor, R.P.; Breij, E.C.; Gritti, G.; Rambaldi, A.; Introna, M.; Parren, P.W.; Beurskens, F.J.; Golay, J. Ibrutinib interferes with the cell-mediated anti-tumor activities of therapeutic CD20 antibodies: Implications for combination therapy. *Haematologica* **2015**, *100*, 77–86. [CrossRef]
17. Feng, M.; Chen, J.Y.; Weissman-Tsukamoto, R.; Volkmer, J.P.; Ho, P.Y.; McKenna, K.M.; Cheshier, S.; Zhang, M.; Guo, N.; Gip, P.; et al. Macrophages eat cancer cells using their own calreticulin as a guide: Roles of TLR and Btk. *Proc. Natl. Acad. Sci. USA* **2015**, *112*, 2145–2150. [CrossRef]
18. Fernandez-Vega, I.; Quiros, L.M.; Santos-Juanes, J.; Pane-Foix, M.; Marafioti, T. Bruton's tyrosine kinase (Btk) is a useful marker for Hodgkin and B cell non-Hodgkin lymphoma. *Virchows Arch.* **2015**, *466*, 229–235. [CrossRef]
19. Martin, P.; Salas, C.; Provencio, M.; Abraira, V.; Bellas, C. Heterogeneous expression of Src tyrosine kinases Lyn, Fyn and Syk in classical Hodgkin lymphoma: Prognostic implications. *Leuk. Lymphoma* **2011**, *52*, 2162–2168. [CrossRef]
20. Hamadani, M.; Balasubramanian, S.; Hari, P.N. Ibrutinib in Refractory Classic Hodgkin's Lymphoma. *N. Engl. J. Med.* **2015**, *373*, 1381–1382. [CrossRef]
21. Badar, T.; Astle, J.; Kakar, I.K.; Zellner, K.; Hari, P.N.; Hamadani, M. Clinical activity of ibrutinib in classical Hodgkin lymphoma relapsing after allogeneic stem cell transplantation is independent of tumor BTK expression. *Br. J. Haematol.* **2020**, *190*, e98–e101. [CrossRef] [PubMed]

22. Cheson, B.D.; Fisher, R.I.; Barrington, S.F.; Cavalli, F.; Schwartz, L.H.; Zucca, E.; Lister, T.A.; Alliance, A.L.; Lymphoma, G.; Eastern Cooperative Oncology, G.; et al. Recommendations for initial evaluation, staging, and response assessment of Hodgkin and non-Hodgkin lymphoma: The Lugano classification. *J. Clin. Oncol.* **2014**, *32*, 3059–3068. [CrossRef] [PubMed]
23. Osa, A.; Uenami, T.; Koyama, S.; Fujimoto, K.; Okuzaki, D.; Takimoto, T.; Hirata, H.; Yano, Y.; Yokota, S.; Kinehara, Y.; et al. Clinical implications of monitoring nivolumab immunokinetics in non-small cell lung cancer patients. *JCI Insight* **2018**, *3*, e59125. [CrossRef] [PubMed]
24. Advani, R.H.; Moskowitz, A.J.; Bartlett, N.L.; Vose, J.M.; Ramchandren, R.; Feldman, T.A.; LaCasce, A.S.; Christian, B.A.; Ansell, S.M.; Moskowitz, C.H.; et al. Brentuximab vedotin in combination with nivolumab in relapsed or refractory Hodgkin lymphoma: 3-year study results. *Blood* **2021**, *138*, 427–438. [CrossRef]
25. Herrera, A.F.; Chen, R.W.; Palmer, J.; Tsai, N.-C.; Mei, M.; Popplewell, L.L.; Nademanee, A.P.; Nikolaenko, L.; McBride, K.; Ortega, R.; et al. PET-Adapted Nivolumab or Nivolumab Plus ICE As First Salvage Therapy in Relapsed or Refractory Hodgkin Lymphoma. *Blood* **2019**, *134* (Suppl. S1), 239. [CrossRef]
26. Armand, P.; Lesokhin, A.; Borrello, I.; Timmerman, J.; Gutierrez, M.; Zhu, L.; Popa McKiver, M.; Ansell, S.M. A phase 1b study of dual PD-1 and CTLA-4 or KIR blockade in patients with relapsed/refractory lymphoid malignancies. *Leukemia* **2021**, *35*, 777–786. [CrossRef]
27. Diefenbach, C.S.; Hong, F.; Ambinder, R.F.; Cohen, J.B.; Robertson, M.J.; David, K.A.; Advani, R.H.; Fenske, T.S.; Barta, S.K.; Palmisiano, N.D.; et al. Ipilimumab, nivolumab, and brentuximab vedotin combination therapies in patients with relapsed or refractory Hodgkin lymphoma: Phase 1 results of an open-label, multicentre, phase 1/2 trial. *Lancet Haematol.* **2020**, *7*, e660–e670. [CrossRef]
28. Younes, A.; Brody, J.; Carpio, C.; Lopez-Guillermo, A.; Ben-Yehuda, D.; Ferhanoglu, B.; Nagler, A.; Ozcan, M.; Avivi, I.; Bosch, F.; et al. Safety and activity of ibrutinib in combination with nivolumab in patients with relapsed non-Hodgkin lymphoma or chronic lymphocytic leukaemia: A phase 1/2a study. *Lancet Haematol.* **2019**, *6*, e67–e78. [CrossRef]
29. Jain, N.; Senapati, J.; Thakral, B.; Ferrajoli, A.; Thompson, P.A.; Burger, J.A.; Basu, S.; Kadia, T.M.; Daver, N.G.; Borthakur, G.; et al. A Phase 2 Study of Nivolumab Combined with Ibrutinib in Patients with Diffuse Large B-cell Richter Transformation of CLL. *Blood Adv.* **2022**. [CrossRef]
30. Manson, G.; Brice, P.; Herbaux, C.; Bouabdallah, K.; Antier, C.; Poizeau, F.; Dercle, L.; Houot, R. Efficacy of anti-PD1 re-treatment in patients with Hodgkin lymphoma who relapsed after anti-PD1 discontinuation. *Haematologica* **2020**, *105*, 2664–2666. [CrossRef]
31. Fedorova, L.V.; Lepik, K.V.; Mikhailova, N.B.; Kondakova, E.V.; Zalyalov, Y.R.; Baykov, V.V.; Babenko, E.V.; Kozlov, A.V.; Moiseev, I.S.; Afanasyev, B.V. Nivolumab discontinuation and retreatment in patients with relapsed or refractory Hodgkin lymphoma. *Ann. Hematol.* **2021**, *100*, 691–698. [CrossRef] [PubMed]
32. Schreck, S.; Friebel, D.; Buettner, M.; Distel, L.; Grabenbauer, G.; Young, L.S.; Niedobitek, G. Prognostic impact of tumour-infiltrating Th2 and regulatory T cells in classical Hodgkin lymphoma. *Hematol. Oncol.* **2009**, *27*, 31–39. [CrossRef] [PubMed]
33. Berglof, A.; Hamasy, A.; Meinke, S.; Palma, M.; Krstic, A.; Mansson, R.; Kimby, E.; Osterborg, A.; Smith, C.I. Targets for Ibrutinib Beyond B Cell Malignancies. *Scand. J. Immunol.* **2015**, *82*, 208–217. [CrossRef] [PubMed]

Disclaimer/Publisher's Note: The statements, opinions and data contained in all publications are solely those of the individual author(s) and contributor(s) and not of MDPI and/or the editor(s). MDPI and/or the editor(s) disclaim responsibility for any injury to people or property resulting from any ideas, methods, instructions or products referred to in the content.

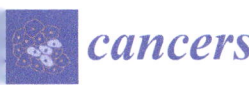

Article

CD8+ Cell Density Gradient across the Tumor Epithelium–Stromal Interface of Non-Muscle Invasive Papillary Urothelial Carcinoma Predicts Recurrence-Free Survival after BCG Immunotherapy

Julius Drachneris [1,2,*], Allan Rasmusson [1,2], Mindaugas Morkunas [2,3], Mantas Fabijonavicius [4], Albertas Cekauskas [3,4], Feliksas Jankevicius [3,4] and Arvydas Laurinavicius [1,2]

[1] Faculty of Medicine, Institute of Biomedical Sciences, Department of Pathology, Forensic Medicine and Pharmacology, Vilnius University, 01513 Vilnius, Lithuania
[2] National Center of Pathology, Affiliate of Vilnius University Hospital Santaros Klinikos, 08406 Vilnius, Lithuania
[3] Institute of Clinical Medicine, Faculty of Medicine, Clinic of Gastroenterology, Nephrourology and Surgery, Vilnius University, 01513 Vilnius, Lithuania
[4] Center of Urology, Vilnius University Hospital Santaros Klinikos, 08410 Vilnius, Lithuania
* Correspondence: julius.drachneris@vpc.lt; Tel.: +370-68502882

Simple Summary: Bacille Calmette–Guerin (BCG) immunotherapy of non-muscle invasive papillary urothelial carcinoma fails in over 30% of cases. In our study, we explore the significance of tumor-infiltrating cytotoxic lymphocytes, assessed by digital analysis and computational methods measuring the cell gradient density profiles across the tumor epithelium–stroma interface, to predict recurrence-free survival in these patients. We analyzed CD8+ cell distribution profiles in the tumor tissue using previously published methods of gradient assessment (center of mass and immunodrop) along with patients' clinical and pathology data. We found that both CD8+ cell gradient indicators were statistically significant prognosticators of recurrence-free survival, and together with clinical and pathological data might be used for improved patient risk stratification. In this context, we propose a prototypic risk assessment system incorporating pathology, patients' history, and CD8+ cell gradient features.

Abstract: Background: Bacille Calmette–Guerin (BCG) immunotherapy is the first-line treatment in patients with high-risk non-muscle invasive papillary urothelial carcinoma (NMIPUC), the most common type of bladder cancer. The therapy outcomes are variable and may depend on the immune response within the tumor microenvironment. In our study, we explored the prognostic value of CD8+ cell density gradient indicators across the tumor epithelium–stroma interface of NMIPUC. Methods: Clinical and pathologic data were retrospectively collected from 157 NMIPUC patients treated with BCG immunotherapy after transurethral resection. Whole-slide digital image analysis of CD8 immunohistochemistry slides was used for tissue segmentation, CD8+ cell quantification, and the assessment of CD8+ cell densities within the epithelium–stroma interface. Subsequently, the gradient indicators (center of mass and immunodrop) were computed to represent the density gradient across the interface. Results: By univariable analysis of the clinicopathologic factors, including the history of previous NMIPUC, poor tumor differentiation, and pT1 stage, were associated with shorter RFS ($p < 0.05$). In CD8+ analyses, only the gradient indicators but not the absolute CD8+ densities were predictive for RFS ($p < 0.05$). The best-performing cross-validated model included previous episodes of NMIPUC (HR = 4.4492, $p = 0.0063$), poor differentiation (HR = 2.3672, $p = 0.0457$), and immunodrop (HR = 5.5072, $p = 0.0455$). Conclusions: We found that gradient indicators of CD8+ cell densities across the tumor epithelium–stroma interface, along with routine clinical and pathology data, improve the prediction of RFS in NMIPUC.

Keywords: computational pathology; digital pathology; artificial intelligence; tumor-infiltrating lymphocytes; anti-tumor immune response; tumor microenvironment; predictive model; immunotherapy

Citation: Drachneris, J.; Rasmusson, A.; Morkunas, M.; Fabijonavicius, M.; Cekauskas, A.; Jankevicius, F.; Laurinavicius, A. CD8+ Cell Density Gradient across the Tumor Epithelium–Stromal Interface of Non-Muscle Invasive Papillary Urothelial Carcinoma Predicts Recurrence-Free Survival after BCG Immunotherapy. *Cancers* **2023**, *15*, 1205. https://doi.org/10.3390/cancers15041205

Academic Editor: Christian Bolenz

Received: 21 December 2022
Revised: 2 February 2023
Accepted: 10 February 2023
Published: 14 February 2023

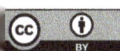

Copyright: © 2023 by the authors. Licensee MDPI, Basel, Switzerland. This article is an open access article distributed under the terms and conditions of the Creative Commons Attribution (CC BY) license (https://creativecommons.org/licenses/by/4.0/).

1. Introduction

Bladder cancer is the tenth most common cancer diagnosed in the world [1], with around three-fourths of the cases being non-muscle-invasive bladder cancer (NMIBC) [2]. Several risk assessment systems have been developed based on traditional tumor properties (grade, stage, size, multifocality, presence of carcinoma in situ, and previous history of recurrence) to support therapy decisions for NMIBC patients [3–6]. For high- and intermediate-risk patients, the main option of adjuvant treatment is intravesical Bacille Calmette–Guérin (BCG) immunotherapy, which has been demonstrated to reduce relapse, progression, and death rates in NMIBC patients [2]. Nevertheless, over 30% of patients experience tumor recurrence after BCG immunotherapy; therefore, better predictive and clinical-decision support tools are in demand [7].

Cancer immunotherapy advances over the last few years are demanding better assessment of the tumor microenvironment [8]. As suggested by Song et al. [9], biological features (high mutational rate, mismatch repair, and DNA damage response deficiencies) of bladder cancer, along with current treatment strategies, make this tumor a good model to understand anti-tumor immune response mechanisms. This led to studies focusing on subsets of cells in the bladder cancer microenvironment, revealing their impact on patient outcomes. However, most of these studies were focused on muscle-invasive bladder cancer (MIBC) [10]. In the subset of NMIBC treated with BCG, evidence for the prognostic significance of specific cell subpopulations has been reported for eosinophils [11], tumor-associated macrophages (TAM) [12–14], dendritic cells [12], tumor-infiltrating lymphocytes (TILs) [13], M1/M2 TAM subsets [15–18], and TIL (T cells subsets, B cells) subpopulations [11,19–22].

TILs were most extensively investigated, revealing potential clinical utility and leading to international initiatives to standardize TIL assessment in a variety of tumors [23,24]. Major progress has been made with novel opportunities brought by digital image analysis (DIA); this has enabled the high-capacity assessment of TILs, also exploring spatial aspects and multiple associations of cell subtypes [25]. As an example, the "Immunoscore" system, proposed by Galon et al. [26] for colorectal cancer, estimates not only the absolute densities of TILs but also their distributions in the tumor compartments. This method was later validated in a large multicentric study [27] and adapted to other tumor types [28]. Recently, Bieri et al. presented a "modified Immunoscore" (mIS) from DIA of tissue microarrays and confirmed their mIS to be an independent prognosticator of clinical outcomes in patients with muscle-invasive bladder cancer [29]. However, in a subsequent study of NMIBC patients, this indicator was only of prognostic significance in the high-risk patient subgroup [22].

Recently, Rasmusson [30] proposed an automated tumor–stroma interface zone (IZ) sampling method, with the subsequent computation of Immunogradient indicators, rather than measuring absolute TIL densities in tumor compartments. This method enables the selective and extensive sampling of the tumor–host interaction area with the quantification of the TIL density gradient across it. These indicators were tested as independent prognostic computational biomarkers in colorectal and breast cancer patients [30–33]. Their performance in the context of immunotherapy has not been investigated.

Non-muscle-invasive papillary urothelial carcinoma (NMIPUC) comprises the vast majority of NMIBC and is defined by papillary structure formation [34]. This specific tumor architecture, along with a lack of conventional invasive growth patterns in the majority of cases, may require a particular approach to assess TILs. Therefore, in this study, we explored the prognostic significance of CD8+ cell density profiles quantified as immunogradient indicators in the delicate architectural context of NMIPUC. We found that a relative decrease in CD8+ cell densities across the narrow range (40 micrometers) of the epithelial–stroma interface was an independent prognostic marker of shorter RFS in the patients after BCG immunotherapy.

2. Materials and Methods

Clinical and pathological data of urinary bladder cancer patients treated with BCG intravesical immunotherapy in Vilnius University Hospital Santaros Klinikos (Vilnius, Lithuania) between 2008 and 2020 (230 in total) were collected. A total of 165 patients with NMIPUC, with a full 6-week BCG induction course and available TUR resection material, were included. After performing tissue sections and IHC (see below), 8 patients with insufficient material were removed from the study. The demographic, clinical, and pathological data of 157 patients are summarized in Table 1. Recurrence-free survival (RFS) time was calculated from the day of the first BCG induction to the date of the first documented tumor recurrence. RFS times were censored after 5 years of follow-up because later recurrences might not represent the true recurrence of a previously diagnosed tumor but the development of a new primary cancer lesion [35].

Table 1. Summary of clinical and pathologic data.

Characteristic	Value (%)
Patients	157 (100%)
Age, years	
Median (range)	69.8 (33–89)
Gender	
Male	128 (81.5%)
Female	29 (18.4%)
RFS time, months	
Median (range)	16.6 (1–174)
Recurrences (BCG failures)	39 (24.8%)
Tumor grade	
G1	5 (3.1%)
G2	67 (42.7%)
G3	85 (54.1%)
pT stage	
Ta	95 (60.5%)
T1	62 (39.5%)
Carcinoma in situ association	8 (5.1%)
Positive reTUR *	58 (36.9%)
Recurrent tumor **	47 (29.9%)
Positive reTUR * or recurrent tumor	90 (57.2%)
Multiple tumors	78 (49.7%)
Tumor size > 30 mm	43 (27.4%)
EORTC risk group	
Intermediate	76 (48.4%)
High	72 (45.9%)
Very High	5 (3.1%)

* NMIPUC identified on repeated transurethral resection; ** not the primary NMIPUC identified on the first transurethral resection.

Archival slides were reviewed by a pathologist (J.D.) who selected the most informative (containing the highest grade and invasive tumor area if present) formalin-fixed paraffin-embedded (FFPE) tissue block. Next, 3 µm tissue sections were stained for CD8 (Dako, clone C8/144B, dilution 1:100, Denmark, using the ultraView Universal DAB Detection kit, Ventana Medical Systems, Oro Valley, AZ, USA) on a Roche Ventana BenchMark ULTRA automated stainer (Ventana Medical Systems, USA).

All CD8 IHC slides were digitized at 20× magnification (0.5 µm per pixel) using an Aperio® AT2 DX scanner (Leica Aperio Technologies, Vista, CA, USA). The HALO® AI (Indica Labs, USA) Densenet v2 classifier was trained using manual annotation provided by the pathologist (J.D.), including the classes 'stroma', 'epithelium', and 'artifacts' (Figure 1A). The latter was added to exclude areas of coagulation that might affect spatial analysis and necrotic areas, hemorrhage, or calcifications. The images were reviewed by a pathologist (J.D.), and epithelial region boundaries shorter than 1000 µm were removed to reduce noise caused by small, incorrectly classified foci. The tissue classification was followed by CD8+ cell segmentation (Figure 1B) and CD8+ cell distribution in the stroma–epithelium interface zone (Figure 1C,D) using HALO® Multiplex IHC and Spatial Analysis modules (Indica Labs, Albuquerque, NM, USA), respectively. The spatial analysis was performed on a 150 μm zone divided into 10 μm width bands in both the epithelial and stromal sides, assigning ranks according to the distance from the epithelium–stroma interface (e.g., rank 1—covering area ranging from the interface (0 distance) to 10 μm; rank 2—from 10 μm to 20 μm; rank 3—from 20 μm to 30 μm, etc.) with a negative or positive rank value assigned to the stromal or to epithelial aspect, respectively (Figure 1E).

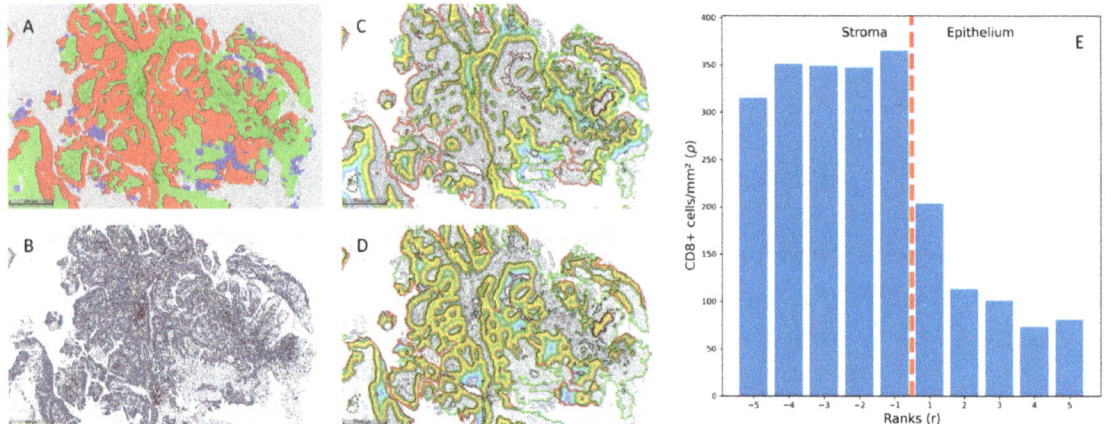

Figure 1. (**A**). Tissue classification results. (**B**). Cell classification results. (**C,D**). Infiltration analysis was performed on stromal and epithelial compartments. The 500 μm measures were added for reference. (**E**). CD8+ cell density distribution by ranks in an example case.

The immunodrop (ID) and center of mass (CM) immunogradient indicators [30] were adapted to the results of the infiltration analysis. ID was calculated as the ratio of CD8+ cell density in a corresponding pair of stromal and epithelial bands (e.g., ID (5) is the ratio between CD8 cell density in the stromal band with rank −5 and the epithelial band with rank 5).

$$\text{ID} = \frac{\rho_{-r}}{\rho_r},$$

where ρ represents CD8+ cell density in the band, and r represents the rank of the band number. CM was calculated as the ratio between the sum of the products of the indices and densities of bands in the IZ and the total sum of CD8+ cell densities in the IZ.

$$\text{CM} = \frac{\sum_{r_i} r_i \times \rho_i}{\sum_{r_i} \rho_i}$$

Additionally, absolute CD8+ cell densities were calculated in the stromal and epithelial compartments and the overall IZ area. To search for the optimal width of the IZ, absolute densities of CD8+ cells and CM gradient indicators were assessed at various IZ widths and ranks, ranging from 20 to 300 μm.

The dataset was randomly split into a training set (117 patients) and a hold-out test set (40 patients) with a similar proportion of patients with tumor recurrence in both sets. The univariable Cox model was used to evaluate the performance of individual features and to select features for multivariable Cox regression. At this point, we had multiple variants of ID, CM, and absolute densities in tumor compartments. The variant with the lowest p-value was selected. For multivariable analysis, we selected factors from univariable analysis with p-value < 0.05, constructing all possible combinations of these variables for modeling. Multivariable Cox regression models using these constellations of variables were then fitted on the training set to select models consisting of independent variables (with p-values of HR for all covariates being <0.05). On these selected models, we performed 5-fold cross-validation using the mean Harrell's C-index on the validation set as a performance indicator. We then selected the best-performing model and tested it on a hold-out test set. The Kaplan–Meier survival estimator was used to investigate the survival of patients stratified according to factors with statistically significant association with recurrence hazard in the univariate Cox analysis, and the log rank test was used for the pairwise comparison of patient survival in groups. For prognosticators with continuous data (ID and CM), we have stratified patients into three equal groups (low, medium, and high). Statistical data analysis was performed using Python libraries (Pandas version 1.3.4, Scikit-learn version 1.0.2 and Lifelines version 0.27.0).

3. Results

3.1. Univariable Cox Regression Analysis

The tumor stage and G3 tumor grade were significantly associated with increased recurrence risk (data summarized in Table 2). Other traditional stratification prognosticators, such as tumor size, concurrent CIS, tumor multifocality and demographic data (age and gender), did not show statistically significant association.

Table 2. Univariable Cox regression results.

Feature	p-Value	HR
Male gender	0.6229	0.7845
Age	0.4051	1.0000
Immunodrop	0.0031	12.2830
Center of mass	0.0082	0.0660
CD8 density epithelial	0.1140	0.9971
CD8 density stromal	0.2718	0.9993
CD8 density overall	0.1659	0.9979
pT1 stage	0.0126	2.6092
G1	0.9959	0.0000
G2	0.0757	0.4773
G3	0.0159	2.7387
Concurrent CIS	0.4793	1.5417
Tumor size > 30 mm	0.5781	0.7686
Multiple tumors	0.4050	1.3858
Positive reTUR *	0.0009	3.6726
Recurrent tumor **	0.3955	1.3945
Positive reTUR * or recurrent tumor	0.0016	5.4702
EORTC Intermediate risk	0.0655	0.4765
EORTC High risk	0.0766	1.9712
EORTC Very high risk	0.2071	2.5514

* NMIPUC identified on repeated transurethral resection; ** not the primary NMIPUC identified on the first transurethral resection.

Both CD8+ cell density gradient indicators (CM and ID) were significantly associated with patient outcomes, while absolute CD8+ cell densities in the stromal, epithelial, and overall IZ compartments failed to show significant association with RFS. The best-performing variation of ID included a ratio of ranks 10–20 μm on stromal and epithelial sides, suggesting that the changes closest to the epithelial–stromal interface are most indicative of patient outcomes. The worse performance of the ID variant using band ranks next to the epithelial–stromal interface (0–10 μm) might be associated with minor inconsistencies in tissue classifier performance. Similarly, the best-performing CM measure was obtained from an IZ covering the 0–20 μm interval from the interface on both epithelial and stromal aspects (ranks −2 to 2).

Of the medical history data, the positive reTUR but not the recurrent tumor was associated with significantly increased recurrence hazard. Interestingly, the combination of these two factors formed an even stronger predictor of BCG failure (the HR of patients having positive reTUR and/or recurrent tumor was 5.4702 in comparison with only having positive reTUR patients HR of 3.6726).

3.2. Multivariable Cox Regression Analysis

A total of 11 multivariable Cox regression models could be obtained from the univariate prognostic features (Table 3). The best-performing model from the 5-fold cross-validation included ID, G3 tumor grade, and positive reTUR or recurrent tumor (Table 4). Other models showed a slightly higher Akaike information criterion (AIC) and lower mean C-index in the validation splits. Some of these models included CM but without the co-occurrence of ID in the same model. The strongest models included the covariates of any medical history parameter with positive anamnesis of a tumor (positive reTUR and/or recurrent tumor), thus showing the high predictive value of this feature.

Table 3. Performance of multivariable Cox regression models (CM—center of mass, ID—immunodrop).

Model Covariates	Mean Validation Set C-Index	AIC
Positive reTUR * or recurrent tumor ** + G3 + ID	0.7837	173.3428
Positive reTUR * or recurrent tumor ** + G3	0.7397	174.6718
Positive reTUR * or recurrent tumor ** + ID	0.7370	174.7917
Positive reTUR * or recurrent tumor ** + pT1 + ID	0.7388	172.5348
Positive reTUR * or recurrent tumor ** + pT1	0.7355	174.4835
Positive reTUR * or recurrent tumor ** + CM	0.7308	174.9942
G3 + ID	0.7028	179.8105
G3 + CM	0.7028	179.8105
Positive reTUR + ID	0.6613	178.3879
pT1 + CM	0.6551	180.2151
pT1 + ID	0.6438	178.4539

* NMIPUC identified on repeated transurethral resection; ** not the primary NMIPUC identified on the first transurethral resection.

Table 4. Best-performing multivariable Cox regression model.

Covariate	p-Value	HR
Positive reTUR * or recurrent tumor **	0.0063	4.4492
G3	0.0457	2.3672
ID	0.0455	5.5072

* NMIPUC identified on repeated transurethral resection; ** not the primary NMIPUC identified on the first transurethral resection.

The best-performing model from the 5-fold cross-validation included ID, G3 tumor grade, and positive reTUR or recurrent tumor (Table 3) (log-likelihood ratio = 22.76, $p < 0.005$). Of note, this model included one anamnestic factor, one histological factor, and one tumor microenvironment factor. The C-index for the test set was 0.7429, slightly lower than the training set C-index of 0.7579, which excludes the possibility of overfitting this model.

3.3. Kaplan–Meier Survival Analysis

Non-parametric survival analyses once again supported our finding from univariable Cox regression analysis, with all six features separating patient groups with statistically significant differences in RFS (Figure 2). The low ID group of patients showed significantly longer RFS, similar to the high CM group, which was expected due to the strong inverse correlation of these indicators. The traditional pathologic factors of tumor stage and grade also separated groups with significantly different RFS. The presence of tumors in reTUR was associated with a significantly shorter RS. However, the combined factor of recurrent tumors and/or the presence of tumors in reTUR extracted a larger group of patients with shorter RFS, resulting in a somewhat better balanced risk stratification.

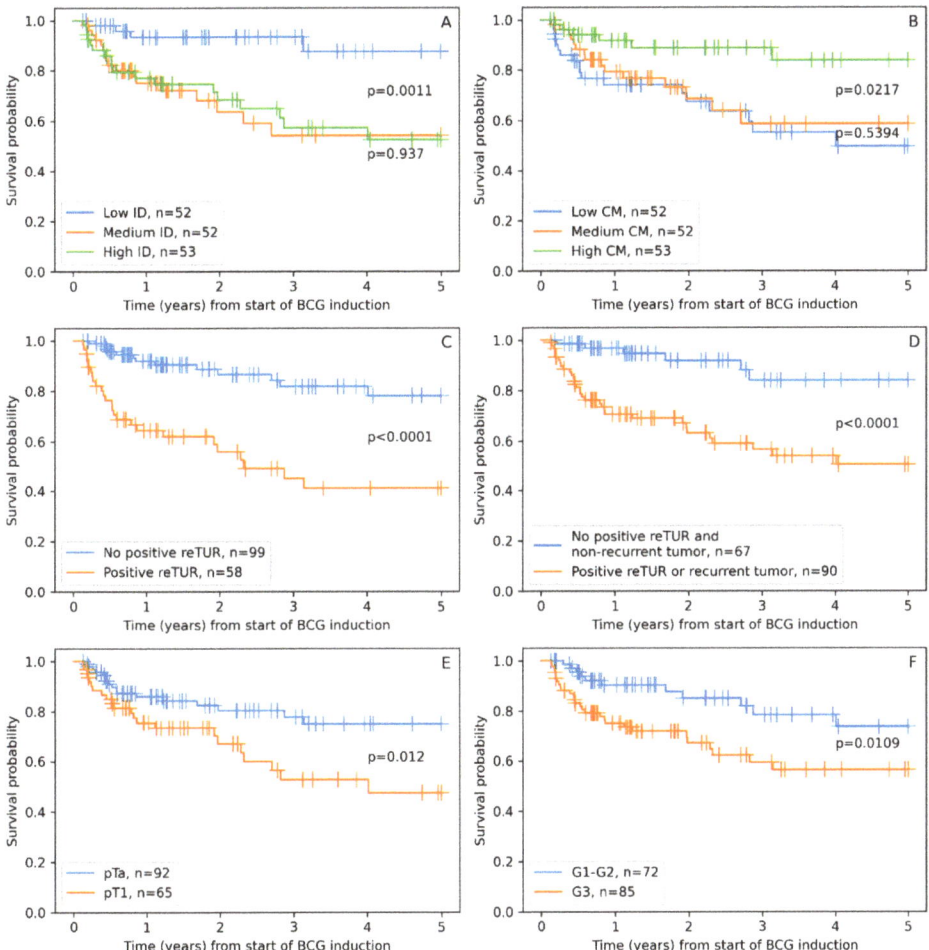

Figure 2. Kaplan–Maier RFS plots stratified according to: (**A**). Immunodrop (ID), (**B**). Center of mass (CM), (**C**). Presence of tumor in reTUR, (**D**). Presence of tumor in repeated transurethral resection (reTUR) or recurrent tumor, (**E**). Tumor stage (pTa vs. pT1), (**F**). Tumor grade (G3 vs. G1–G2).

Additionally, we constructed a combined risk assessment score based on three independent factors included in the best-performing Cox regression model. A score of 1 was added for each G3 tumor grade, positive reTUR or recurrent tumor, and medium or high ID. For the final stratification, patients having 0 or 1 point were assigned to the "low recurrence risk score" group, thus forming a more balanced patient distribution between groups; patients with 2 points were assigned to the "intermediate recurrence risk score" group; and patients with 3 points to the "high recurrence risk score" group. This scoring system enabled statistically significant risk stratification in regard to RFS (Figure 3).

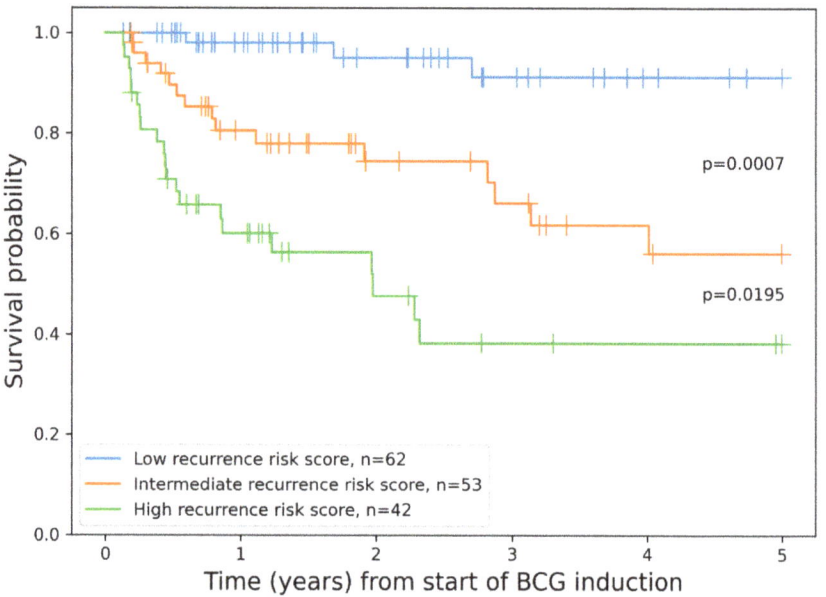

Figure 3. Kaplan–Meier plot of RFS grouped by combined model for patient risk assessment.

4. Discussion

Our study reveals that CD8+ cell density gradient indicators, ID and CM, were significantly associated with the RFS of patients treated with BCG immunotherapy for NMIPUC, highlighting the importance of the spatial distribution of CD8+ cells across the tumor interface. Similar work published recently by Bieri et al. [22,29] explored the prognostic significance of TILs in bladder cancer by introducing the mIS concept for the assessment of TILs in the tumor tissue. In both of their studies, mIS enabled significant risk stratification only in subsets of patients (progression-free survival and cancer-specific survival stratification in MIBC after cystectomy—the AJCC stage IIIa group, RFS stratification in NMIPUC treated with BCG—EORTC high-risk group). In contrast, the CD8+ Immunogradient indicators provided significant stratification in the entire cohort of our patients.

An important advantage of our method is that it generates the CD8+ cell density data from the epithelium–stroma interface with high selectivity and capacity while also maintaining the spatial context of the tumor–host interaction area. In the univariate analyses, best-performing variants of both CM and ID were generated from the IZ within the range of 20 μm into both the stromal and epithelial aspects. DIA performed a precise selection of areas of interest and, paired with the high-throughput nature of the method in WSI, enabled an optimized solution to assess tissue immune response in this tumor with a peculiar papillary microarchitecture. In contrast to other tumor types, where immunogradient indicators and Immunoscore were found to be prognostic, NMIPUC, in most cases, does not have a wide invasive border. Instead, tumor–host interaction takes place in a very thin, elongated, papillary tumor structure, requiring a more delicate approach. Our study shows that this can be achieved with AI-based pixel-level tissue classification with subsequent computational immunohistochemistry assessment.

Another important observation emerging from our study is that CD8+ cell density gradient indicators were significant prognosticators of RFS, while none of the absolute CD8+

cell densities in any tumor tissue compartment showed a significant impact. This further supports the importance of spatial analytics to study tumor microenvironments rather than relying on the quantification of cell densities in tumor tissue compartments. Whereas all patients in our cohort received BCG immunotherapy, our computational models enable the assessment of RFS probability and, with an appropriate study design, can be tested as predictive biomarkers for immunotherapy modalities.

Based on three independent prognostic factors in our best-performing multivariable Cox regression model after cross-validation procedures, we constructed a scoring system which, importantly, combines clinical, pathology, and immune response features. The model enables RFS probability assessment by assigning the patients after BCG immunotherapy into three risk categories (Figure 3). To compare our model to the current routine risk assessment strategy, we simulated the performance of the EORTC risk stratification algorithm (REF) in our patient cohort. The EORTC risk groups provided statistically significant differences only between intermediate and very high-risk groups (p = 0.0448), while other pairwise differences did not reach statistical significance (intermediate vs. high p = 0.1698, high vs. very high p = 0.1073). This "underperformance" of the EORTC scheme might be explained by some shift toward more aggressive tumors in our patients, eligible for BCG immunotherapy. Additionally, the impact of BCG on RFS and/or the limited sample size of our study remains to be considered. Nevertheless, we found that our scoring scheme was best-performing in our patient cohort and remains to be tested for its potential in clinical decision making.

The evidence on the use of early radical cystectomy for high-risk non-muscle-invasive bladder cancer that can be performed upfront or in a delayed setting after BCG failure remains controversial [36]. However, many recent reports have shown that in patients with BCG-unresponsive HGT1 disease, cancer-specific and overall survival were lower after delayed (>2 years) versus early radical cystectomy [37–39]. However, the retrospective series suggested that in patients with T1G3 tumors, there was only a small difference in recurrence rate between the BCG-treated and the non-BCG-treated group (70 vs. 75%) [40]. Nearly 40% of patients in our study harbored HGT1 disease and, therefore, were less likely to respond to BCG therapy than high-grade Ta tumors. In this context, any improvement of pretreatment prognostic stratification may have very high clinical importance, improving oncological outcomes in significant numbers of patients or/and sparing them from excess radical cystectomy.

Our study has some limitations. Small inconsistencies in our tissue classifier performance caused some misclassified epithelial areas in the stroma which required some manual data curation. It was performed in a standardized manner, nevertheless, making the DIA not entirely automated. Another issue in urothelial tumors is the cytological similarity of the malignant and nonmalignant urothelium, which is why the interface zone in our study includes any urothelium. Therefore, all tissue has been classified as 'stroma' or 'epithelium'. However, to reduce the impact of data derived from normal mucosa, we have selected tissue samples for the study with a predominance of tumor epithelium over normal urothelium.

5. Conclusions

Our study reveals an independent informative value of CD8+ cell density gradient across the epithelium–stroma interface to predict RFS in patients with NMIPUC treated with BCG immunotherapy. Importantly, absolute CD8+ cell densities in the tumor epithelia or stroma compartments did not reveal any prognostic impact. This further supports the advantage of immunogradient indicators to assess patterns of infiltrating immune cell distribution in the tumor microenvironment. Combining CD8+ immunogradient with the patient's history of reTUR and histological grade of the tumor, we propose a risk assessment score to predict RFS in patients with NMIPUC after BCG immunotherapy.

Author Contributions: Conceptualization, F.J., A.L., A.C., A.R., M.M. and J.D.; methodology, A.R., M.M. and J.D.; software, J.D.; validation, J.D.; formal analysis, J.D.; investigation, A.C., M.F. and J.D.; resources, F.J., A.L. and A.C.; data curation, M.F. and J.D.; writing—original draft preparation, J.D.; writing—review and editing, A.L., A.R. and F.J.; visualization, J.D., F.J. and A.L.; project administration, F.J. and A.L.; funding acquisition, F.J. All authors have read and agreed to the published version of the manuscript.

Funding: This research was funded by a grant (No. S-MIP-21-31) from the Research Council of Lithuania.

Institutional Review Board Statement: The study was conducted in accordance with the Declaration of Helsinki and approved by the Vilnius Regional Biomedical Research Ethics Committee (research permit No. 2021/11-1394-867 issued on 5 November 2021).

Informed Consent Statement: Patient consent was waived by the Lithuanian Bioethics Committee according to the International Ethical Guidelines for Health-related Research Involving Humans [41].

Data Availability Statement: Data presented in this study can be obtained from the author on request. These data are not available to the public due to permit restrictions.

Conflicts of Interest: The authors declare no conflict of interest.

References

1. Bray, F.; Ferlay, J.; Soerjomataram, I.; Siegel, R.L.; Torre, L.A.; Jemal, A. Global Cancer Statistics 2018: GLOBOCAN Estimates of Incidence and Mortality Worldwide for 36 Cancers in 185 Countries. *CA Cancer J. Clin.* **2018**, *68*, 394–424. [CrossRef] [PubMed]
2. Babjuk, M.; Burger, M.; Čapoun, O.; Cohen, D.; Compérat, E.; Escrig, J.L.D.; Gontero, P.; Liedberg, F.; Masson-Lecomte, A.; Mostafid, H.; et al. European Association of Urology Guidelines on Non-Muscle-Invasive Bladder Cancer (Ta, T1, and Carcinoma in Situ). *Eur. Urol.* **2021**, *81*, 75–94. [CrossRef] [PubMed]
3. Cambier, S.; Sylvester, R.J.; Collette, L.; Gontero, P.; Brausi, M.A.; van Andel, G.; Kirkels, W.J.; Silva, F.C.D.; Oosterlinck, W.; Prescott, S.; et al. EORTC Nomograms and Risk Groups for Predicting Recurrence, Progression, and Disease-Specific and Overall Survival in Non–Muscle-Invasive Stage Ta–T1 Urothelial Bladder Cancer Patients Treated with 1–3 Years of Maintenance Bacillus Calmette-Guérin. *Eur. Urol.* **2016**, *69*, 60–69. [CrossRef] [PubMed]
4. Sylvester, R.J.; van der Meijden, A.P.M.; Oosterlinck, W.; Witjes, J.A.; Bouffioux, C.; Denis, L.; Newling, D.W.W.; Kurth, K. Predicting Recurrence and Progression in Individual Patients with Stage Ta T1 Bladder Cancer Using EORTC Risk Tables: A Combined Analysis of 2596 Patients from Seven EORTC Trials. *Eur. Urol.* **2006**, *49*, 466–477. [CrossRef]
5. Lammers, R.J.M.; Hendriks, J.C.M.; Rodriguez Faba, O.R.F.; Witjes, W.P.J.; Palou, J.; Witjes, J.A. Prediction Model for Recurrence Probabilities after Intravesical Chemotherapy in Patients with Intermediate-Risk Non-Muscle-Invasive Bladder Cancer, Including External Validation. *World J. Urol.* **2016**, *34*, 173–180. [CrossRef]
6. Fernandez-Gomez, J.; Madero, R.; Solsona, E.; Unda, M.; Martinez-Piñeiro, L.; Gonzalez, M.; Portillo, J.; Ojea, A.; Pertusa, C.; Rodriguez-Molina, J.; et al. Predicting Nonmuscle Invasive Bladder Cancer Recurrence and Progression in Patients Treated with Bacillus Calmette-Guerin: The CUETO Scoring Model. *J. Urol.* **2009**, *182*, 2195–2203. [CrossRef]
7. Kamat, A.M.; Roger, L.; Li, R.; O'Donnell, M.A.; Choyke, P.L.; Black, P.C.; Rouprêt, M.; Catto, J.W.F.; Comperat, E.; Ingersoll, M.A.; et al. Predicting Response to Intravesical Bacillus Calmette-Guérin Immunotherapy: Are We There Yet? A Systematic Review. *Eur. Urol.* **2018**, *73*, 738–748. [CrossRef]
8. Sadeghi Rad, H.; Monkman, J.; Warkiani, M.E.; Ladwa, R.; O'Byrne, K.; Rezaei, N.; Kulasinghe, A. Understanding the Tumor Microenvironment for Effective Immunotherapy. *Med. Res. Rev.* **2021**, *41*, 1474–1498. [CrossRef]
9. Song, D.; Powles, T.; Shi, L.; Zhang, L.; Ingersoll, M.A.; Lu, Y.-J. Bladder Cancer, a Unique Model to Understand Cancer Immunity and Develop Immunotherapy Approaches. *J. Pathol.* **2019**, *249*, 151–165. [CrossRef]
10. Schneider, A.K.; Chevalier, M.F.; Derré, L. The Multifaceted Immune Regulation of Bladder Cancer. *Nat. Rev. Urol.* **2019**, *16*, 613–630. [CrossRef]
11. Pichler, R.; Gruenbacher, G.; Culig, Z.; Brunner, A.; Fuchs, D.; Fritz, J.; Gander, H.; Rahm, A.; Thurnher, M. Intratumoral Th2 Predisposition Combines with an Increased Th1 Functional Phenotype in Clinical Response to Intravesical BCG in Bladder Cancer. *Cancer Immunol. Immunother.* **2017**, *66*, 427–440. [CrossRef]
12. Takayama, H.; Nishimura, K.; Tsujimura, A.; Nakai, Y.; Nakayama, M.; Aozasa, K.; Okuyama, A.; Nonomura, N. Increased Infiltration of Tumor Associated Macrophages Is Associated with Poor Prognosis of Bladder Carcinoma in Situ after Intravesical Bacillus Calmette-Guerin Installation. *J. Urol.* **2009**, *181*, 1894–1900. [CrossRef]
13. Sjödahl, G.; Lövgren, K.; Lauss, M.; Chebil, G.; Patschan, O.; Gudjonsson, S.; Månsson, W.; Fernö, M.; Leandersson, K.; Lindgren, D.; et al. Infiltration of $CD3^+$ and $CD68^+$ Cells in Bladder Cancer Is Subtype Specific and Affects the Outcome of Patients with Muscle-Invasive Tumors. *Urol. Oncol.-Semin. Orig. Investig.* **2014**, *32*, 791–797. [CrossRef]
14. Ajili, F.; Kourda, N.; Darouiche, A.; Chebil, M.; Boubaker, S. Prognostic Value of Tumor-Associated Macrophages Count in Human Non-Muscle-Invasive Bladder Cancer Treated by BCG Immunotherapy. *Ultrastruct. Pathol.* **2013**, *37*, 56–61. [CrossRef]

15. Miyake, M.; Tatsumi, Y.; Gotoh, D.; Ohnishi, S.; Owari, T.; Iida, K.; Ohnishi, K.; Hori, S.; Morizawa, Y.; Itami, Y.; et al. Regulatory T Cells and Tumor-Associated Macrophages in the Tumor Microenvironment in Non-Muscle Invasive Bladder Cancer Treated with Intravesical Bacille Calmette-Guérin: A Long-Term Follow-Up Study of a Japanese Cohort. *Int. J. Mol. Sci.* **2017**, *18*, 2186. [CrossRef]
16. Lima, L.; Oliveira, D.; Tavares, A.; Amaro, T.; Cruz, R.; Oliveira, M.J.; Ferreira, J.A.; Santos, L. The Predominance of M2-Polarized Macrophages in the Stroma of Low-Hypoxic Bladder Tumors Is Associated with BCG Immunotherapy Failure. *Urol. Oncol.-Semin. Orig. Investig.* **2014**, *32*, 449–457. [CrossRef]
17. Suriano, F.; Santini, D.; Perrone, G.; Amato, M.; Vincenzi, B.; Tonini, G.; Muda, A.O.; Boggia, S.; Buscarini, M.; Pantano, F.; et al. Tumor Associated Macrophages Polarization Dictates the Efficacy of BCG Instillation in Non-Muscle Invasive Urothelial Bladder Cancer. *J. Exp. Clin. Cancer Res.* **2013**, *32*, 87. [CrossRef]
18. Boström, M.M.; Irjala, H.; Mirtti, T.; Taimen, P.; Kauko, T.; Ålgars, A.; Jalkanen, S.; Boström, P.J. Tumor-Associated Macrophages Provide Significant Prognostic Information in Urothelial Bladder Cancer. *PLoS ONE* **2015**, *10*, e0133552. [CrossRef]
19. Winerdal, M.E.; Marits, P.; Winerdal, M.; Hasan, M.N.; Rosenblatt, R.; Tolf, A.; Selling, K.; Sherif, A.; Winqvist, O. FOXP3 and Survival in Urinary Bladder Cancer. *BJUI* **2011**, *108*, 1672–1678. [CrossRef]
20. Pichler, R.; Fritz, J.; Zavadil, C.; Schäfer, G.; Culig, Z.; Brunner, A. Tumor-Infiltrating Immune Cell Subpopulations Influence the Oncologic Outcome after Intravesical Bacillus Calmette-Guérin Therapy in Bladder Cancer. *Oncotarget* **2016**, *7*, 39916–39930. [CrossRef]
21. Nunez-Nateras, R.; Castle, E.P.; Protheroe, C.A.; Stanton, M.L.; Ocal, T.I.; Ferrigni, E.N.; Ochkur, S.I.; Jacobsen, E.A.; Hou, Y.X.; Andrews, P.E.; et al. Predicting Response to Bacillus Calmette-Guérin (BCG) in Patients with Carcinoma in Situ of the Bladder. *Urol. Oncol.-Semin. Orig. Investig.* **2014**, *32*, 45.e23–45.e30. [CrossRef] [PubMed]
22. Bieri, U.; Enderlin, D.; Buser, L.; Wettstein, M.S.; Eberli, D.; Moch, H.; Hermanns, T.; Poyet, C. Modified Immunoscore Improves the Prediction of Progression-Free Survival in Patients with Non-Muscle-Invasive Bladder Cancer: A Digital Pathology Study. *Front. Oncol.* **2022**, *12*, 964672. [CrossRef] [PubMed]
23. Hendry, S.; Salgado, R.; Gevaert, T.; Russell, P.A.; John, T.; Thapa, B.; Christie, M.; van de Vijver, K.; Estrada, M.V.; Gonzalez-Ericsson, P.I.; et al. Assessing Tumor-infiltrating Lymphocytes in Solid Tumors: A Practical Review for Pathologists and Proposal for a Standardized Method From the International Immunooncology Biomarkers Working Group: Part 1: Assessing the Host Immune Response, TILs in Invasive Breast Carcinoma and Ductal Carcinoma In Situ, Metastatic Tumor Deposits and Areas for Further Research. *Adv. Anat. Pathol.* **2017**, *24*, 235–251. [CrossRef] [PubMed]
24. Hendry, S.; Salgado, R.; Gevaert, T.; Russell, P.A.; John, T.; Thapa, B.; Christie, M.; van de Vijver, K.; Estrada, M.V.; Gonzalez-Ericsson, P.I.; et al. Assessing Tumor-Infiltrating Lymphocytes in Solid Tumors: A Practical Review for Pathologists and Proposal for a Standardized Method from the International Immuno-Oncology Biomarkers Working Group: Part 2: TILs in Melanoma, Gastrointestinal Tract Carcinomas, Non-Small Cell Lung Carcinoma and Mesothelioma, Endometrial and Ovarian Carcinomas, Squamous Cell Carcinoma of the Head and Neck, Genitourinary Carcinomas, and Primary Brain Tumors. *Adv. Anat. Pathol.* **2017**, *24*, 311–335. [CrossRef]
25. Steele, K.E.; Tan, T.H.; Korn, R.; Dacosta, K.; Brown, C.; Kuziora, M.; Zimmermann, J.; Laffin, B.; Widmaier, M.; Rognoni, L.; et al. Measuring Multiple Parameters of CD8+ Tumor-Infiltrating Lymphocytes in Human Cancers by Image Analysis. *J. Immunother. Cancer* **2018**, *6*, 20. [CrossRef]
26. Galon, J.; Pagès, F.; Marincola, F.M.; Angell, H.K.; Angell, H.K.; Thurin, M.; Lugli, A.; Zlobec, I.; Berger, A.; Bifulco, C.; et al. Cancer Classification Using the Immunoscore: A Worldwide Task Force. *J. Transl. Med.* **2012**, *10*, 205. [CrossRef]
27. Pagès, F.; Mlecnik, B.; Marliot, F.; Bindea, G.; Ou, F.S.; Ou, F.-S.; Bifulco, C.; Bifulco, C.; Lugli, A.; Zlobec, I.; et al. International Validation of the Consensus Immunoscore for the Classification of Colon Cancer: A Prognostic and Accuracy Study. *Lancet* **2018**, *391*, 2128–2139. [CrossRef]
28. Angell, H.K.; Bruni, D.; Barrett, J.C.; Herbst, R.; Galon, J. The Immunoscore: Colon Cancer and Beyond. *Clin. Cancer Res.* **2020**, *26*, 332–339. [CrossRef]
29. Bieri, U.; Buser, L.; Wettstein, M.S.; Eberli, D.; Saba, K.; Moch, H.; Hermanns, T.; Poyet, C. Modified Immunoscore Improves Prediction of Survival Outcomes in Patients Undergoing Radical Cystectomy for Bladder Cancer—A Retrospective Digital Pathology Study. *Diagnostics* **2022**, *12*, 1360. [CrossRef]
30. Rasmusson, A.; Zilenaite, D.; Nestarenkaite, A.; Augulis, R.; Laurinaviciene, A.; Ostapenko, V.; Poskus, T.; Laurinavicius, A. Immunogradient Indicators for Antitumor Response Assessment by Automated Tumor-Stroma Interface Zone Detection. *Am. J. Pathol.* **2020**, *190*, 1309–1322. [CrossRef]
31. Zilenaite, D.; Rasmusson, A.; Augulis, R.; Besusparis, J.; Laurinaviciene, A.; Plancoulaine, B.; Ostapenko, V.; Laurinavicius, A. Independent Prognostic Value of Intratumoral Heterogeneity and Immune Response Features by Automated Digital Immunohistochemistry Analysis in Early Hormone Receptor-Positive Breast Carcinoma. *Front. Oncol.* **2020**, *10*, 950. [CrossRef]
32. Nestarenkaite, A.; Fadhil, W.; Rasmusson, A.; Susanti, S.; Hadjimichael, E.; Laurinaviciene, A.; Ilyas, M.; Laurinavicius, A. Immuno-Interface Score to Predict Outcome in Colorectal Cancer Independent of Microsatellite Instability Status. *Cancers* **2020**, *12*, 2902. [CrossRef]
33. Radziuviene, G.; Rasmusson, A.; Augulis, R.; Grineviciute, R.B.; Zilenaite, D.; Laurinaviciene, A.; Ostapenko, V.; Laurinavicius, A. Intratumoral Heterogeneity and Immune Response Indicators to Predict Overall Survival in a Retrospective Study of HER2-Borderline (IHC 2+) Breast Cancer Patients. *Front. Oncol.* **2021**, *11*, 774088. [CrossRef]

34. WHO Classification of Tumours Editorial Board. *Urinary and Male Genital Tumours*; International Agency for Research on Cancer: Lyon, France, 2022; ISBN 978-92-832-4512-4.
35. Bryan, R.T.; Collins, S.I.; Daykin, M.C.; Zeegers, M.P.; Cheng, K.; Wallace, D.M.A.; Sole, G.M. Mechanisms of Recurrence of Ta/T1 Bladder Cancer. *Ann. R. Coll. Surg. Engl.* **2010**, *92*, 519–524. [CrossRef]
36. Diamant, E.; Roumiguié, M.; Ingels, A.; Parra, J.; Vordos, D.; Bajeot, A.-S.; Chartier-Kastler, E.; Soulié, M.; de la Taille, A.; Rouprêt, M.; et al. Effectiveness of Early Radical Cystectomy for High-Risk Non-Muscle Invasive Bladder Cancer. *Cancers* **2022**, *14*, 3797. [CrossRef]
37. Jäger, W.; Thomas, C.; Haag, S.; Hampel, C.; Salzer, A.; Thüroff, J.W.; Wiesner, C. Early vs. Delayed Radical Cystectomy for 'High-Risk' Carcinoma Not Invading Bladder Muscle: Delay of Cystectomy Reduces Cancer-Specific Survival. *BJU Int.* **2011**, *108*, E284–E288. [CrossRef]
38. Canter, D.; Egleston, B.; Wong, Y.-N.; Smaldone, M.C.; Simhan, J.; Greenberg, R.E.; Uzzo, R.G.; Kutikov, A. Use of Radical Cystectomy as Initial Therapy for the Treatment of High-Grade T1 Urothelial Carcinoma of the Bladder: A SEER Database Analysis. *Urol. Oncol. Semin. Orig. Investig.* **2013**, *31*, 866–870. [CrossRef]
39. Tully, K.H.; Roghmann, F.; Noldus, J.; Chen, X.; Häuser, L.; Kibel, A.S.; Sonpavde, G.P.; Mossanen, M.; Trinh, Q.-D. Quantifying the Overall Survival Benefit with Early Radical Cystectomy for Patients with Histologically Confirmed T1 Non–Muscle-Invasive Bladder Cancer. *Clin. Genitourin. Cancer* **2020**, *18*, e651–e659. [CrossRef]
40. Shahin, O.; Thalmann, G.N.; Rentsch, C.; Mazzucchelli, L.; Studer, U.E. A Retrospective Analysis of 153 Patients Treated With or Without Intravesical Bacillus Calmette-Guerin for Primary Stage T1 Grade 3 Bladder Cancer: Recurrence, Progression and Survival. *J. Urol.* **2003**, *169*, 96–100. [CrossRef] [PubMed]
41. Council for International Organizations of Medical Sciences (CIOMS). *International Ethical Guidelines for Health-Related Research Involving Humans*; Council for International Organizations of Medical Sciences (CIOMS): Geneva, Switzerland, 2016.

Disclaimer/Publisher's Note: The statements, opinions and data contained in all publications are solely those of the individual author(s) and contributor(s) and not of MDPI and/or the editor(s). MDPI and/or the editor(s) disclaim responsibility for any injury to people or property resulting from any ideas, methods, instructions or products referred to in the content.

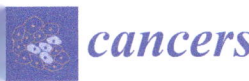

Article

A Case Study of Chimeric Antigen Receptor T Cell Function: Donor Therapeutic Differences in Activity and Modulation with Verteporfin

Jiyong Liang [1,2], Dexing Fang [1], Joy Gumin [1], Hinda Najem [3,4], Moloud Sooreshjani [3,4], Renduo Song [1], Aria Sabbagh [1], Ling-Yuan Kong [1], Joseph Duffy [3,4], Irina V. Balyasnikova [3,4], Seth M. Pollack [5], Vinay K. Puduvalli [2] and Amy B. Heimberger [3,4,6,*]

[1] Department of Neurosurgery, The University of Texas MD Anderson Cancer Center, Houston, TX 77030, USA
[2] Department of Neuro-Oncology, The University of Texas MD Anderson Cancer Center, Houston, TX 77030, USA
[3] Department of Neurological Surgery, Feinberg School of Medicine, Northwestern University, Chicago, IL 60611, USA
[4] Malnati Brain Tumor Institute of the Lurie Comprehensive Cancer Center, Feinberg School of Medicine, Northwestern University, Chicago, IL 60611, USA
[5] Department of Cancer Biology, Feinberg School of Medicine, Northwestern University, Chicago, IL 60611, USA
[6] Department of Neurosurgery, Northwestern University, Simpson Querrey Biomedical Research Center, 303 E. Superior Street, 6-516, Chicago, IL 60611, USA
* Correspondence: amy.heimberger@northwestern.edu; Tel.: +1-312-503-3805

Simple Summary: The loss of tumor antigens prevents the immune system from recognizing and destroying cancer cells. Immune cells can remove these antigens and express them on their surface. Other immune cells becoming confused, kill the anti-tumor immune cells. By blocking this process using a drug commonly used to treat a variety of eye conditions, we were able to restore anti-tumor immune responses for impaired T cells in mouse models of brain cancer.

Abstract: Background: Chimeric antigen receptor (CAR) T cells have recently been demonstrated to extract and express cognate tumor antigens through trogocytosis. This process may contribute to tumor antigen escape, T cell exhaustion, and fratricide, which plays a central role in CAR dysfunction. We sought to evaluate the importance of this effect in epidermal growth factor receptor variant III (EGFRvIII) specific CAR T cells targeting glioma. Methods: EGFRvIII-specific CAR T cells were generated from various donors and analyzed for cytotoxicity, trogocytosis, and in vivo therapeutic activity against intracranial glioma. Tumor autophagy resulting from CAR T cell activity was evaluated in combination with an autophagy inducer (verteporfin) or inhibitor (bafilomycin A1). Results: CAR T cell products derived from different donors induced markedly divergent levels of trogocytosis of tumor antigen as well as PD-L1 upon engaging target tumor cells correlating with variability in efficacy in mice. Pharmacological facilitation of CAR induced-autophagy with verteporfin inhibits trogocytic expression of tumor antigen on CARs and increases CAR persistence and efficacy in mice. Conclusion: These data propose CAR-induced autophagy as a mechanism counteracting CAR-induced trogocytosis and provide a new strategy to innovate high-performance CARs through pharmacological facilitation of T cell-induced tumor death.

Keywords: trogocytosis; epidermal growth factor receptor variant III; chimeric antigen receptor T cells; autophagy; phagocytosis; glioblastoma

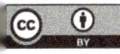

1. Introduction

Trogocytosis is a process whereby cell surface molecules are transferred to effector T cells through the immunologic synapse, often by antigen-presenting cells (APCs). While this process has long been recognized as a critical aspect of functional immunity [1], it has recently emerged as a potentially important cause of chimeric antigen receptor (CAR) T cell dysfunction [2,3]. CAR T cells are generated by transducing a T cell with a CAR construct containing a tumor antigen recognition domain linked to the constant regions of a signaling T cell receptor. The CAR T cell then recognizes the tumor antigen with high specificity in a non-MHC-restricted manner that is independent of antigen processing [4]. During CAR-induced trogocytosis, the CAR T cells can uptake cognate antigens from the surface of target cells, allowing the escape of target cells through localized antigen loss at the immunologic synapse and fratricide of CAR T cells once target antigen becomes expressed on the CAR T cell surface [2]. Overstimulation of the effector CAR T cells may also lead to the development of an exhausted phenotype.

We have been developing EGFRvIII-specific CAR T cells for the treatment of glioma and hypothesize that trogocytosis could potentially play a role in the development of antigen loss, and T cell exhaustion previously reported [5,6]. CAR T cell-mediated tumor killing is often oversimplified as instantaneous perforin-induced lysis of tumor cells. In fact, there is a complex process of autophagy induced by T cells [7], which may actually oppose trogocytosis by mediating the degradation of endocytic substrates in tumor targets. Previously, we demonstrated that verteporfin acts as an autophagy inducer and promotes autophagosome formation and autophagy flux, as shown by increases in LC3-II, decreases in p62, and autophagy-mediated degradation [8]. The purpose of this study was to ascertain if pharmacological facilitation of autophagy with verteporfin inhibits trogocytosis of the EGFRvIII tumor antigen by CAR T cells and to determine if this increases their persistence and efficacy in mice.

2. Materials and Methods
2.1. Cell Lines

The U87 cell line was obtained from the American Type Culture Collection. The K562 EGFRvIII clone 27 (activating and antigen-presenting cells, aAPCs) with stable expression of 41BB-L, CD86, CD64, tCD19, and membrane-tethered IL-15 was a gift from Dr. Laurence Cooper at MD Anderson Cancer Center. K562 cells were maintained in RPMI1640 supplemented with 10% fetal bovine serum (FBS). U87-EGFRvIII-Zeomycin cells were a gift from Dr. Oliver Bogler at MD Anderson Cancer Center and were cultured in complete Dulbecco's Modified Eagle Medium (DMEM) containing 10% FBS and 2mM glutamax at 37 °C and in an atmosphere of 95% air/5% CO_2.

2.2. EGFRvIII CAR Engineering

As previously described [5], the EGFRvIII CAR was engineered by fusing the CSF2RA signal peptide, scFvs of monoclonal antibodies 139 with a Whitlow linker inserted between the light and heavy chains, the IgG4 extracellular stalk, and the CD28 and CD3-zeta intracellular signaling domains. The plasmid encoding for CAR was then co-transfected with the Sleeping Beauty (SB) plasmid. CAR+ T cells were stimulated in a 1:2 ratio with the irradiated EGFRvIII+ K562 in the presence of 30 ng/mL IL-21. For in vivo trafficking, Firefly luciferase was cloned in frame to the C terminus of the EGFRvIII CAR construct with a P2A self-cleavage linker. Human donor T cells were transfected by electroporation with the CAR-P2A-ffLUC SB transposon along with the SB11 transposase.

2.3. T Cells Isolation, Transfection, and Ex Vivo CAR Expansion

Peripheral blood mononuclear cells (PBMCs) from healthy donors were obtained from the Gulf Coast Regional Blood Bank and isolated using Ficoll-Paque (GE Healthcare, Chicago, IL, USA) per the manufacturer's protocol. The PBMCs were either freshly used or cryopreserved and thawed immediately before use. CD3+ T cell selection was performed using the Human Pan T cell isolation microbeads (Miltenyi Biotec, San Diego, CA) per the manufacturer's protocol. The cells were then allowed to rest for 2 h before CAR nucleofection using Amaxa Nucleofector 2B (Lonza, Basel, Switzerland). Briefly, 20×10^6 CD3+ cells were suspended in 100 µL of human T cell electroporation buffer (Lonza, Basel, Switzerland), 10 µg of CAR plasmid, and 5 µg of SB11 transposase (a gift from Amer Najjar at the MD Anderson Cancer Center) and then electroporated using program U-014. Immediately after electroporation, the cells were transferred to a prewarmed recovery medium (phenol-free RPMI medium, 20% FBS, and 2 mM glutamax) for 24 h. The cells were then counted and phenotyped by flow cytometry to determine the percentage of CAR expression. Cells were harvested for initial stimulation with 100 Gy-irradiated aAPCs at a 1:2 ratio (CAR$^+$: aAPC) in the presence of 30 ng/mL IL-21 in RPMI1640 medium supplemented with 10% FBS. Cytokines were replenished every other day for 7 days. Subsequent expansion after 7 days was performed with a weekly iteration of aAPC stimulation and the addition of 50 U/mL IL-2 and 30 ng/mL IL-21 every other day.

2.4. Glioma and CAR T Cell Co-Culture

Ex vivo expanded EGFRvIII CAR T cells were added to target (U87-EGFRvIII) glioma cells at indicated cell ratios.

2.5. Flow Cytometry Analysis and Trogocytosis Assay

For direct flow cytometry, up to 10^6 cells were stained with mAbs (Supplementary Table S1) in FACS buffer (PBS, 2% FBS, 0.05% sodium azide) for 30 min in the dark at 4 °C. Data were collected on a FACS Celesta (BD Biosciences, San Jose, CA, USA) using the FACSDiva software (version 8.0.1, BD Biosciences, San Jose, CA, USA). All data were analyzed using FlowJo software (version 10.7, TreeStar, Ashland, OR, USA). CAR T cells were exposed to target tumor cells at a 1:1 ratio and then harvested and probed with an EGFRvIII primary antibody (V3980, NSJ Bioreagents, San Diego, CA, USA) and a secondary antibody tagged with PE or APC followed by flow cytometry analysis.

2.6. Evaluation of T Cell Efficacy in Intracranial Glioma Xenografts

Animal experiments were carried out according to regulations from the Institutional Animal Care and Use Committee (IACUC) at MD Anderson Cancer Center (ACUF 00001544-RN00). Both female and male NOD.Cg-PrkdcscidIL2Rγtm1Wjl/Sz (NSG, Jackson Laboratory, Bar Harbor, ME) mice aged 6–8 weeks were anesthetized by intraperitoneal injection using a cocktail of 10 mg/mL ketamine and 0.5 mg/mL xylazine at a dose of 0.1 mL/10 g. A guide screw was surgically implanted 2.5 mm to the right of the coronal suture and 1 mm posterior to the bregma at a depth of 3 mm. Two weeks after surgery, intracranial tumors were established by implantation of 250,000 U87-EGFRvIII-Zeomycin in 5 µL PBS through the guide screw. The CAR infiltration in the tumor was serially imaged using Xenogen IVIS Spectrum (Caliper Life Sciences, Hopkinton, MA, USA) 10 min after intraperitoneal injection of 3 mg D-luciferin potassium salt (cat. # MB000102-R70170, Syd Labs, Natick, MA). CAR flux (photons/s/cm^2/steradian) was measured using Living Image software (version 2.50, Caliper Life Sciences, Hopkinton, MA, USA) in a delineated region encompassing the entire cranium. Mice were sorted into treatment groups 4 days after tumor implantation. The mice were treated on day 5 with 4×10^6 EGFRvIII CAR T cells in 5 µL of PBS administered intracranially through the guide screw and treated per the designated schemas. Mice were treated with verteporfin (10 mg/Kg) via intraperitoneal injection. Mice were sacrificed when they displayed progressive weight loss of >25%, rapid weight loss of >10% within 48 h, hind limb paralysis, or any two of the following clinical symptoms of illness: ataxia, hunched posture, or irregular respiration rate.

2.7. Statistical Analyses

Statistical analyses were performed in GraphPad Prism, version 8.0. Data were examined for normality through boxplots and QQ plots prior to the application of linear statistical models. Statistical analyses of in vitro assays were performed using one-way ANOVA, two-way ANOVA, or unpaired T-test, as indicated in the figure legends. Analyses of in vivo tumor BLI imaging were performed using two-way ANOVA with repeated measures and Sidak's post hoc test for multiple comparisons. Survival analysis of the mice was performed using the log-rank (Mantel-Cox) test. Significance of the findings is defined as follows: ns = not significant, $p >= 0.05$; * $p < 0.05$; ** $p < 0.01$; *** $p < 0.001$; **** $p < 0.0001$.

3. Results

3.1. Differential Trogocytosis and Efficacy in CAR Products

Our group has a long-standing interest in trying to analyze why different donors exhibit different CAR T cell activity despite identical cell manufacturing procedures using the same CAR construct. We hypothesized that trogocytosis might play a differential role in CAR T cell dysfunction and contribute to donor differences in CAR activity. As part of this effort, we sought to identify two dichotomized CAR T cell products that have significant differences in trogocytosis. Much higher levels of EGFRvIII were detected on the surface of CAR T cells of Donor 1 relative to other donors (Figure 1A). As a control, we confirmed that EGFRvIII was detected abundantly at basal levels on target tumor cells expressing EGFRvIII but not on antigen naïve CARs (Figure 1B).

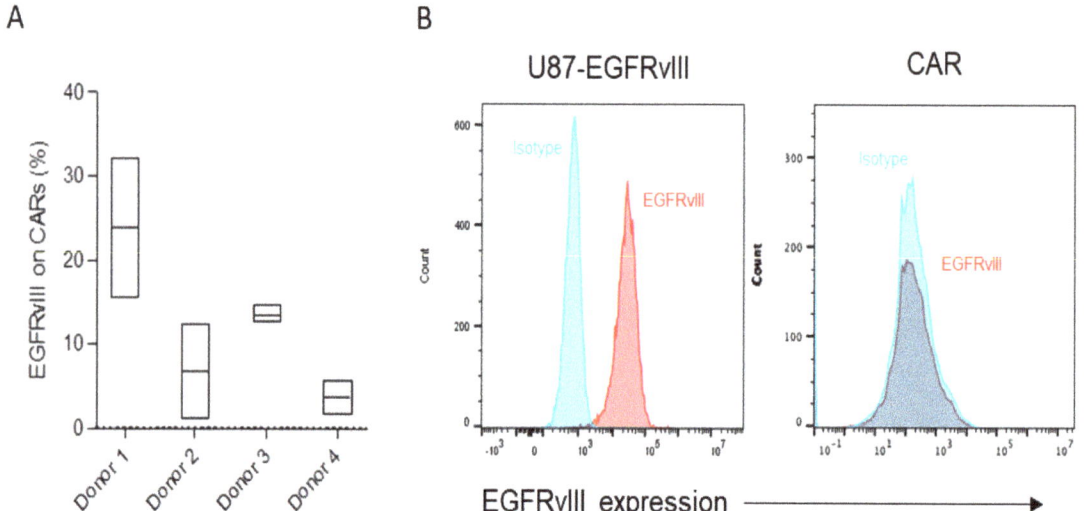

Figure 1. (**A,B**) Trogocytic EGFRvIII expression was gated on CAR+ cells analyzed in triplicate following co-culture with targets (U87-EGFRvIII) for 2 h. The gate was set based on CAR T cells without a target and then plotted based on the range of expression on flow cytometry. (**B**) A representative flow cytometry analysis of baseline EGFRvIII expression on target tumor (U87-EGFRvIII) and EGFRvIII CAR T cells.

To further characterize two dichotomized CAR T cell products, two donors were selected and labeled "donor 1" and "donor 2." Donor 1 CAR T cells resulted in minimal therapeutic effect in vivo compared with the relatively higher level of potency of Donor 2 (40% long-term survivors) (Figure 2A), as well as in the U87EGFRvIII tumor line in vitro (Figure 2B; $p = 0.0001$).

To ascertain if the phenotypic composition might account for the difference between products, the CAR product was profiled. Both donors exhibited CAR lineage skewing towards the CD8+ population with an expansion-dependent loss of the CD4+ population. This skewing was observed regardless of initial CD8:CD4 ratios (Figure 3A), suggesting that T cell phenotype was not a key variable explaining their differences in therapeutic response. Furthermore, CARs of both donors expressed T cell exhaustion markers PD-1, TIM-3, and LAG-3 on day 28 of ex vivo expansion, with Donor 2 CAR T cells expressing relatively higher levels of these markers despite their higher therapeutic efficacy (Figure 3B,C). In contrast, Donor 1, but not Donor 2 CAR T cells, expressed CD57, the T cell senescence marker, at a higher level (Figure 3B,C). Thus, expansion-induced CAR lineage skewing and expression of exhaustion markers alone were insufficient to explain donor variations in CAR efficacy.

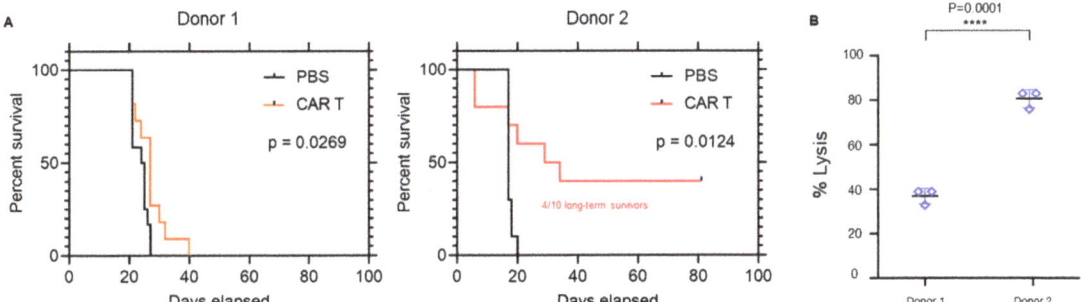

Figure 2. Donor differences in CAR activity and trogocytosis. (**A**) Representative survival curves of mice bearing U87-EGFRvIII tumors treated with EGFRvIII CARs engineered from Donor 1 and Donor 2 (n = 10/group). (**B**) Target tumor cell (U87-EGFRvIII) lysis following co-culture with EGFRvIII CARs (E:T 5:1) from Donors 1 and 2 for 24 h. **** $p = 0.0001$.

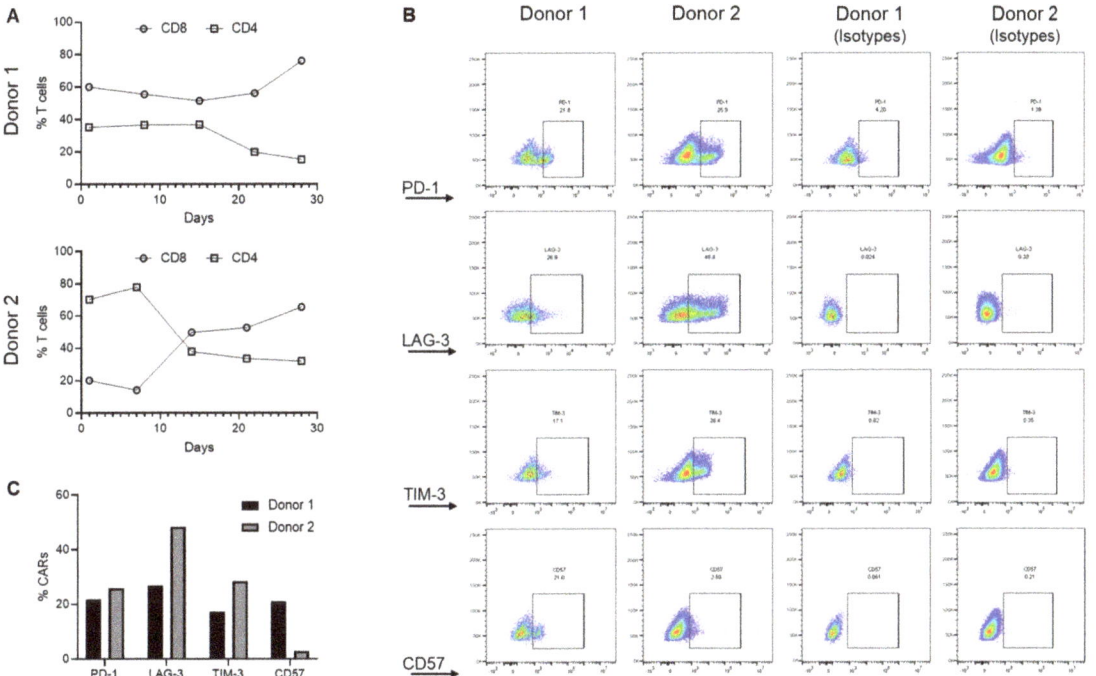

Figure 3. Donor lineage skewing and the expression of exhaustion markers. (**A**) Changes in CD8 and CD4 cells during ex vivo expansion of EGFRvIII CAR T cells. (**B,C**) Expression of T cell exhaustion (PD-1, TIM3, and LAG3) and senescence (CD57) markers on CAR T cells. These data summarize the analysis generated from two different donors (Donor 1 and Donor 2) and are representative of a triplicate analysis.

3.2. Autophagy Antagonizes Trogocytosis and Increases Target Killing

The trogosome cargos are likely processed through the endosome systems, where cargo is either recycled to the cell surface or sorted for lysosomal and autophagy-dependent degradation (Figure 4). Through assessment of the trogocytosis kinetics, we found expression of EGFRvIII on CAR T cells was maximal at 2 h and declined by 4 h (Figure 5A). We recently reported that verteporfin activates the autophagy pathway and that PD-L1 is degraded as part of this process [8]. We hypothesized that verteporfin might induce autophagy to counter trogocytosis through increased degradation of EGFRvIII. Indeed, we found the level of EGFRvIII expression was reduced in co-cultures treated with verteporfin (Figure 5B).

Next, we assayed the effect of verteporfin treatment on CAR-mediated target cell killing. Verteporfin, whether alone or in co-treatment with CARs, was found to have no effect on target cell viability at lower E:T ratios. However, at a ratio of 5:1 E:T, Donor 1 CAR killing ability was markedly increased when treated with verteporfin (Figure 5C). Verteporfin did not affect the cytotoxic activity of Donor 2 CARs (Figure 5D) that had lower levels of trogocytosis.

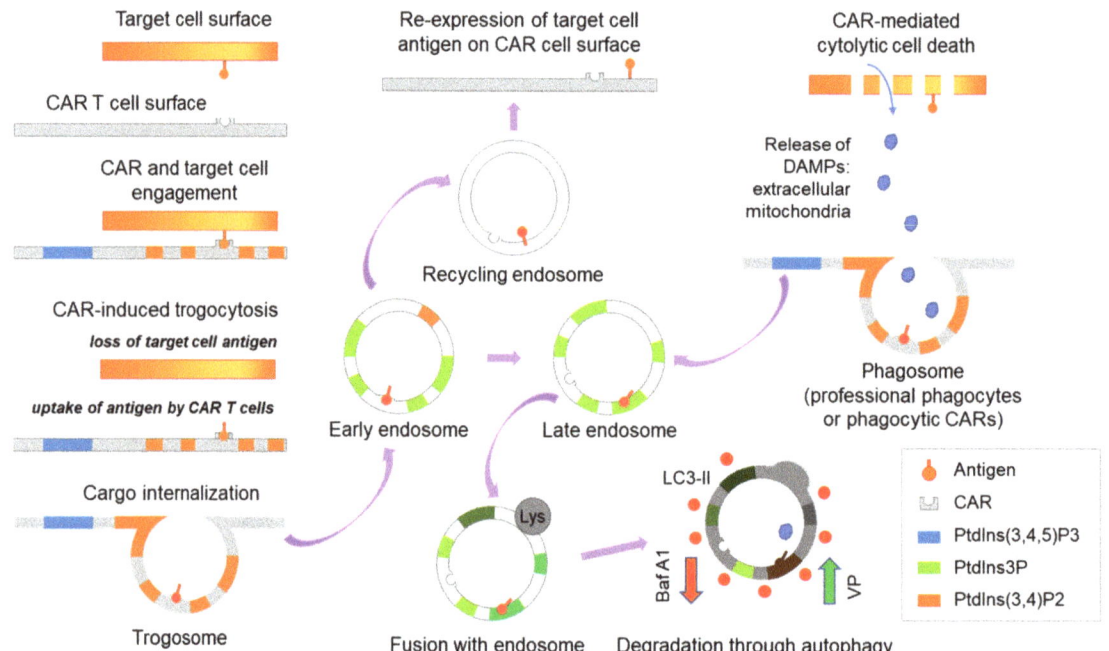

Figure 4. Scheme demonstrating CAR-induced trogocytosis. Trogocytosis occurs upon CAR-target engagement resulting in the expression of the target tumor antigen on CAR T cells. Following extraction by CAR T cells, the tumor antigen is internalized and processed through the endosome system and then is either recycled to the cell surface or shuttled to late endosomes and subsequently degraded through lysosome and autophagy-dependent mechanisms. Activation and inhibition of autophagy may regulate trogocytosis and modulate CAR T cell function. In addition, trogocytosis may interface with phagocytosis. Baf A1, bafilomycin A1, an inhibitor of vacuolar ATPase and autophagy; VP, verteporfin, an activator of selective autophagy; DAMPs, damage-associated molecular patterns.

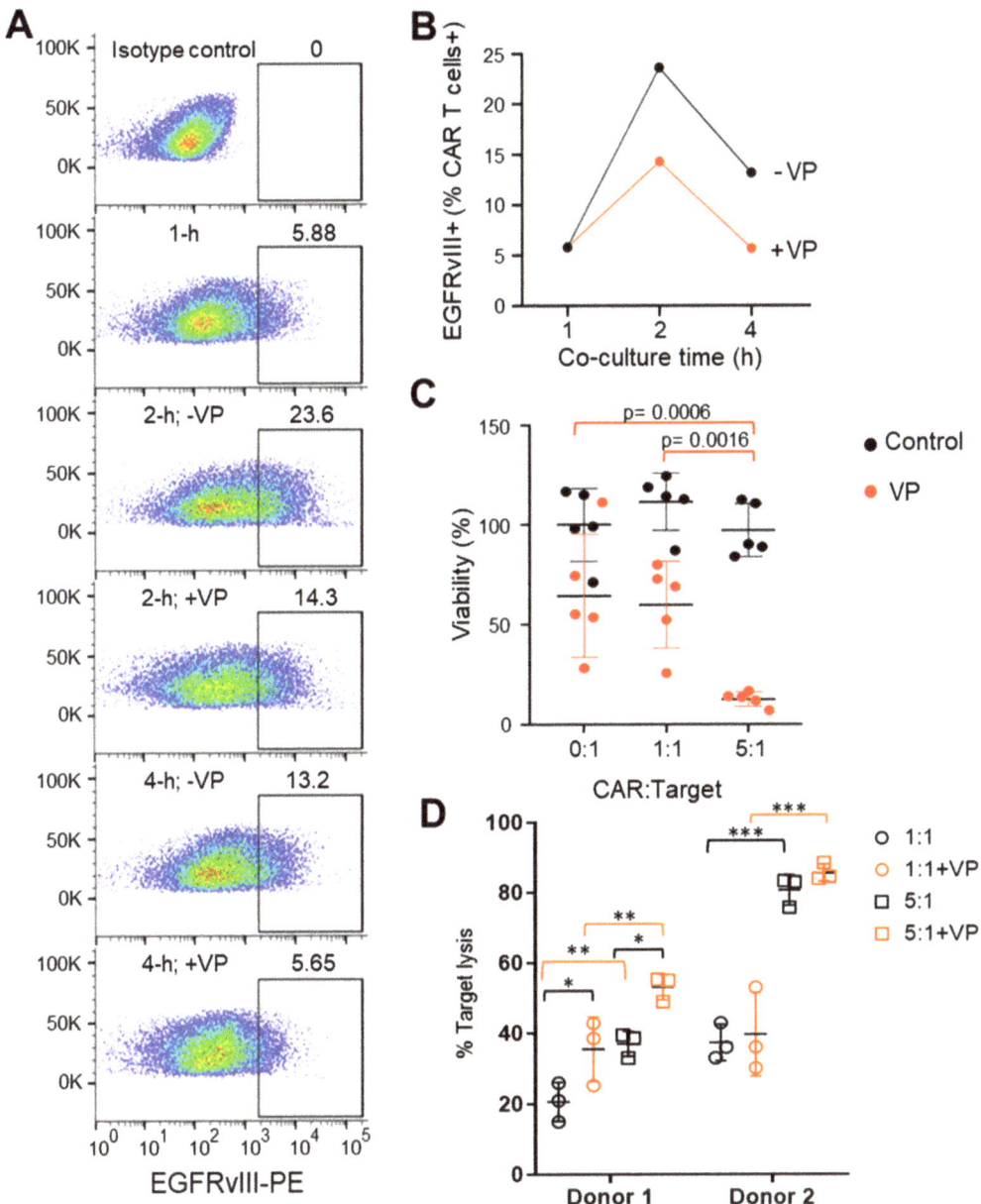

Figure 5. Verteporfin inhibits CAR-induced trogocytosis and increases CAR activity. (**A**) Representative flow cytometry example of EGFRvIII expression on Donor 1 CAR prior to or following co-culture with targets (U87-EGFRvIII) in the absence (-) or presence (+) of verteporfin (VP). The gate is set against the isotype control and was conducted in triplicate. (**B**) Summarized kinetic data from A of CAR T cell EGFRvIII expression in the absence and presence of VP. (**C**) Target (U87-EGFRvIII) cell viability treated with Donor 1 CARs in the absence (control; black circles) or presence of verteporfin (VP; red circles) for 24 h. A Two-way ANOVA test and Turkey's multiple comparisons were conducted with no statistical significance between the control groups (black circles). Statistical significance

between the VP-treated groups (red circles): $p = 0.0006$ (0:1 vs. 5:1), $p = 0.0016$ (1:1 vs. 5:1). (**D**) CAR-mediated lysis of target (U87-EGFRvIII) cells treated with EGFRvIII CARs derived from Donor 1 and Donor 2 at 1:1 and 5:1 ratio in the absence (-VP) or presence (+VP) of verteporfin for 24 h. * $p < 0.05$; ** $p < 0.01$; *** $p < 0.001$ (unpaired *t*-test). For Donor 1: $p = 0.039$ (1:1 vs. 1:1+VP), $p = 0.0312$ (5:1 vs. 5:1+VP), $p = 0.0145$ (1:1 vs. 5:1), $p = 0.0117$ (1:1+VP vs. 5:1+VP). For Donor 2: not significant (1:1 vs. 1:1+VP), not significant (5:1 vs. 5:1+VP), $p = 0.0001$ (1:1 vs. 5:1), $p = 0.0001$ (1:1+VP vs. 5:1+VP).

3.3. CAR-Induced Autophagy Mediates Degradation of Cross-Transferred PD-L1

Because the immune checkpoint ligand PD-L1 and other proteins can be transferred to T cells and monocytes from antigen-presenting and cancer cells [9,10], we next evaluated whether such proteins were transferred to the CAR T cells in our system. At baseline, PD-L1 is not expressed on primary T cells (Figure 6A), on CAR T cells expanded on PD-L1-feeders (Figure 6B), or on anti-CD3/CD28 dynabeads (Figure 6C). Although PD-L1 is almost never observed on circulating T cells in any normal physiologic circumstance, there are some circumstances where this has been observed [11,12]. To be sure that the PD-L1 expression on the CAR T effectors was indeed a product of trogocytosis rather than a result of an inducible mechanism (such as IFN-γ) that can sometimes be responsible for increases in PD-L1 expression in target tumor cells, expression profiling was performed in the setting of IFN-γ. As would be expected, PD-L1 was not detected on CAR T cells either treated with IFN-γ or following exposure to CAR-target condition media in the absence of targets (Figure 6C) and was only detected on CARs in the presence of targets (Figure 6D). To examine the impact on trogocytic PD-L1 uptake by CAR T cells, we inhibited autophagy using the drug bafilomycin. Indeed, enhanced PD-L1 uptake was observed with its use (Figure 6E). Furthermore, bafilomycin-related autophagy inhibition was also more potent in Donor 2 compared to Donor 1 (Figure 6E), suggesting counteracting mechanisms of trogocytosis and autophagy (Figure 4).

3.4. Verteporfin Increases CAR T Cell Persistence and Efficacy

To improve CAR persistence in the GBM tumor microenvironment, we sought to determine whether autophagy counters trogocytosis in vivo. We first assayed the abundance of CAR T cells in the brain of U87-EGFRvIII tumor-bearing mice treated with or without verteporfin. The bioluminescence (BLI) CAR T cell signal was only detected in CAR-infused tumors (Figure 7A). Although there was no significant difference in CAR retention noted one day after infusion, verteporfin-treated mice maintained significantly higher levels of CAR signal ten days after infusion (Figure 7B; $p < 0.0001$).

We hypothesized that the impact of verteporfin on improving CAR T cell function and persistence is independent of any activity it might exert on the tumor cells themselves in vivo. To test this, we evaluated the dysfunctional Donor 1 CAR T cells in combination with verteporfin. Consistent with our previous study [8], verteporfin alone did not exert any therapeutic effect (Figure 8A). However, treatment with the combination of verteporfin and Donor 1 CAR T cells extended the survival of EGFRvIII+ tumor-bearing mice relative to both PBS and monotherapy with CAR T cells (Figure 8B; $p = 0.02$).

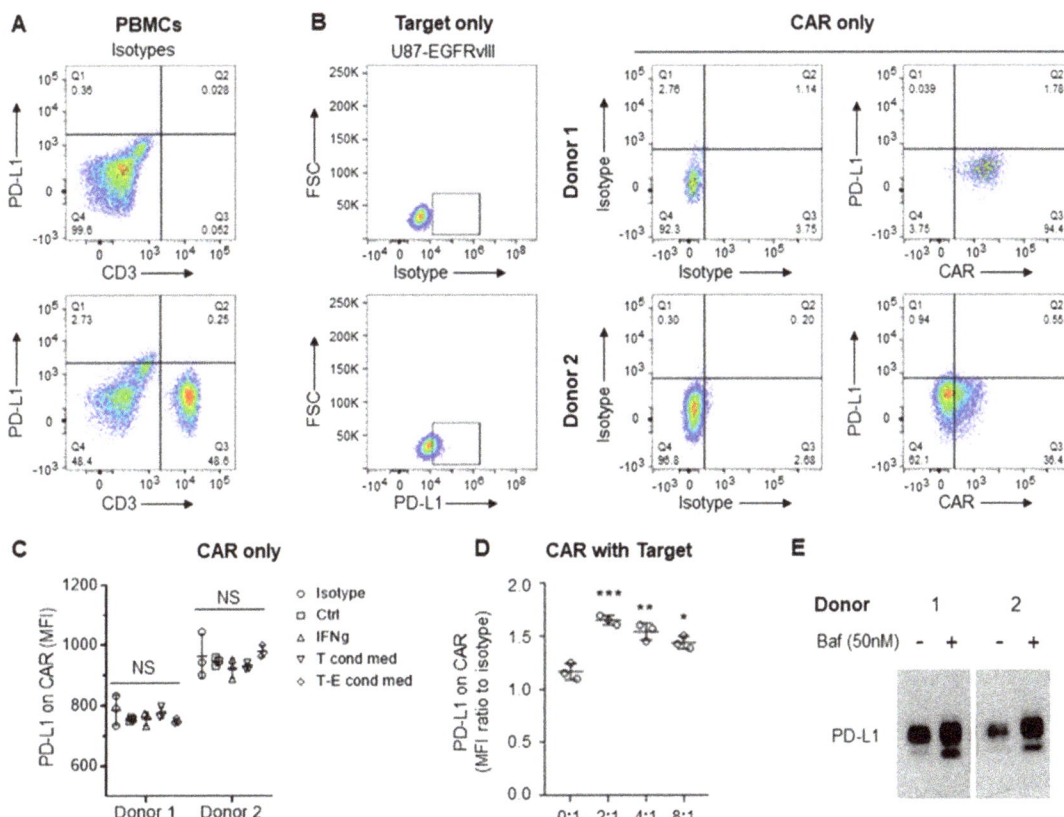

Figure 6. Expression of PD-L1 on target tumor but not on CAR T cells. (**A**) Flow cytometry analysis of baseline PD-L1 expression on CD3+ primary T cells from peripheral blood mononuclear cells (PBMCs). Analysis was conducted in triplicates. (**B**) Flow cytometry analysis of target tumor (U87-EGFRvIII) and EGFRvIII CAR T cells. (**C,D**) Summary of flow cytometry analysis of PD-L1 levels (MFI, mean fluorescence intensity) on CAR T cells expanded on anti-CD3/CD28 dynabeads (Ctl), treated with interferon γ (IFNγ, 5 ng/ml), exposed to condition media from the target (T cond med) or target-CAR (T-E = 2:1) conditioned media (**D**). Summarized flow cytometry analysis of PD-L1 on CARs after co-culture with target tumor for 20 h, taken from biological replicates of Donor 1. Targets and CARs are distinct populations gated on SCC/FSC, GFP (targets), and CAR (CD3). * $p < 0.05$; ** $p < 0.01$; *** $p < 0.001$ relative to no target. (**E**) Western blot analysis of PD-L1 expression on EGFRvIII-specific CARs generated by Donors 1 and 2 following CAR-target co-culture for 20 h in the absence (-) or presence (+) of bafilomycin (Baf). Original flow cytometry see Supplementary Figure S1. Original blots see Supplementary Figure S2.

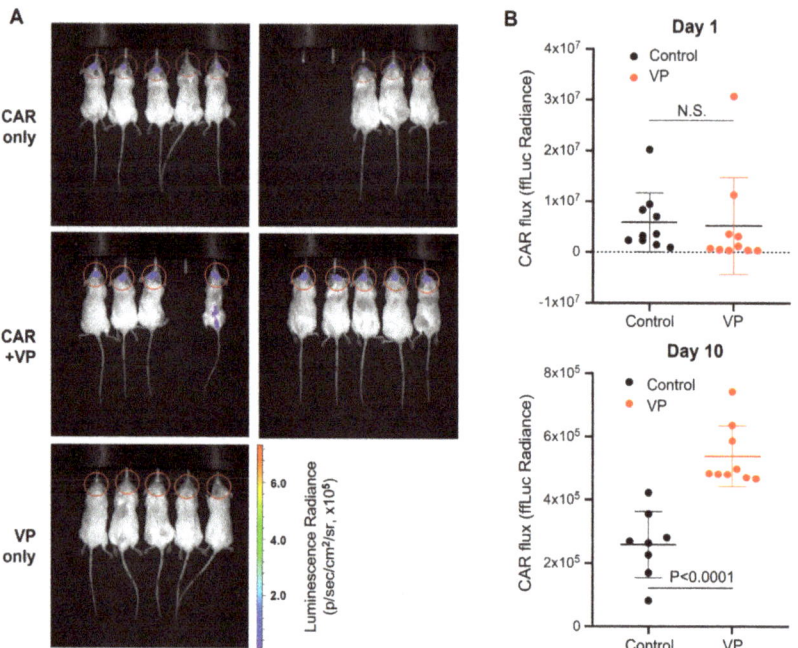

Figure 7. Verteporfin increases CAR persistence in tumors. (**A**) BLI of the CAR signals was assayed on day 10 after infusion with and without verteporfin. (**B**) Summarized data of firefly bioluminescence (ffLuc) imaging of CAR signal acquired on day 1 (infusion) and day 10 after infusion into U87-EGFRvII tumors (implanted on day 4) with and without treatment of verteporfin for 3 days prior to CAR infusion.

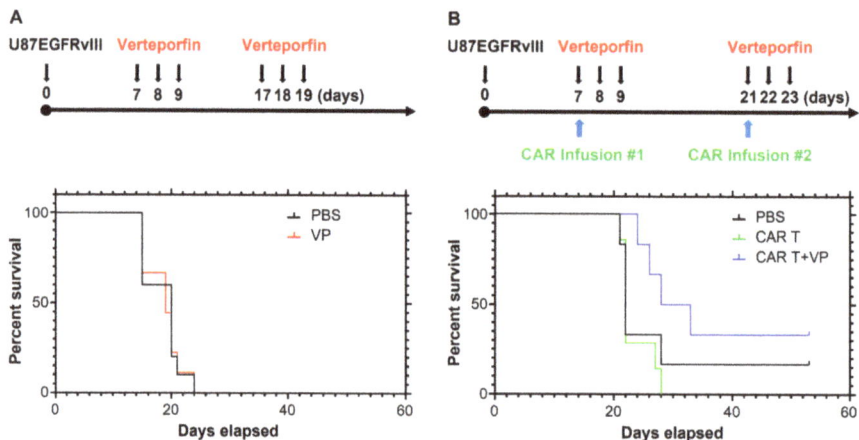

Figure 8. Verteporfin reverses CAR dysfunction. (**A**) Treatment schema and survival curves of mice bearing U87-EGFRvII tumor treated with or without verteporfin, median survival 17 days (PBS and VP). (**B**) Treatment schema and survival curves of mice bearing U87-EGFRvIII tumors treated with Donor 1 CAR with or without verteporfin, median survival 22 (PBS), 22 (CAR T), and 30.5 days (CAR T+VP). If the mouse was moribund or dead, it did not receive the second CAR treatment.

4. Discussion

Trogocytosis is a newly recognized mechanism underlying CAR T cell dysfunction leading to tumor antigen escape, T cell exhaustion, and CAR T cell fratricide [2]. Here we confirm that trogocytosis occurs in the stimulation of EGFRvIII CAR T cells but surprisingly find that it is variable between donors. As might be expected, we find that the amount of trogocytosis is inversely associated with CAR efficacy in a murine glioma model. Notably, CAR-induced trogocytosis also mediates the cross-transfer of the immune checkpoint ligand PD-L1 in addition to tumor antigens in this system. Thus, efforts to reduce trogocytosis may enhance CAR function and improve efficacy. Through activation of CAR T cell-induced autophagy, verteporfin inhibits trogocytosis, increases CAR persistence in vivo, and improves the efficacy of CAR T cells targeting EGFRvIII+ tumors in vivo. CAR expression levels have been previously found to be inversely associated with CAR function, with higher CAR expression increasing CAR signaling and dysfunction [13–16]. Consistent with these findings, CAR levels were found to be lower in representative Donor 1 relative to Donor 2, which may contribute to increased CAR activity and be linked to differences in trogocytosis, which is a CAR-dependent process. Furthermore, this study suggests that varying amounts of trogocytosis following CAR T cell target recognition is an important factor creating differences in CAR T cell function and therapeutic efficacy between donors.

Other pharmacological strategies that could be considered for the inhibition of trogocytosis include phosphoinositide 3-kinase (PI3K) inhibitors [2,17,18]. However, non-selective effects on T cell viability and function may be problematic. More selective PI3K inhibitors may resolve this problem [19,20]. Ultimately genetic modulation of this pathway in CAR T cells will likely be the path forward. Our findings suggest that trogocytosis can be counteracted by verteporfin-facilitated autophagy, pushing the downstream pathway into late-endosome formation and degradation of the target cell antigens instead of its re-expression on the cell surface by recycling endosomes (Figure 4), offering a strategy to circumvent some of the limitations associated with targeting trogocytosis. Although our findings might be specific to the model system used in this study, both trogocytosis and autophagy are universal cell processes. Thus, the specific use of verteporfin for other CAR T cells, such as those targeting IL13RA2, GD2 [21], and others [22,23], will need to be tested to validate these findings.

T cells were isolated and expanded from healthy donors and then engineered to express the full CAR construct. This CAR system requires the presence of a stimulating cell line for CAR T cell proliferation and expansion [24]. The CAR expression in Donor 1 was higher than in Donor 2. However, in vivo cytotoxicity of the CAR T cells from Donor 2 was higher than Donor 1. It should be noted that higher levels of CAR expression are not always associated with increased CAR function. Instead, higher CAR expression can be associated with tonic CAR signaling, which causes exhaustion and impairs CAR T cell function and persistence [13–16]. Our findings appear to be consistent with these data.

Although tumor antigens seem particularly susceptible to transfer through CAR-induced trogocytosis [2], the full extent of adjacent membrane proteins transferred through the trogosome remains undetermined [25–28] because, in the CAR system we used, a non-targeting CAR T cell as a control was not feasible. As such, we evaluated whether other targets could be involved in trogocytosis. In addition to CAR-induced trogocytosis of cognate tumor antigen, we documented cross-cell transfer of the immune checkpoint ligand PD-L1 from tumor cells to CAR T cells. This observation may be a function of verteporfin regulating the turnover of receptors more generally. The acquisition of PD-L1 in T cells has previously been shown to inhibit effector function in circulating T cells [11,12]. To our knowledge, this is the first description of PD-L1 expression on CAR T cells acquired through trogocytosis. The functional immunological consequences of this finding will be a focus of future studies. Since PD-1 is overexpressed by exhausted T cells, its engagement with PD-L1 expressing CAR T cells is expected to activate the immune checkpoint and may also represent an underlying mechanism of fratricide as a consequence of CAR-induced trogocytosis.

While trogocytosis is markedly different between these two donors, there are undoubtedly many factors that may explain the difference in the effector functions of CAR-T cells identified between these two donors, including promotor polymorphism of immune stimulatory cytokines and HLA matching. As opposed to standard CAR-T cell therapies that are used clinically, this model is an allogeneic therapy in an immunocompromised mouse model. The endogenous T cell receptor for donor 1 and donor 2 have not been deleted, so differential alloreactivity between these two donors is a confounder for analysis. While this first study establishes the phenomenon, a larger study with more donors will be needed to estimate exactly how big a factor trogocytosis is in CAR T product variability. It is also important to note that verteporfin has multiple biological and cellular effects. It is also possible that verteporfin is altering CAR turnover or proliferation. As such, it is unclear if the results are exclusively due to verteporfin via its effect on trogocytosis. Additional mechanistic studies are required to elucidate exactly how autophagy activation by verteporfin is associated with the inhibition of trogocytosis. Moreover, there are intrinsic effects of verteporfin on glioma cells [29]. Ultimately, strategies that genetically manipulate these functions in CAR-T cells will likely be evaluated and may be the preferred approach moving forward. Notably, there are additional hurdles that will need to be considered that influence CAR anti-tumor activity, such as distribution in the tumor microenvironment and tumor-mediated immune suppression [30,31].

Our prior study showed that the photodynamic agent verteporfin induces autophagy and selective degradation of the PD-L1 immune checkpoint ligand at clinically achievable concentrations [8]. Although verteporfin can aggregate in glioblastoma cells [32] and has a photodynamic effect leading to extensive protein cross-linking, this would not be applicable in non-illuminated solid tumors.

5. Conclusions

This study provides further evidence that verteporfin-induced autophagy, independent of its photodynamic property, plays a role in antagonizing CAR-induced trogocytosis and might also be promoting the phagocytic activity of CAR T cells. By inducing autophagy to allow clearance of trogosome cargo, verteporfin counteracts the recycling of cargo to the cell membrane. Given its trogocytosis-dependent and -independent drug actions, verteporfin may be particularly effective in counteracting both tumor antigen and PD-L1 trogocytosis in PD-L1+ target tumor cells [26].

Supplementary Materials: The following supporting information can be downloaded at: https://www.mdpi.com/article/10.3390/cancers15041085/s1, Figure S1: Gating strategy for detecting CART cells and acquisition of EGFRvIII (vIII) expression from target co-culture; Table S1: Table listing the antibody name, tag, catalog number, and vendor used in all flow cytometry and western blot experiments. Figure S2: Original blots.

Author Contributions: Conception and design: J.L., D.F. and A.B.H. Development of methodology: J.L., D.F., J.G., A.S. and L.-Y.K. Acquisition of data (provided animals, acquired, and managed patients, provided facilities, etc.): D.F., J.L., J.G., R.S. and A.S. Analysis, and interpretation of data (e.g., statistical analysis, biostatistics, computational analysis): J.L. and D.F. Writing, review, and/or revision of the manuscript: J.L., D.F., H.N., M.S., J.D., I.V.B., S.M.P., V.K.P. and A.B.H. Administrative, technical, or material support (i.e., reporting or organizing data, constructing databases): A.B.H. All authors have read and agreed to the published version of the manuscript.

Funding: Funding was provided by the ReMission Alliance, NIH grants RO1CA120813, RO1NS120547, P50CA221747, and P30CA060553, the Traver Walsh Foundation, the Anne C. Brooks and Anthony D. Bullock Foundation, and the MD Anderson Cancer Center Provost Fund.

Institutional Review Board Statement: The animal study protocol was approved by the Institutional Review Board of MD Anderson Cancer Center (ACUF 00001544-RN00).

Informed Consent Statement: Not applicable.

Data Availability Statement: All data is presented in this article.

Acknowledgments: The authors thank Audria Patrick for assisting in manuscript preparation.

Conflicts of Interest: The authors declare that the research was conducted in the absence of any commercial or financial relationships that could be construed as a potential conflict of interest.

References

1. Miyake, K.; Karasuyama, H. The Role of Trogocytosis in the Modulation of Immune Cell Functions. *Cells* **2021**, *10*, 1255. [CrossRef]
2. Hamieh, M.; Dobrin, A.; Cabriolu, A.; Van Der Stegen, S.J.C.; Giavridis, T.; Mansilla-Soto, J.; Eyquem, J.; Zhao, Z.; Whitlock, B.M.; Miele, M.M.; et al. CAR T cell trogocytosis and cooperative killing regulate tumour antigen escape. *Nature* **2019**, *568*, 112–116. [CrossRef]
3. Miao, L.; Zhang, Z.; Ren, Z.; Tang, F.; Li, Y. Obstacles and Coping Strategies of CAR-T Cell Immunotherapy in Solid Tumors. *Front. Immunol.* **2021**, *12*, 687822. [CrossRef]
4. Land, C.A.; Musich, P.R.; Haydar, D.; Krenciute, G.; Xie, Q. Chimeric antigen receptor T-cell therapy in glioblastoma: Charging the T cells to fight. *J. Transl. Med.* **2020**, *18*, 428. [CrossRef]
5. Caruso, H.G.; Tanaka, R.; Liang, J.; Ling, X.; Sabbagh, A.; Henry, V.K.; Collier, T.L.; Heimberger, A.B. Shortened ex vivo manufacturing time of EGFRvIII-specific chimeric antigen receptor (CAR) T cells reduces immune exhaustion and enhances antiglioma therapeutic function. *J. Neuro-Oncol.* **2019**, *145*, 429–439. [CrossRef]
6. O'Rourke, D.M.; Nasrallah, M.P.; Desai, A.; Melenhorst, J.J.; Mansfield, K.; Morrissette, J.J.; Maus, M.V. A single dose of peripherally infused EGFRvIII-directed CAR T cells mediates antigen loss and induces adaptive resistance in patients with recurrent glioblastoma. *Sci. Transl. Med.* **2017**, *9*, eaaa0984. [CrossRef]
7. Macian, F. Autophagy in T Cell Function and Aging. *Front. Cell Dev. Biol.* **2019**, *7*, 213. [CrossRef]
8. Liang, J.; Wang, L.; Wang, C.; Shen, J.; Su, B.; Marisetty, A.L.; Heimberger, A.B. Verteporfin Inhibits PD-L1 through Autophagy and the STAT1-IRF1-TRIM28 Signaling Axis, Exerting Antitumor Efficacy. *Cancer Immunol. Res.* **2020**, *8*, 952–965. [CrossRef]
9. Gary, R.; Voelkl, S.; Palmisano, R.; Ullrich, E.; Bosch, J.J.; Mackensen, A. Antigen-Specific Transfer of Functional Programmed Death Ligand 1 from Human APCs onto CD8+ T Cells via Trogocytosis. *J. Immunol.* **2012**, *188*, 744–752. [CrossRef]
10. Kawashima, M.; Carreras, J.; Higuchi, H.; Kotaki, R.; Hoshina, T.; Okuyama, K.; Kotani, A. PD-L1/L2 protein levels rapidly increase on monocytes via trogocytosis from tumor cells in classical Hodgkin lymphoma. *Leukemia* **2020**, *34*, 2405–2417. [CrossRef]
11. Jacquelot, N.; Roberti, M.P.; Enot, D.P.; Rusakiewicz, S.; Ternès, N.; Jegou, S.; Woods, D.M.; Sodré, A.L.; Hansen, M.; Meirow, Y.; et al. Predictors of responses to immune checkpoint blockade in advanced melanoma. *Nat. Commun.* **2017**, *8*, 592. [CrossRef]
12. Brochez, L.; Meireson, A.; Chevolet, I.; Sundahl, N.; Ost, P.; Kruse, V. Challenging PD-L1 expressing cytotoxic T cells as a predictor for response to immunotherapy in melanoma. *Nat. Commun.* **2018**, *9*, 2921. [CrossRef]
13. Long, A.H.; Haso, W.M.; Shern, J.F.; Wanhainen, K.M.; Murgai, M.; Ingaramo, M.; Smith, J.P.; Walker, A.J.; Kohler, M.E.; Venkateshwara, V.R.; et al. 4-1BB costimulation ameliorates T cell exhaustion induced by tonic signaling of chimeric antigen receptors. *Nat. Med.* **2015**, *21*, 581–590. [CrossRef] [PubMed]
14. Eyquem, J.; Mansilla-Soto, J.; Giavridis, T.; van der Stegen, S.J.C.; Hamieh, M.; Cunanan, K.M.; Odak, A.; Gönen, M.; Sadelain, M. Targeting a CAR to the TRAC locus with CRISPR/Cas9 enhances tumour rejection. *Nature* **2017**, *543*, 113–117. [CrossRef] [PubMed]
15. Gomes-Silva, D.; Mukherjee, M.; Srinivasan, M.; Krenciute, G.; Dakhova, O.; Zheng, Y.; Cabral, J.M.; Rooney, C.M.; Orange, J.S.; Brenner, M.K.; et al. Tonic 4-1BB Costimulation in Chimeric Antigen Receptors Impedes T Cell Survival and Is Vector-Dependent. *Cell Rep.* **2017**, *21*, 17–26. [CrossRef] [PubMed]
16. Ajina, A.; Maher, J. Strategies to Address Chimeric Antigen Receptor Tonic Signaling. *Mol. Cancer Ther.* **2018**, *17*, 1795–1815. [CrossRef]
17. Martínez-Martín, N.; Fernández-Arenas, E.; Cemerski, S.; Delgado, P.; Turner, M.; Heuser, J.; Irvine, D.J.; Huang, B.; Bustelo, X.R.; Shaw, A.; et al. T Cell Receptor Internalization from the Immunological Synapse Is Mediated by TC21 and RhoG GTPase-Dependent Phagocytosis. *Immunity* **2011**, *35*, 208–222. [CrossRef]
18. Dopfer, E.P.; Minguet, S.; Schamel, W.W. A New Vampire Saga: The Molecular Mechanism of T Cell Trogocytosis. *Immunity* **2011**, *35*, 151–153. [CrossRef]
19. Okkenhaug, K.; Vanhaesebroeck, B. PI3K in lymphocyte development, differentiation and activation. *Nat. Rev. Immunol.* **2003**, *3*, 317–330. [CrossRef]
20. Stock, S.; Übelhart, R.; Schubert, M.-L.; Fan, F.; He, B.; Hoffmann, J.-M.; Wang, L.; Wang, S.; Gong, W.; Neuber, B.; et al. Idelalisib for optimized CD19-specific chimeric antigen receptor T cells in chronic lymphocytic leukemia patients. *Int. J. Cancer* **2019**, *145*, 1312–1324. [CrossRef]
21. Prapa, M.; Chiavelli, C.; Golinelli, G.; Grisendi, G.; Bestagno, M.; Di Tinco, R.; Dall'Ora, M.; Neri, G.; Candini, O.; Spano, C.; et al. GD2 CAR T cells against human glioblastoma. *Npj Precis. Oncol.* **2021**, *5*, 93. [CrossRef]
22. Karschnia, P.; Teske, N.; Thon, N.; Subklewe, M.; Tonn, J.C.; Dietrich, J.; von Baumgarten, L. Chimeric Antigen Receptor T Cells for Glioblastoma: Current Concepts, Challenges, and Future Perspectives. *Neurology* **2021**, *97*, 218–230. [CrossRef]
23. Maggs, L.; Cattaneo, G.; Dal, A.E.; Moghaddam, A.S.; Ferrone, S. CAR T Cell-Based Immunotherapy for the Treatment of Glioblastoma. *Front. Neurosci.* **2021**, *15*, 662064. [CrossRef]

24. Caruso, H.G.; Hurton, L.V.; Najjar, A.; Rushworth, D.; Ang, S.; Olivares, S.; Mi, T.; Switzer, K.; Singh, H.; Huls, H.; et al. Tuning Sensitivity of CAR to EGFR Density Limits Recognition of Normal Tissue While Maintaining Potent Antitumor Activity. *Cancer Res* **2015**, *75*, 3505–3518. [CrossRef]
25. Dance, A. Core Concept: Cells nibble one another via the under-appreciated process of trogocytosis. *Proc. Natl. Acad. Sci. USA* **2019**, *116*, 17608–17610. [CrossRef]
26. Bettadapur, A.; Miller, H.W.; Ralston, K.S. Biting Off What Can Be Chewed: Trogocytosis in Health, Infection, and Disease. *Infect. Immun.* **2020**, *88*, e00930-19. [CrossRef]
27. Zeng, Q.; Schwarz, H. The role of trogocytosis in immune surveillance of Hodgkin lymphoma. *Oncoimmunology* **2020**, *9*, 1781334. [CrossRef]
28. Tekguc, M.; Wing, J.B.; Osaki, M.; Long, J.; Sakaguchi, S. Treg-expressed CTLA-4 depletes CD80/CD86 by trogocytosis, releasing free PD-L1 on antigen-presenting cells. *Proc. Natl. Acad. Sci. USA* **2021**, *118*, e2023739118. [CrossRef]
29. Kuramoto, K.; Yamamoto, M.; Suzuki, S.; Sanomachi, T.; Togashi, K.; Seino, S.; Kitanaka, C.; Okada, M. Verteporfin inhibits oxidative phosphorylation and induces cell death specifically in glioma stem cells. *FEBS J.* **2020**, *287*, 2023–2036. [CrossRef]
30. Boccalatte, F.; Mina, R.; Aroldi, A.; Leone, S.; Suryadevara, C.M.; Placantonakis, D.G.; Bruno, B. Advances and Hurdles in CAR T Cell Immune Therapy for Solid Tumors. *Cancers* **2022**, *14*, 5108. [CrossRef]
31. Di Cintio, F.; Bo, M.D.; Baboci, L.; De Mattia, E.; Polano, M.; Toffoli, G. The Molecular and Microenvironmental Landscape of Glioblastomas: Implications for the Novel Treatment Choices. *Front. Neurosci.* **2020**, *14*, 603647. [CrossRef] [PubMed]
32. Calori, I.R.; Caetano, W.; Tedesco, A.C.; Hioka, N. Self-aggregation of verteporfin in glioblastoma multiforme cells: A static and time-resolved fluorescence study. *Dye. Pigment.* **2020**, *182*, 108598. [CrossRef]

Disclaimer/Publisher's Note: The statements, opinions and data contained in all publications are solely those of the individual author(s) and contributor(s) and not of MDPI and/or the editor(s). MDPI and/or the editor(s) disclaim responsibility for any injury to people or property resulting from any ideas, methods, instructions or products referred to in the content.

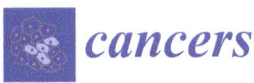

Article

Chemotherapeutics Used for High-Risk Neuroblastoma Therapy Improve the Efficacy of Anti-GD2 Antibody Dinutuximab Beta in Preclinical Spheroid Models

Sascha Troschke-Meurer [1], Maxi Zumpe [1], Lena Meißner [1], Nikolai Siebert [1], Piotr Grabarczyk [2], Hannes Forkel [2], Claudia Maletzki [3], Sander Bekeschus [4] and Holger N. Lode [1,*]

[1] Department of Pediatric Oncology and Hematology, University Medicine Greifswald, Ferdinand-Sauerbruch Strasse 1, 17475 Greifswald, Germany
[2] Department of Internal Medicine, Clinic III—Hematology, Oncology, University Medicine Greifswald, Ferdinand-Sauerbruch Strasse 1, 17475 Greifswald, Germany
[3] Department of Medicine, Clinic III—Hematology, Oncology, Palliative Medicine, Rostock University Medical Center, Ernst-Heydemann-Str. 6, 18057 Rostock, Germany
[4] ZIK Plasmatis, Leibniz Institute for Plasma Science and Technology (INP), Felix-Hausdorff-Str. 2, 17489 Greifswald, Germany
* Correspondence: lode@uni-greifswald.de; Tel.: +49-3834-86-6300; Fax: +49-3834-86-6410

Simple Summary: We investigated the effects of chemotherapeutics used for the frontline treatment of newly diagnosed high-risk neuroblastoma patients in combination with anti-GD2 antibody ch14.18/CHO (dinutuximab beta, DB) in the presence of immune cells in preclinical models of neuroblastoma. The combined treatment showed an up-to-17-fold-stronger and GD2-specific cytotoxic effect compared to the controls treated with chemotherapy alone in the presence or absence of immune cells. These findings further support a clinical evaluation of DB in combination with frontline induction therapy for high-risk neuroblastoma patients.

Abstract: Anti-disialoganglioside GD2 antibody ch14.18/CHO (dinutuximab beta, DB) improved the outcome of patients with high-risk neuroblastoma (HR-NB) in the maintenance phase. We investigated chemotherapeutic compounds used in newly diagnosed patients in combination with DB. Vincristine, etoposide, carboplatin, cisplatin, and cyclophosphamide, as well as DB, were used at concentrations achieved in pediatric clinical trials. The effects on stress ligand and checkpoint expression by neuroblastoma cells and on activation receptors of NK cells were determined by using flow cytometry. NK-cell activity was measured with a CD107a/IFN-γ assay. Long-term cytotoxicity was analyzed in three spheroid models derived from GD2-positive neuroblastoma cell lines (LAN-1, CHLA 20, and CHLA 136) expressing a fluorescent near-infrared protein. Chemotherapeutics combined with DB in the presence of immune cells improved cytotoxic efficacy up to 17-fold compared to in the controls, and the effect was GD2-specific. The activating stress and inhibitory checkpoint ligands on neuroblastoma cells were upregulated by the chemotherapeutics up to 9- and 5-fold, respectively, and activation receptors on NK cells were not affected. The CD107a/IFN-γ assay revealed no additional activation of NK cells by the chemotherapeutics. The synergistic effect of DB with chemotherapeutics seems primarily attributed to the combined toxicity of antibody-dependent cellular cytotoxicity and chemotherapy, which supports further clinical evaluation in frontline induction therapy.

Keywords: ADCC; carboplatin; chemoimmunotherapy; cisplatin; cyclophosphamide; dinutuximab beta; etoposide; neuroblastoma; vincristine

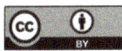

1. Introduction

Neuroblastoma is the leading cancer-related cause of death in children [1]. Despite intensive multimodal treatment options, the long-term event-free survival is still only

50% [2]. Neuroblastoma cells highly express the tumor-associated antigen disialoganglioside GD2, which can be targeted with the monoclonal antibody (mAb) dinutuximab beta (DB, ch14.18/CHO). Although this therapy has increased the overall survival of patients (pts) with high-risk neuroblastoma (HR-NB) at 5 years by 15% [3], new treatment options are needed to further improve the outcome.

One promising approach is the combination of antibody treatment with chemotherapy. In a prospective randomized trial conducted by the Children's Oncology Group (COG) in patients with relapsed or refractory neuroblastoma, pts treated with dinutuximab (ch14.18/SP2/0) combined with irinotecan, temozolomide, and granulocyte-macrophage stimulating factor (GM-CSF) showed an objective response rate of 41.5% [4]. In a non-randomized study, anti-GD2 antibody hu14.18K322A was combined with six cycles of the COG induction chemotherapy and granulocyte-macrophage colony-stimulating factor and low-dose interleukin-2 (IL-2) in newly diagnosed high-risk neuroblastoma patients [5]. The end-of-induction partial response and complete response rate were 97%, and no patients experienced progressive disease during induction, suggesting an improvement over historical control.

However, the use of the anti-GD2 antibody DB during the European neuroblastoma chemotherapy induction regimen has not been evaluated yet [6]. The main mechanism of action of a DB-based immunotherapy is the induction of antibody-dependent cellular cytotoxicity (ADCC), and the combination of such chemotherapeutics with DB might have differential effects on antitumor efficacy.

Chemotherapeutics kill tumor cells by means of genotoxic stress or prevention of mitosis, resulting in apoptosis, senescence, and immunogenic cell death.

Studies showed that the mere reduction of the tumor cell mass during chemotherapy improves the immunological antitumor response [7]. Additionally, an increasing body of evidence suggests that an innate immune response is crucial for the antitumor activity of chemotherapeutics [8–10], as they induce immunogenic cell death that can increase antigen presentation and elicit a cytotoxic T-cell response [11]. In this context, the PD-1 immune checkpoint blockade improved CD8+ T-cell effector functions during chemotherapy [12].

Immunological advantages of chemotherapy also emerge from an increased visibility of tumor cells to the immune system mediated by stress ligand expression, and NK cells are the main effector cells that kill tumor cells upon stress-ligand recognition [13,14]. Stress ligands can bind NK-cell-specific activating receptors such as NKp30 (receptor for B7-H6) and NKG2D (receptor for ULBPs and MICA/B) and therefore tip the balance toward NK-cell stimulation [15]. Accordingly, it has been shown that chemotherapy-induced B7-H6 sensitizes leukemia and solid tumor cells for NK-cell-mediated cytotoxicity [16].

Importantly, agents used in European neuroblastoma induction regimens rapid COJEC and GPOH [6,17], such as cisplatin and vincristine, induced B7-H6 and ULBP expression in cell lines, e.g., multiple myeloma and human embryonic kidney cells (HEK293) [13,16]. In line with that, the combination treatment of cisplatin and NK cells has proven to overcome the chemotherapy resistance of cancer cells by inducing ULBP stress ligands in vitro [18]. Despite the fact that chemotherapeutics have been considered to be immune-inhibitory agents, there is evidence that NK cells are functional during chemotherapy [19]. Therefore, chemoimmunotherapy might be an excellent tool for enhancing antitumor efficacy during induction therapy in HR-NB.

However, the beneficial effects of chemotherapeutics combined with the antitumor effects of therapeutic antibodies (ADCC) may be counter-regulated by inducing immune checkpoints on tumor cells. We and others have shown that ADCC and also chemotherapies induce PD-L1 expression, leading to inhibited antibody-mediated tumor killing [20,21]. A chemoimmunotherapy therefore might be hindered by tumor cells harnessing immune checkpoint pathways to escape immune surveillance [18].

Due to the mode of action of chemotherapies, a long-term analysis of antitumor activity of chemotherapeutics is imperative [22]. We therefore established a live-cell neuroblastoma spheroid model to assess long-term chemotherapeutic effects. A spheroid model is a

3-dimensional (3D) spherical aggregation of tumor cells that represent a complex tumor environment and architecture including zones of proliferation at the outside and quiescent cells in the inside [23–25]. Therefore, spheroid models provide a more clinically relevant model regarding chemotherapy diffusion, angiogenesis, tumor invasion and chemotherapy resistance compared to 2D models [23,26–30].

We used the described spheroid model, to test the hypothesis that combining chemotherapeutic agents used in induction therapy regimens for pts with HR-NB with DB can enhance antitumor efficacy and determined their effect on activating and inhibitory receptors and ligands on target and effector cells.

2. Materials and Methods

2.1. Cell Culture

The human NB cell line LA-N-1 was cultured in RPMI (PAN BIOTECH, P04–016520) supplemented with 4.5 g/L glucose, 2 mM stable glutamine, 10% FCS and 100 U/mL penicillin, and 0.1 mg/mL streptomycin ($1\times$ P/S; PAN BIO- 485 TECH, P06–07100). The human NB cell lines CHLA-20 and CHLA-136 were cultured in IMDM (PAN BIOTECH, P04–20250) supplemented with 4 mM stable glutamine, 20% FCS, $1\times$ ITS (BD Biosciences, 3220669), and $1\times$ P/S. Human PBMCs (peripheral blood mononuclear cells) were isolated from whole blood concentrates without serum of healthy donors, using the Pancoll separating method (human, density 1.077 g/mL, BIOTECH, P04-60500). PBMCs were cultured in RPMI supplemented with 10% FCS, 50 µM, 100 IU/mL, IL-2, β-mercaptoethanol, and $1\times$ P/S for 72 h prior to the experiments.

2.2. Chemotherapy and Antibodies for Cytotoxicity Assay

Tumor cells were treated with drug concentrations of carboplatin (2 µg/mL), cisplatin (1 µg/mL), etoposide (0.1–1 µg/mL), vincristine (0.05 µg/mL), and 4-HPC (2 µg/mL), as achieved in pediatric pharmacokinetic studies [5,31–35]. Cells were washed 24 h after the start of treatment. Solutions of chemotherapeutics were produced by the university pharmacy Greifswald and used within 28 days. The antibody DB was used at a concentration of 10 µg/mL in line with concentrations achieved in clinical trials [36]. DB was purchased from EUSA Pharma (UK), and rituximab from Roche (Switzerland).

2.3. Stable Transduction of Tumor Cells Using Lentiviral Vectors

For recombinant lentivirus production, a second-generation lentiviral vector system was used. The non-confluent Lenti-X™ 293T cells were co-transfected with purified pVSV-G-envelope-expressing plasmid (Addgene, Watertown, MA, USA), psPAX2 (Addgene, Watertown, MA, USA) vector encoding virus polymerase and packaging genes, and lentiviral vector pWPXL (Addgene, Watertown, MA, USA) coding for a near-infrared reporter (NIR) (iRFP680). The transfection of Lenti-X™ 293T cells was conducted by using CalPhos Mammalian Transfection Kit (Takara Bio Europe, Saint-Germain-en-Laye, France) according to the manufacturer's instructions. For transduction, 8 mg/mL Polybrene (Merck KGaA, Darmstadt, Germany) and lentiviral supernatants were added to the target cells. Target cells were cultured under cell culture conditions, and after 72 h, they were tested for the successful transduction of the IncuCyte® SX5 live-cell analysis system (Sartorius, Göttingen, Germany).

2.4. Long-Term Live-Cell Spheroid Viability Assay and Treatment Conditions

To yield three-dimensional (3D) tumor spheroids, we used ultra-low attachment plates (ULA plates, S-BIO PrimeSurface®, MS-90384UZ) that were precoated with a hydrophilic polymer facilitating spontaneous self-assembly by preventing cellular attachment to the surface. This method was recently shown to be the best approach for studying the efficacy of drugs with respect to spheroid maintenance and reproducibility of results [37]. A total of 3000 iRFP680-positive neuroblastoma cells were seeded into ULA 384-well plates. For CHLA-136, we additionally used 0.5% Matrigel to improve spheroid formation. Cells were centrifuged at 150× g for 10 min and incubated for 72 h at 37 °C and 5% CO_2. Spheroids were treated with the respective chemotherapeutic compound for 24 h, followed by the addition of 22,500 PBMCs with and without the anti-GD2 antibody DB and incubation for a further 216 h under cell culture conditions.

Image acquisition was performed every 8 h for 240 h (10 days), using the IncuCyte® SX5 live-cell analysis system. Spheroid viability was calculated as the ratio of integrated spheroid fluorescence intensity of every time point to fluorescence at baseline (0 h). Experiments were performed in six replicates, and viability is reported in %±SEM.

2.5. Flow Cytometry

2.5.1. Validation of Near Infrared Reporter (NIR) as Viability Marker

To validate NIR fluorescence (680 nm) from stable transduced NB tumor cells as the viability marker, flow cytometry analyses were performed by using 40,6-diamino-2-phenylindole (DAPI) (Merck KGaA, Darmstadt, Germany). For these analyses, 50% of the cells were lysed (65 °C, 5 min) to obtain samples with live and dead cells in an equal amount. Next, cells were incubated with a 0.1 mg/mL DAPI solution (Sigma-Aldrich, D9542) for 5 min prior to acquisition. For each sample, 20,000 cells were analyzed by using a BD CANTO II cytometer and FACS Diva software (BD Biosciences, San Jose, CA, USA). Data were analyzed with FlowJo V10 software (Ashland, OR, USA) analyzing the frequency of NIR- and DAPI-positive and -negative cells of all single cells.

2.5.2. Stress-Ligand Abundance on Chemotherapy-Treated Tumor Cells

For the analysis of the stress ligand abundance of chemotherapy-treated tumor cells, 1×10^6 live neuroblastoma cells were seeded into Petri dishes in 10 mL of respective medium and cultured for one day (37 °C/5% CO_2). Cells were treated with chemotherapy as described above and washed after 24 h. After 72 h, 1×10^6 live cells were washed and treated with Zombie NIR™ Fixable Viability Dye (Biolegend, RT, San Diego, CA, USA) according to the manufactures protocol. The cells were then incubated with the following antibodies: anti-human B7-H6-APC (mouse IgG1, clone 875001), ULBP-1-PerCP (mouse IgG2a, clone 170818), ULBP-2/5/6-Alexa Fluor® 405 (mouse IgG2a, clone 165903), ULBP-3-PE (mouse IgG2a, clone 166510) all from R & D Systems, 1:20 diluted, and MICA/MICB-PE-Cy7 (Biolegend, mouse IgG2a,κ, clone 6D4, 1:20). A total of 20,000 live cells were measured per sample. Due to chemotherapy-related changes of the autofluorescence, we determined the expression level of respective antigen according to the following formula: MFI of stained sample—MFI of unstained sample.

2.5.3. Immune Checkpoint Ligand Abundance on Chemotherapy-Treated Tumor Cells

Immune checkpoint ligand expression analysis by tumor cells was performed in analogy to the stress ligand expression analysis detailed above, using the following antibodies: anti-human CD80-BV421 (Biolegend, mouse IgG1,κ, clone 2D10, 1:20), CD86-PerCP-Vio 700 (Miltenyi Biotec, Bergisch Gladbach, REA968, 1:50), CD112-APC (Miltenyi Biotec, REA1195, 1:50), CD155-PE-Vio 770 (Miltenyi Biotec, REA1081, 1:50), Galectin-9-PE (Miltenyi Biotec, REA435, 1:50), and CD274 (PD-L1)-Vio Bright B515 (Miltenyi Biotec, REA1197, 1:50). The mouse IgG1,κ antibody-BV421 (Biolegend, clone MOPC-21) and respective REA controls (Miltenyi Biotec, REA293) were used as isotype controls.

2.5.4. NK Cell Activation after Chemotherapy Treatment

For the analysis of activating receptor expression by cytotoxic NK cells (CD3-; CD56dim), 5×10^6 human PBMCs were treated with the respective chemotherapeutic compound and incubated for 72 h (37 °C/5% CO_2). Then cells were harvested and 1×10^6 live cells were washed with wash buffer, followed by incubation with 10 µL of Tandem Signal Enhancer (Miltenyi Biotec). Incubation with the following antibodies in a total volume of 100 µL was conducted for 20 min at RT: CD3-VioGreen (REA613, 1:200), CD56-APC-Vio770 (REA196, 1:200), CD226-VioBlue (REA1040, 1:50); CD335 (NKp46)-Vio Bright B515

(REA808, 1:50), CD337 (NKp30)-PE (REA823, 1:75), CD336 (NKp44)-APC (REA1163, 1:75), and CD314 (NKG2D)-PE-Vio 770 (REA1228, 1:75), all from Miltenyi Biotec. As isotype controls served respective REA controls (Miltenyi Biotec, REA293). To exclude dead cells from analysis, 0.25 µg propidium iodide solution was added prior to acquisition. At least 20,000 CD3−/CD56+ cells were analyzed for each sample.

2.5.5. CD107a Degranulation Assay

First, 0.25×10^6 tumor cells LAN-1 and CHLA-20 and respective B7-H6 knockout cells generated as described below were seeded into a 24-well plate in 1 mL RPMI. After 24 h, cells were treated with etoposide (LAN-1) and carboplatin (CHLA-20) and washed after 24 h. After a further 48 h, medium was removed, and 2×10^6 PBMCs, including 2 µL Brefeldin A (Invitrogen, Waltham, MA, USA), 2 µL Monensin (Invitrogen), 1 µg/µL DB, and 2 µL CD107a-VBV515 (Miltenyi Biotec, REA792) in a total volume of 1 mL RPMI, were added. PBMCs without tumor cells and DB served as the control. Cells were incubated for 5 h under cell culture conditions. Then cells were stained by using Viobility™ 405/452 Fixable Dye (1:100 in 1× PBS, 15 min). Cells were fixed by using Inside Stain Kit (Miltenyi Biotec, 130-090-477) according to manufacturer's guidelines. A total of 10 µL of Tandem Signal Enhancer was added prior to cell-surface staining with CD3-VioGreen (REA613, 1:200), CD16-PerCP-Vio770 (REA423, 1:50), and CD56-APC-Vio770 (REA196, 1:200), all from Miltenyi Biotec and CD45-PE-Cy7 (BD Biosciences, mouse IgG1, clone J33, 1:300). After permeabilization, using an Inside Stain Kit, intracellular staining with INF-γ-APC (REA600, 1:50, 100 µL, 20 min) was performed. At least 20,000 CD45+/CD3−/CD56+ cells were analyzed for each sample.

2.6. CRISPR/CAS9 B7-H6 Knockout in Tumor Cells

To delete B7-H6 (NCR3LG1 locus), 1×10^6 tumor cells were transfected by using SF Cell Line Solution (Lonza, Switzerland) and program FF-120. Following DNA target sequences of the NCR3LG1, crRNAs were used: 5'-GTGTGTGGTACGGCATGCGT-3', 5'- TCACGTCTATGGGTATCACC-3', and 5'-CACCAAGAGGCATTCCGACC-3'. Successful abrogation of B7-H6 was shown via flow cytometry analysis and stable deletion was confirmed regularly (every four weeks).

2.7. Statistics

Differences between the groups were assessed by using ANOVA with Dunnett's post hoc test, if the assumption of normality was met (Shapiro–Wilk Test). Due to donor-dependent variability of PBMCs-dependent antitumor toxicity, the significant difference between the groups was analyzed by using repeated measurement ANOVA for individual data points. Statistical analysis was performed by using GraphPad Prism (version 9.4.1 for Windows, GraphPad Software, San Diego, CA, USA). Viability data are presented as mean ± SEM (standard error of the mean), and flow cytometry data are shown as individual data point with mean and SEM indicated.

3. Results

3.1. Establishment of a Long-Term Real-Time Viability Assay

We developed a long-term viability assay by using live-cell image acquisition and fluorescent tumor cells. First, the neuroblastoma cell lines LAN-1, CHLA-136, and CHLA-20 were transduced by using a lentiviral expression system to yield stable expression of the fluorescent near-infrared protein iRFP680 (NIR) used as viability staining [38]. Stable expression was confirmed by flow cytometry up to one month after transduction. Only cell lines with over 95% NIR+ cells were used. The correlation between viability and NIR-fluorescence status was confirmed with DAPI staining and analyzed by flow cytometry (Figure 1). NIR-fluorescence was an accurate marker for viability in over 95% of tumor cells analyzed (99.3%, 99.6%, and 97.6% were NIR+ and DAPI- or NIR- and DAPI+, for LAN-1, CHLA-20, and CHLA-136, respectively) (Figure 1A). Importantly, we found that the effects of chemotherapeutics used in concentrations realistic in the clinical setting were only measurable from day four after the start of the treatment, showing the requirement for long-term assays to assess effects (Figures 1B and 2A, cisplatin, Video S1–S3 for cisplatin + ADCC and controls in LAN-1).

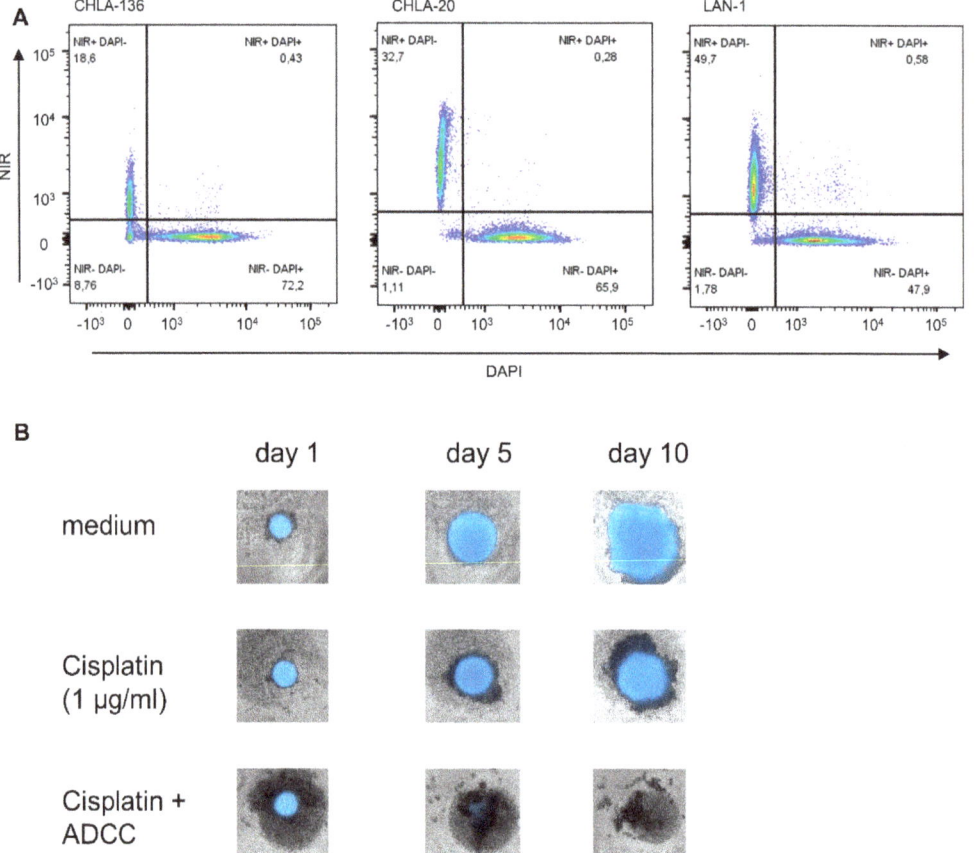

Figure 1. Establishment of a live-cell assay for analysis of long-term chemoimmunotherapeutic effects on tumor cell viability. (**A**) Flow cytometric analysis of neuroblastoma cells transduced to yield NIR-fluorescence (680 nm) used as viability marker. NIR+ cells were lysed, mixed with living cells, and subsequently stained with DAPI to confirm the correct discrimination of live and dead cells, using the NIR fluorescence. About 99.5% of live and dead cells could be correctly identified by using NIR-fluorescence: NIR-positive cells (live) were DAPI-negative, and NIR-negative cells (dead) were DAPI-positive. (**B**) Representative picture showing loss or gain of spheroid fluorescence intensity under therapy.

3.2. Effects of Chemotherapeutics on Antibody-Dependent Cellular Cytotoxicity (ADCC)

We investigated how chemotherapeutics affect the ADCC with DB (10 µg/mL) and effector cells (PBMCs (7.5×10^4 cells)) against established tumor spheroids generated from the three cell lines, using real-time viability assay over 10 days.

The chemotherapeutics used at clinically relevant concentrations combined with DB and effector cells (ADCC condition) had an up-to-17-fold-higher long-term antitumoral effect in this model ($p = 0.0029$). ADCC conditions also showed a delayed tumor growth that was stronger compared to the controls of chemotherapeutics combined with effector cells only (without DB; antibody-independent cellular cytotoxicity (AICC); see Figures 2 and 3).

This clearly indicates a DB-dependent and GD2 specific effect. The viability curves of AICC with and without chimeric isotype control (rituximab) were not different.

There was a differential pattern of efficacy depending on the cell line used to establish the spheroids. For instance, the chemoimmunotherapy with platin agents (cisplatin and carboplatin) significantly improved the antitumoral effects compared to chemotherapy alone or compared to chemotherapy with effector cell only (AICC) in LAN-1 and CHLA-20 spheroids, but to a lesser extent in CHLA-136 spheroids (3.6-, 2.8-, and 2.0-fold decrease in viability (at 10 d) versus AICC in combination with cisplatin, respectively; for overview, see Table 1). Cyclophosphamide significantly increased ADCC in LAN-1- and CHLA-20 spheroids but not in CHLA-136 (1.6-, 1.6-, and 0.8-fold decrease in viability compared to AICC + cyclophosphamide, respectively; see Figure 2A, right panel). This might be attributable to higher resistance of CHLA-136 against cyclophosphamide compared to LAN-1 and CHLA-20 (Figure 2C, right panel).

Table 1. Overview of viability in %±SEM after 240 h of respective treatment. Viability was calculated as total integrated NIR intensity after 240 h divided by total integrated NIR intensity at 0 h. Statistical difference was assessed by using repeated measure ANOVA; ** $p < 0.01$ vs. and * $p < 0.05$ for ADCC + chemotherapy vs. AICC + chemotherapy.

Cell Line	Therapeutics	Viability ± SEM (240 h in %Compared to 0 h)					Fold Decrease in Viability of ADCC + Chemotherapy vs.			p-Value
		Medium	Chemo.	ADCC	AICC + Chemo.	ADCC + Chemo.	Chemo.	ADCC	AICC + Chemo.	
LAN-1	carboplatin	1120 ± 96	877 ± 128	352 ± 106	615 ± 150	199 ± 85	4.4	1.8	3.1	** 0.0075
	cisplatin	1222 ± 107	399 ± 62	302 ± 119	276 ± 52	84 ± 58	4.7	3.6	3.3	** 0.0059
	4-HPC	962 ± 127	503 ± 48	426 ± 126	434.7 ± 87	265 ± 65	1.9	1.6	1.6	* 0.0317
	etoposide	930 ± 53	146 ± 29	309 ± 59	113 ± 27	17 ± 8	8.3	17.6	6.4	* 0.0178
	vincristine	1211 ± 95	397 ± 91	352 ± 107	306 ± 90	115 ± 47	3.5	3.1	2.7	* 0.0337
CHLA-20	carboplatin	958 ± 47	330 ± 75	428 ± 47	449 ± 69	100 ± 44	3.3	4.2	4.5	* 0.0204
	cisplatin	938 ± 41	399 ± 66	460 ± 77	387 ± 69	138 ± 61	2.9	3.3	2.8	** 0.0097
	4-HPC	673 ± 41	408 ± 19	409 ± 66	319 ± 3.2	204 ± 6.4	2.0	2.0	1.6	* 0.0013
	etoposide	917 ± 40	762 ± 71	436 ± 67	587 ± 78	413 ± 49	1.8	1.1	1.4	0.0653
	vincristine	1039 ± 62	765 ± 77	479 ± 64	579 ± 50	261 ± 72	2.9	1.8	2.2	** 0.0040
CHLA-136	carboplatin	454 ± 33	348 ± 31	248 ± 64	228 ± 39	164 ± 43.6	2.1	1.5	1.4	** 0.0045
	cisplatin	415 ± 54	304 ± 31	192 ± 77	188 ± 100	93 ± 46	3.3	2.1	2.0	0.1796
	4-HPC	334 ± 53	327 ± 26	100 ± 67	93 ± 48	110 ± 57	0.9	1.0	0.8	0.9215
	etoposide	400 ± 24	203 ± 16.4	227 ± 52	105 ± 15	54 ± 19.6	3.7	4.6	2.9	0.0954
	vincristine	414 ± 34	358 ± 33	305 ± 77	233 ± 24	230 ± 42	1.6	1.1	1.0	0.9995

Chemoimmunotherapy with etoposide was highly effective against LAN-1 and CHLA-136 spheroids (6.4- and 2.9-fold decrease in viability compared to AICC in combination with etoposide; see Figure 3A,C), whereas CHLA-20 spheroids were too sensitive to etoposide with PBMCs to allow for a differentiation between chemoimmunotherapy with AICC and ADCC, even at low concentrations of etoposide (0.1 µg/mL, 1.4-fold decrease; see Figure 3B). Chemoimmunotherapy with vincristine was significantly more effective in LAN-1 and CHLA-20 spheroids, but not in CHLA-136-spheroids (Figure 3A–C) (2.7-, 2.2-, and 1.0-fold decrease in viability compared to AICC + vincristine, respectively; see Figure 3A–C, right panel).

In conclusion, chemotherapeutics used in induction regimens combined with DB and effector cells showed superior effects against neuroblastoma spheroids compared to the respective controls.

3.3. Chemotherapy-Induced Stress Ligands on Tumor Cells

To further investigate the reasons for the observed improved antitumor effects of chemoimmunotherapy compared to monotherapy controls, we investigated the induction of stress ligands involved in NK-cell activation (B7-H6, ULBP 1–3 and MICA/B) three days after chemotherapy, using flow cytometry.

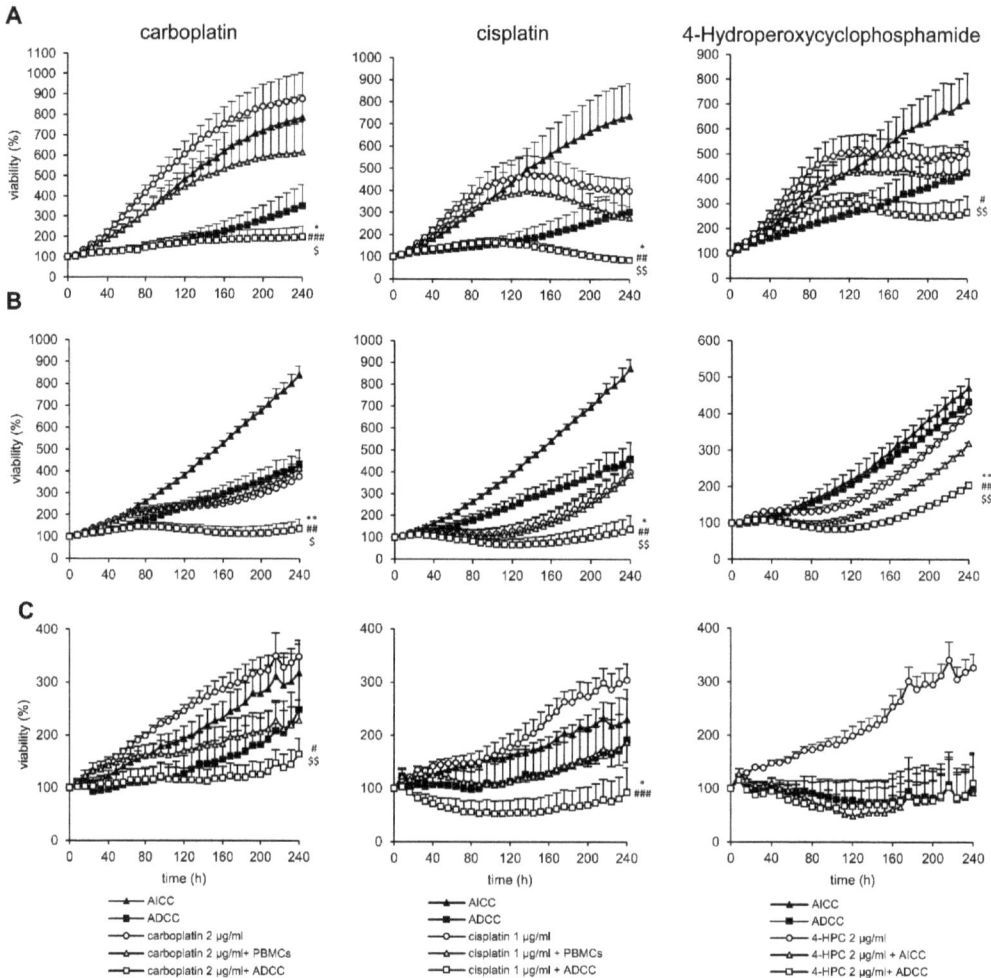

Figure 2. Impact of 2 μg/mL carboplatin and 1 μg/mL cisplatin and cyclophosphamide (4-Hydroperoxycyclophosphamide) on ADCC against the chemotherapy resistant cell line (**A**) LAN-1, (**B**) CHLA-20, and (**C**) CHLA-136. Tumor cells were transduced with a gene coding for near-infrared fluorescent protein (iRFP680) to track viability. To establish stable spheroids, 3000 tumor cells/well were seeded into a 384-well plate and cultivated for three days under cell culture conditions. Spheroids were then treated with their respective chemotherapies, which were removed after 24 h, or PBMCs or the anti-GD2 antibody DB and incubated for a further seven days. Viability was calculated as total integrated spheroid fluorescence of the respective time point divided by the total fluorescence at time point 0 h. Graphs show viability of spheroids treated with or without chemotherapy (black line, white or black marker, respectively), PBMCs alone (solid triangle), ADCC (solid square). Data are shown as means from four independent experiments (performed in six replicates) ± SEM. Endpoint (240 h). Viability data of ADCC (*), chemotherapy (#), and chemotherapy + AICC ($) vs. chemotherapy + ADCC were compared by using repeated measures ANOVA; ** $p < 0.01$; * $p < 0.05$ vs. ADCC; ### $p < 0.001$; ## $p < 0.01$; # $p < 0.05$ vs. chemotherapy; $$ $p < 0.01$; $ $p < 0.05$ vs. chemotherapy + ADCC.

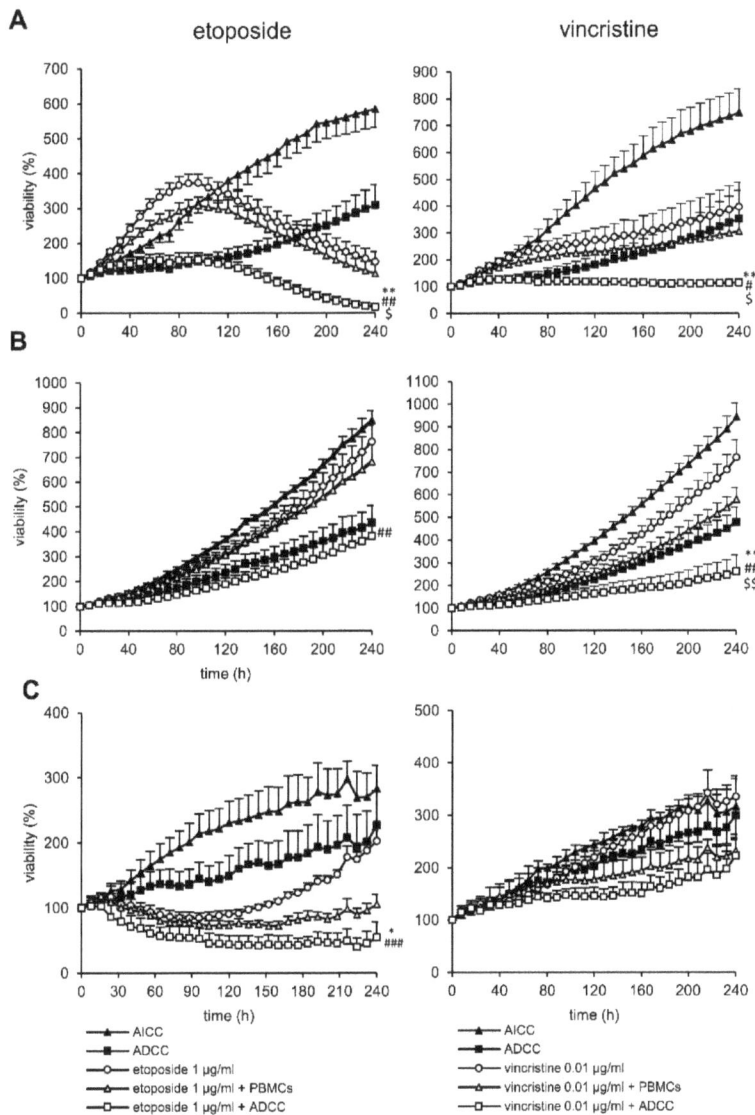

Figure 3. Impact of 0.1 (CHLA-20) –1 µg/mL etoposide (LAN-1 and CHLA-136) and 0,05 µg/mL vincristine on ADCC against the chemotherapy resistant neuroblastoma cells (**A**) LAN-1, (**B**) CHLA-20, and (**C**) CHLA-136. Tumor cells were transduced with a gene coding for near-infrared fluorescent protein (iRFP680) to track viability. To establish stable spheroids, 3000 tumor cells/well were seeded into a 384-well plate and cultivated for three days under cell culture conditions. Spheroids were then treated with respective chemotherapy, which was removed after 24 h, or PBMCs or with the anti-GD2 antibody DB, and incubated for a further seven days. Viability was calculated as total integrated spheroid fluorescence of the respective time point divided by the total fluorescence at time point 0 h. Graphs show viability of spheroids treated with or without chemotherapy (black line, white or black marker, respectively), PBMCs alone (solid triangle), ADCC (solid square). Data are shown as means from four independent experiments ± SEM. Endpoint (240 h). Viability data of ADCC (*), chemotherapy (#), and chemotherapy + AICC ($) vs. chemotherapy + ADCC were compared by using repeated measures ANOVA; ** $p < 0.01$; * $p < 0.05$ vs. ADCC; ### $p < 0.001$; ## $p < 0.01$; # $p < 0.05$ vs. chemotherapy; $$ $p < 0.01$; $ $p < 0.05$ vs. chemotherapy + ADCC.

All cell lines showed a measurable B7-H6 (NKp30 ligand) but low ULBP and MICA/B (NKG2D ligands) baseline cell surface abundance (Figure 4). The pattern of chemotherapy-dependent induction of stress ligands was cell-line specific. In LAN-1, the NKp30 ligand B7-H6 was significantly increased by cisplatin, etoposide, and cyclophosphamide treatment compared to controls (2.3-, 2.0-, and 1.5-fold; $p < 0.0001$, <0.0001, and $p = 0.0111$, respectively), in CHLA-20 by carboplatin, cisplatin, and etoposide (1.2-, 1.2-, and 1.4-fold, $p = 0.024$, 0.0041, and 0.113, respectively) and in CHLA-136 by cisplatin (1.3-fold, $p = 0.0129$) (Figure 4A). This is in line with a higher level of antitumor toxicity by DB, immune cells, and platin compounds compared to the platin compounds and AICC (Figure 2).

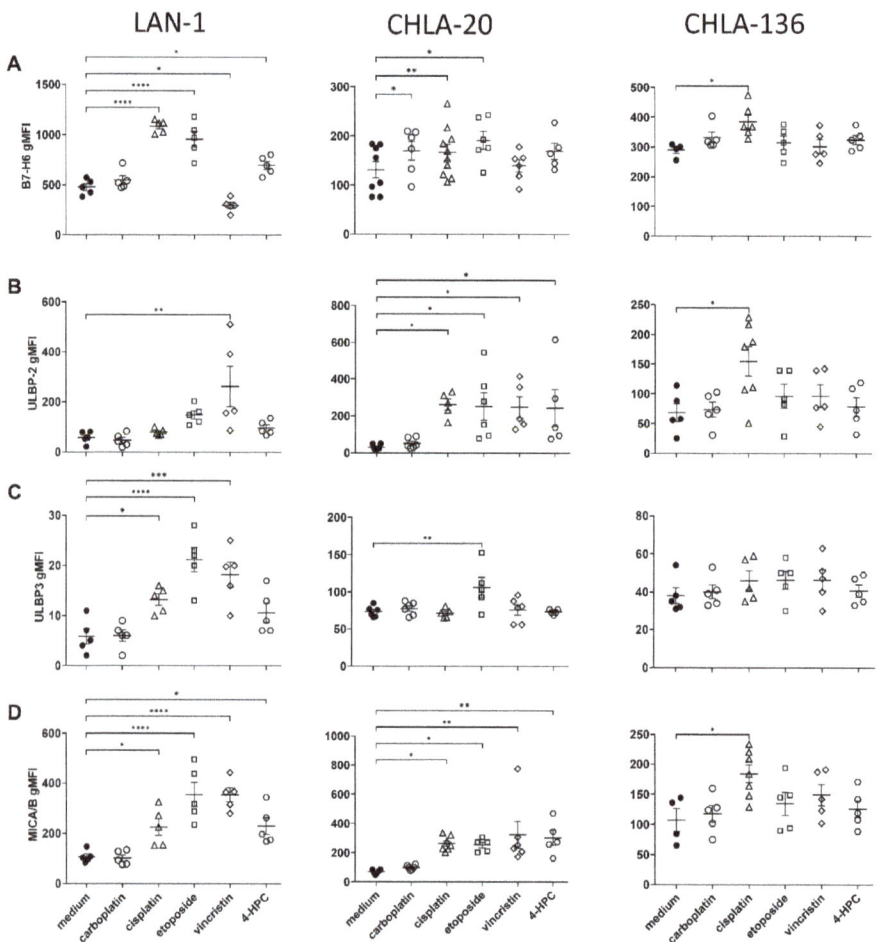

Figure 4. Chemotherapy-induced stress-ligand surface abundance on tumor cells: 1×10^6 tumor cells treated for 24 h under cell culture conditions with either carboplatin (2 µg/mL, open circles), cisplatin (1 µg/mL, open triangles) etoposide (0.5 µg/mL, open squares), vincristine (0.05 µg/mL, open diamonds), or the cyclophosphamide metabolite 4-hydroperoxycyclophosphamide (1 µg/mL, open hexagons). After 72 h of culturing, LAN-1 (left panel), CHLA-20 (center), and CHLA-136 (right panel) were analyzed for surface abundance of (**A**) B7-H6, (**B**) ULBP2, (**C**) ULBP-3, and (**D**) MICA/B, using flow cytometry. Data represent at least five biological replicates. Means and SEM are indicated as black lines and error bars, respectively. For statistical analysis, ANOVA with appropriate post hoc test was used; * $p < 0.05$, ** $p < 0.01$, *** $p < 0.001$, and **** $p < 0.0001$ vs. untreated control (medium).

We found a differential induction of the NKG2D ligands ULBP2, ULBP-3, and MICA/B in all three cell lines (Figure 4B–D). Interestingly, all chemotherapeutics except carboplatin significantly increased ULBP-2 and MICA/B in CHLA-20 and in LAN-1 (up to 4.5- (vincristine) and 3.3- (etoposide) and up to 9- (cisplatin) and 4.5-fold (cyclophosphamide). We mainly observed effects on ULBP3 abundance after cisplatin, etoposide, and vincristine treatment (up to 3.6-fold increase).

Overall, most chemotherapeutics elicited a stress response in LAN-1 and in CHLA-20. However, only cisplatin significantly affected CHLA-136 stress-ligand surface abundance (B7-H6, ULBP-2, and MICA/B, up to 2.3-fold increase).

3.4. Chemotherapy Increased Immune Checkpoint Ligand Surface Abundance

We investigated chemotherapy effects on the expression of PD-L1 (PD-1), CD86 (CTLA-4), CD155 (TIGIT), and Gal-9 (TIM-3) immune checkpoint ligands by neuroblastoma cells (Figure 5). In LAN-1, etoposide showed the strongest effects on all checkpoint ligands analyzed (2.6-, 4.1-, 3.3-, and 5.2-fold increase for PD-L1, CD86, CD155, and Gal-9, $p < 0.0001$ respectively). Cisplatin had a significant impact on PD-L1, CD155, and Gal-9 but not on CD86 (2.3-, 2.7-, and 3.1-fold increase; $p = 0.0115$, $p < 0.0001$, and $p = 0.0998$), vincristine significantly elevated CD86 and Gal9 expression (3.0- and 3.3-fold increase; $p = 0.0002$ and $p < 0.0001$), whereas cyclophosphamide increased the expression of CD155 and Gal-9 (2.1- and 3.1-fold increase, $p < 0.0001$).

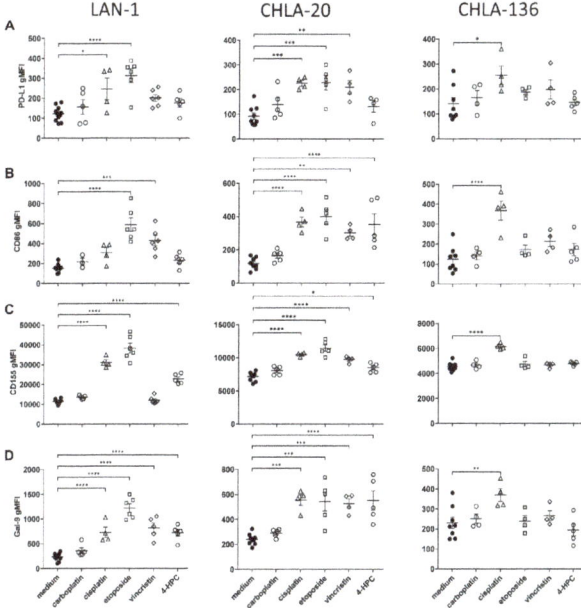

Figure 5. Chemotherapy-induced immune-checkpoint ligand-cell surface abundance on tumor cells. 1×10^6 tumor cells treated for 24 h under cell culture conditions with either carboplatin (2 µg/mL, open circles), cisplatin (1 µg/mL, open triangles), etoposide (0.5 µg/mL, open squares), vincristine (0.05 µg/mL, open diamonds), or the cyclophosphamide metabolite 4-HPC (1 µg/mL, open hexagons). After 72 h of culturing, LAN-1 (left panel), CHLA-20 (center), and CHLA-136 (right panel) were analyzed for surface abundance of (**A**) PD-L1, (**B**) CD86, (**C**) CD155, and (**D**) Gal-9, using flow cytometry. Data represent at least five biological replicates. Means and SEM are indicated as black lines and error bars, respectively. For statistical analysis, ANOVA with appropriate post hoc test was used; * $p < 0.05$ vs., ** $p < 0.01$, *** $p < 0.001$, and **** $p < 0.0001$ versus untreated control (medium).

CHLA-20 cells also revealed a strong induction of immune checkpoints by all chemotherapeutics, except for carboplatin (up to 2.4-fold increase, cisplatin, Gal-9, $p = 0.0002$; see Figure 5A–D). Interestingly, and in line with the stress-ligand results, we only observed a cisplatin-dependent rise in PD-L1, CD86, CD155, and Gal9 surface abundance on CHLA-136 tumor cells (1.7-, 2.8-, 1.6-, and 1.3-fold increase; $p = 0.0222$, $p < 0.0001$, $p < 0.0001$, and $p = 0.0093$, respectively).

These data indicate that checkpoint ligand expression also correlates with the tumor stress response following chemotherapy.

3.5. Effects of Chemotherapy on Activating NK Cell Receptors

To further evaluate the immunological effects of chemotherapy on NK cells, we determined the percentage of cytotoxic NK cells (CD56^{dim}) in lymphocytes and measured activating NK cell receptors (NKp30, NKp44, NKG2D, and CD226) for the reported stress ligands by flow cytometry. Etoposide and cyclophosphamide significantly reduced cytotoxic NK cell abundance compared to the medium control (1.64 ± 0.26%, 0.89 ± 0.17% vs. 8.17 ± 0.73% in live lymphocytes, respectively; see Figure 6A), whereas vincristine treatment significantly increased the NK-cell number (10.04 ± 1.7%, Figure 6A). Most chemotherapeutics did not affect stress-ligand receptors (Figure 6B,C). However, etoposide and cyclophosphamide significantly increased NKp44 expression (1.66- and 2.2-fold increase; see Figure 6B,D), whereas NKp46 and CD226 were significantly decreased by etoposide and vincristine treatment (1.41- and 1.47-fold decrease, respectively; see Figure 6B,C,E).

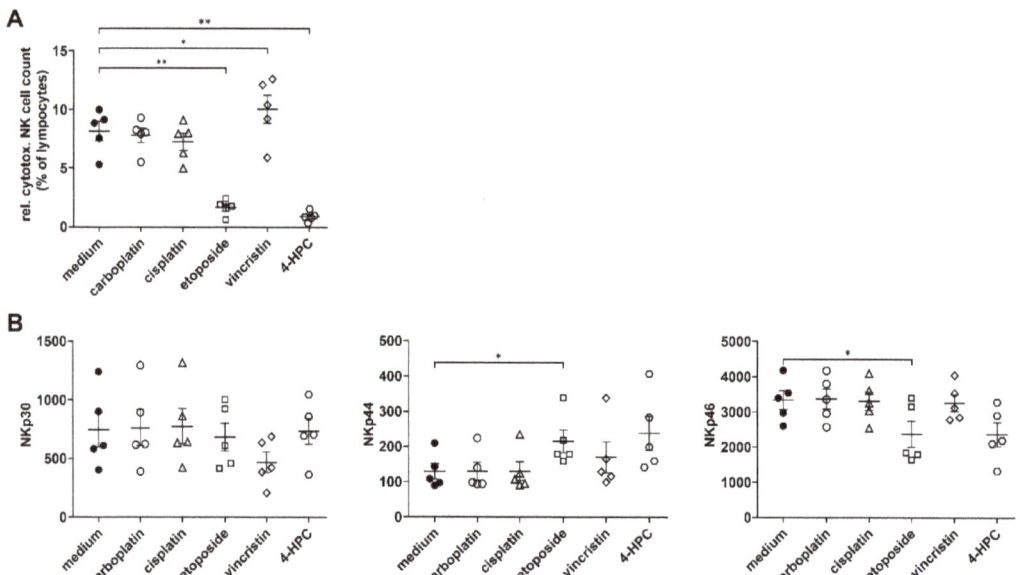

Figure 6. *Cont.*

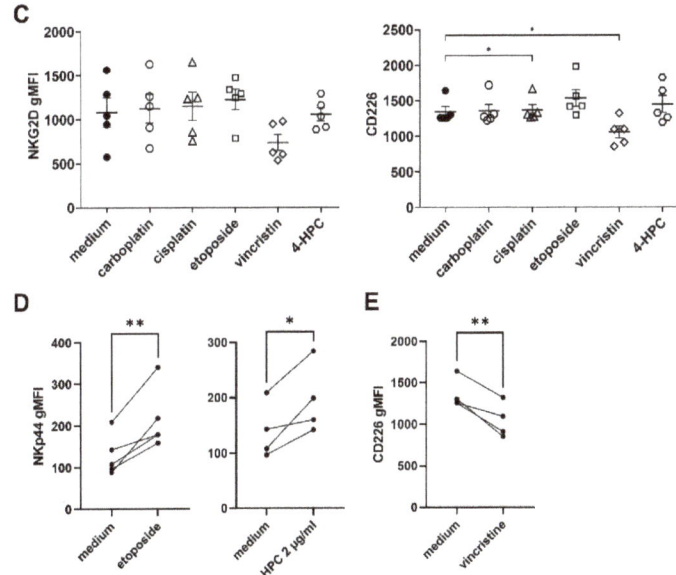

Figure 6. Impact of chemotherapy on percentage of (**A**) cytotoxic NK cells of lymphocytes and NK-cell-specific activating receptors. (**B–E**) 5×10^6 PBMCs were treated for 24 h under cell culture conditions with either carboplatin (2 µg/mL, open circles), cisplatin (1 µg/mL, open triangles), etoposide (0.5 µg/mL, open squares), vincristine (0.05 µg/mL, open diamonds), or the cyclophosphamide metabolite (4-HPC, 1 µg/mL, open hexagons). After 72 h of culturing, cells were analyzed for NKp30, NKp44, NKp46, NKG2D, and CD226 expression, using flow cytometry. (**A**) Relative number of cytotoxic NK cells (CD3$^-$, CD56^{dim}) in lymphocytes. (**B–E**) Geometric mean fluorescence intensity (gMFI) of respective activating receptor of cytotoxic NK cells after chemotherapy. Data represent at least four biological replicates. Means and SEM are indicated as black lines and error bars, respectively. For statistical analysis, repeated measures ANOVA with appropriate post hoc test was used; * $p < 0.05$ vs., ** $p < 0.01$ versus untreated control (medium).

In conclusion, etoposide and cyclophosphamide increased the activating receptor NKp44, and vincristine increased the number of cytotoxic NK cells, indicating an immunological impact of etoposide, cyclophosphamide, and vincristine on NK cells.

3.6. Role of Stress Ligands in Chemotherapy-Mediated Antitumor Efficacy of the Anti-GD2 Treatment

B7-H6 stress ligand and NKp30 receptor engagement have been shown to play a crucial role in NK-cell activation. Therefore, we deleted the B7-H6 gene in LAN-1 and CHLA-20 cells to investigate the role of B7-H6 interaction in the cytotoxicity of chemoimmunotherapy in our model (Figure 7).

Since chemoimmunotherapy with carboplatin showed a strong effect compared to ADCC controls (Figure 2B) and carboplatin exclusively increased B7-H6 surface abundance (Figure 4A, center), we tested the hypothesis that a B7-H6 knockout (KO) in CHLA-20 cells will reverse some of the beneficial effects of the carboplatin-based chemoimmunotherapy. Additionally, we investigated the impact of a B7-H6-KO in LAN-1 cells treated with etoposide-based chemoimmunotherapy, as this was highly effective (Figure 3A), and etoposide treatment activated all stress ligands analyzed in wild-type LAN-1 cells (Figure 4A–C left panel).

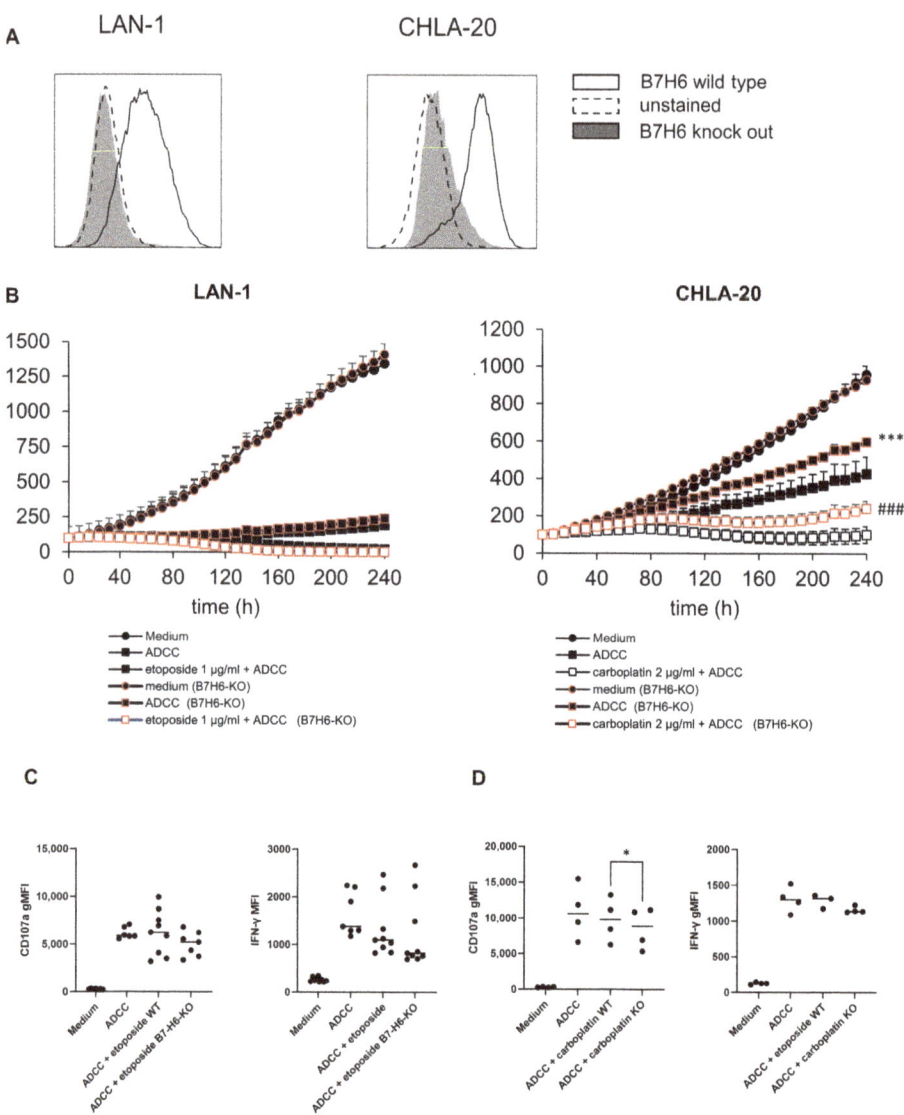

Figure 7. Role of chemotherapy-induced stress ligands in NK cell activation. B7H6 was deleted by using CRISPR/CAS9 system, and (**A**) successful knock out was confirmed by flow cytometry. The data represent means of at least three independent experiments. (**B**) Graphs show viability of spheroids treated with or without chemotherapy (black line, white or black marker, respectively), PBMCs alone (solid triangle), ADCC (solid square). Viability data for B7-H6-KO cells are shown with red bordered markers. (**C**,**D**) CD107a and IFN-γ degranulation assay was performed after 24 h chemotherapy with etoposide (**C**, LAN-1) and carboplatin (**D**, CHLA-20) and three days overall incubation. Then 5×10^6 PBMCs were co-incubated with 1×10^6 tumor cells, followed by flow cytometric analysis of NK cells (CD45$^+$, CD3$^-$, CD56^{dim}), using degranulation (CD107a) and activation marker (IFN-γ). Difference between viability after 240 h ADCC (wild type) vs. ADCC (B7-H6-KO) and ADCC (wild type) + chemotherapy vs. ADCC + chemotherapy (B7-H6-KO) was assessed by using paired t-test. (**A**) *** $p < 0.001$ vs. ADCC and $^{\#\#\#}$ $p \leq 0.001$ vs. chemoimmunotherapy (wild type). (**B**) *** $p < 0.001$ vs. ADCC and $^{\#\#\#}$ $p < 0.001$ vs. chemoimmunotherapy. (**D**) * $p < 0.05$ vs. chemoimmunotherapy (wild type).

Indeed, we found that the B7-H6-KO of CHLA-20 cells significantly reversed the chemoimmunotherapy effect of cisplatin, carboplatin and vincristine compared to the wildtype control (Figure 7B, right panel; and Supplementary Figure S1). Since the viability was also improved under ADCC conditions in B7-H6 KO-cells, the effect was mainly attributable to the B7-H6-KO.

In contrast, LAN-1 cells did not show any dependency on B7-H6 (Figure 7B left panel). In summary, we found a partial B7-H6-dependency in CHLA-20 but not in LAN-1 maybe due to strong checkpoint induction after chemoimmunotherapy (Figure 2A–D, left panel).

3.7. Antibody-Mediated NK Cell Activation

To further investigate whether checkpoint- and stress-ligand-induction affect NK cell activation, we measured the activation of NK cells by means of degranulation (CD107a) and IFN-γ production, using flow cytometry, as described in the Materials and Methods section. For that, we cultured the PBMCs of healthy donors for 5 h with DB and LAN-1- and CHLA-20 tumor cells (wild type and B7-H6-KO) pretreated with etoposide and carboplatin, respectively. The ADCC conditions showed a strong NK cell degranulation (CD107a) and activation (IFN-γ) (Figure 7).

The chemotherapy-treated tumor cells did not enhance NK cell activation compared to untreated LAN-1 and CHLA-20 cells (Figure 7C,D). Indeed, the activation of NK cells against LAN-1 with B7-H6-KO was markedly, but not significantly, decreased, and against CHLA-20, B7-H6-KO was significantly reduced (Figure 6C, $p = 0.0831$; and Figure 7D, $p = 0.0265$). Overall, we could not observe a stronger activation of NK cells by chemotherapy-treated compared to untreated tumor cells.

4. Discussion

We evaluated the effects of chemotherapeutics currently used in the standard induction regimen to treat patients with HR-NB in combination with the anti-GD2 antibody DB against spheroids generated from tumor cells derived from patients with progressive disease. Antitumor efficacy of chemoimmunotherapy was superior compared to the chemotherapy or DB in the presence of immune effector cells (ADCC) alone (up to 17-fold decrease in viability compared to ADCC; see Figures 5 and 6 and Table 1). Our data provide preclinical proof-of-concept for a combined use of chemotherapy with anti-GD2 antibodies against neuroblastoma.

We developed a spheroid viability assay that allowed us to measure the long-term effects of the chemotherapeutic compound at clinically relevant concentrations (Figure 1). Live-cell microscopy using fluorescent tumor cells provides the advantage of undisturbed long-term viability analysis. Our approach circumvents the common problem of short-term viability assays that lead to EC50 values that are too high to be achieved in patients [22]. Additionally, a spheroid represents a model that is closer to the clinical reality compared to 2D models [26]. The architecture of a spheroid provides a nutrition and oxygen gradient that can result in the development of cancer-stem-like cells that represent a chemotherapy resistant subgroup of high clinical relevance [39]. However, this model can be further improved by incorporating multiple cell types, such as cancer-associated fibroblast and myeloid-derived suppressor cells to mimic an inhibitory tumor microenvironment [30]. The spheroid model used here is limited, as it does not reflect anti-angiogenic effects of chemotherapy and the role of fluidic shear stress in metastasis [28,40,41]. Despite these limitations, we have shown that a long-term spheroid viability assay is an appropriate tool to analyze combined effects of chemotherapy with antibody-dependent NK-cell-mediated tumor-cell lysis (Figures 2 and 3).

NK cells are the main effector cells mediating the effect of DB, and the activation of NK cells depends on an equilibrium of inhibitory receptors [42], such as killer-cell immunoglobulin-like receptors (KIRs) and PD-1, as well as activating receptors, such as NKGD2 and NKp30 [15], binding to the stress ligands ULBPs and MICA/B, as well as B7-H6, respectively.

The induction of stress ligands on neuroblastoma cells (Figure 4) and, to a lesser extent, of activating receptors on NK cells (Figure 6) might explain the synergistic efficacy of the chemoimmunotherapy (Figures 2 and 3). In line with that, it has been shown that B7-H6 sensitizes HEK293 cells for NK cell-mediated cytotoxicity [16]. Since NKp30 plays a crucial role in NK-cell activation and tumor surveillance, the increased expression of its cognate ligand B7-H6 by chemotherapeutics enhances NK cell-mediated ADCC against tumor cells [43].

However, we also found a chemotherapy-dependent induction of the checkpoint ligand expression on neuroblastoma, namely PD-L1, CD86, CD155, and Gal-9 (up to 5-fold increase vs. control; see Figure 5). Checkpoint ligand expression correlates with poor survival attributed to inhibition of immune surveillance [44]. This observation suggests that we consider checkpoint inhibitors in chemoimmunotherapy concepts. Another limiting aspect for chemoimmunotherapy may be the effects of chemotherapy on NK cell viability that might directly impact the efficacy of an ADCC-based immunotherapy. For instance, in a clinical study in acute lymphoblastic leukemia that also includes vincristine treatment, the total lymphocyte rate was reduced 18 months after maintenance chemotherapy [45]. Here, platin agents did not negatively affect cytotoxic NK cell count and vincristine even increased the NK cell to lymphocyte ratio (Figure 6A). In contrast, etoposide and cyclophosphamide reduced the number of cytotoxic NK cells (Figure 6A). However, etoposide and cyclophosphamide significantly increased the activating receptor NKp44 levels on cytotoxic NK-cells (Figure 6B,D). Importantly, NKp44, but not NKp30 and NKp46, is an activation marker for cytotoxic NK cells (Figure 6B,D) [46,47].

This underlines the ambiguous effect of chemotherapy with beneficial but also detrimental consequences for immunotherapy, which is dependent on a functional immune effector cells [48]. In light of the encouraging in vitro effects observed here, it remains crucial to evaluate this concept in patients.

In addition to effects of chemotherapy on NK cells and the role of immune checkpoint pathways, the inhibitory tumor microenvironment and inhibitory leukocyte populations have to be considered for a more comprehensive picture of a DB-based chemoimmunotherapy in HR-NB.

Despite a substantial increase of checkpoint ligands during chemotherapy (Figure 5), we could demonstrate that chemoimmunotherapy with DB improved efficacy in our models (Figures 2 and 3). Regardless of the much weaker stress response in CHLA-136 spheroids compared to LAN-1 and CHLA-20 spheroids, chemoimmunotherapy with cisplatin and etoposide was more effective compared to the monotherapies. CHLA-136 spheroids showed higher resistance toward cyclophosphamide and vincristine, and, consequently, these agents did not further improve the ADCC effect.

Finally, we observed that ADCC was partially B7-H6-stress-ligand dependent (Figure 7B). However, we could not find evidence to support the hypothesis that chemotherapy-induced stress ligands improved ADCC (Figure 7C). This might be attributable to the observed strong induction of checkpoint ligand expression found in tumor cells after chemotherapy. Accordingly, we and others showed that PD-L1 was also elevated by ADCC and IFN-γ via JAK/STAT signaling [49]. On top of that, chemotherapy can increase NFκB-signaling, which, in turn, can elevate PD-L1 expression [50,51]. Intriguingly, NFκB is a transcription factor that also positively regulates GD3-synthase and, therefore, GD2-abundance in cancer stem cells [52]. Increased NFκB expression might therefore lead to higher GD2 abundance and increased susceptibility toward anti-GD2 treatment, which is subject to further research.

5. Conclusions

In conclusion, chemotherapy used in European chemotherapy induction regimens for HR-NB combined with antibody-based immunotherapy can effectively eradicate tumor spheroids derived from relapsed/refractory patients. Our results encourage the implementation of DB in the induction therapy in future clinical trials.

Supplementary Materials: The following supporting information can be downloaded at https://www.mdpi.com/xxx/s1. Figure S1: B7-H6-KO results for CHLA-20. Video S1: Spheroid viability medium control. Video S2: Spheroid viability during cisplatin chemotherapy. Video S3: Spheroid viability during chemoimmunotherapy (cisplatin + ADCC).

Author Contributions: Conceptualization, H.N.L. and S.T.-M.; Methodology, S.T.-M., P.G., H.F., C.M., M.Z. and S.B.; Validation, S.T.-M. and H.N.L.; Formal Analysis, S.T.-M. and L.M.; Investigation, S.T.-M. and L.M.; Resources, H.N.L.; Data Curation, M.Z. and N.S.; Writing—Original Draft Preparation, S.T.-M.; Writing—Review and Editing, H.N.L., N.S., M.Z., P.G., H.F., C.M., S.B. and L.M.; Visualization, S.T.-M.; Supervision, H.N.L.; Project Administration, S.T.-M.; Funding Acquisition, S.T.-M., H.N.L. and N.S. All authors have read and agreed to the published version of the manuscript.

Funding: This research was funded by H.W. & J. Hector Stiftung, Germany, under Grant M2116; and Deutsche Forschungsgemeinschaft, under Grant SI 2147.

Institutional Review Board Statement: All procedures involving human participants were in accordance with the ethical standards of the institutional and national research committee and with the 1964 Helsinki declaration and its later amendments or comparable ethical standards. Blood samples were provided by the department of transfusion medicine of the University Medicine Greifswald. Informed consent was obtained from all participants (Ethics Board of the Medical Faculty of the University Greifswald, approval code number: BB 014/14, 24 January 2014).

Informed Consent Statement: Informed consent was obtained from all subjects involved in the study.

Data Availability Statement: The data that support the findings of this study are available from the corresponding author (H.L) upon reasonable request.

Conflicts of Interest: The authors declare no conflict of interest.

References

1. Park, J.R.; Eggert, A.; Caron, H. Neuroblastoma: Biology, Prognosis, and Treatment. *Hematol./Oncol. Clin. N. Am.* **2010**, *24*, 65–86. [CrossRef] [PubMed]
2. Ladenstein, R.; Pötschger, U.; Pearson, A.D.; Brock, P.; Luksch, R.; Castel, V.; Yaniv, I.; Papadakis, V.; Laureys, G.; Malis, J.; et al. Busulfan and melphalan versus carboplatin, etoposide, and melphalan as high-dose chemotherapy for high-risk neuroblastoma (HR-NBL1/SIOPEN): An international, randomised, multi-arm, open-label, phase 3 trial. *Lancet Oncol.* **2017**, *18*, 500–514. [CrossRef] [PubMed]
3. Ladenstein, R.; Pötschger, U.; Valteau-Couanet, D.; Luksch, R.; Castel, V.; Ash, S.; Laureys, G.; Brock, P.; Michon, J.M.; Owens, C.; et al. Investigation of the Role of Dinutuximab Beta-Based Immunotherapy in the SIOPEN High-Risk Neuroblastoma 1 Trial (HR-NBL1). *Cancers* **2020**, *12*, 309. [CrossRef] [PubMed]
4. Mody, R.; Alice, L.Y.; Naranjo, A.; Zhang, F.F.; London, W.B.; Shulkin, B.L.; Parisi, M.T.; Diccianni, M.B.; Hank, J.A.; Felder, M.; et al. Irinotecan, Temozolomide, and Dinutuximab With GM-CSF in Children With Refractory or Relapsed Neuroblastoma: A Report From the Children's Oncology Group. *J. Clin. Oncol.* **2020**, *38*, 2160–2169. [CrossRef]
5. Van de Velde, M.E.; Panetta, J.C.; Wilhelm, A.J.; van den Berg, M.H.; van der Sluis, I.M.; van den Bos, C.; Abbink, F.C.; van den Heuvel-Eibrink, M.M.; Segers, H.; Chantrain, C.; et al. Population Pharmacokinetics of Vincristine Related to Infusion Duration and Peripheral Neuropathy in Pediatric Oncology Patients. *Cancers* **2020**, *12*, 1789. [CrossRef]
6. Ladenstein, R.; Valteau-Couanet, D.; Brock, P.; Yaniv, I.; Castel, V.; Laureys, G.; Malis, J.; Papadakis, V.; Lacerda, A.; Ruud, E.; et al. Randomized Trial of prophylactic granulocyte colony-stimulating factor during rapid COJEC induction in pediatric patients with high-risk neuroblastoma: The European HR-NBL1/SIOPEN study. *J. Clin. Oncol.* **2010**, *28*, 3516–3524. [CrossRef]
7. Danna, E.A.; Sinha, P.; Gilbert, M.; Clements, V.K.; Pulaski, B.A.; Ostrand-Rosenberg, S. Surgical removal of primary tumor reverses tumor-induced immunosuppression despite the presence of metastatic disease. *Cancer Res.* **2004**, *64*, 2205–2211. [CrossRef]
8. Zitvogel, L.; Apetoh, L.; Ghiringhelli, F.; André, F.; Tesniere, A.; Kroemer, G. The anticancer immune response: Indispensable for therapeutic success? *J. Clin. Investig.* **2008**, *118*, 1991–2001. [CrossRef]
9. Zitvogel, L.; Apetoh, L.; Ghiringhelli, F.; Kroemer, G. Immunological aspects of cancer chemotherapy. *Nat. Rev. Immunol.* **2008**, *8*, 59–73. [CrossRef]
10. Zitvogel, L.; Kepp, O.; Kroemer, G. Immune parameters affecting the efficacy of chemotherapeutic regimens. *Nat. Rev. Clin. Oncol.* **2011**, *8*, 151–160. [CrossRef]
11. Beyranvand Nejad, E.; van der Sluis, T.C.; van Duikeren, S.; Yagita, H.; Janssen, G.M.; van Veelen, P.A.; Melief, C.J.; van der Burg, S.H.; Arens, R. Tumor Eradication by Cisplatin Is Sustained by CD80/86-Mediated Costimulation of CD8+ T Cells. *Cancer Res.* **2016**, *76*, 6017–6029. [CrossRef] [PubMed]

12. Mathew, M.; Enzler, T.; Shu, C.A.; Rizvi, N.A. Combining chemotherapy with PD-1 blockade in NSCLC. *Pharmacol. Ther.* **2018**, *186*, 130–137. [CrossRef] [PubMed]
13. Zingoni, A.; Fionda, C.; Borrelli, C.; Cippitelli, M.; Santoni, A.; Soriani, A. Natural Killer Cell Response to Chemotherapy-Stressed Cancer Cells: Role in Tumor Immunosurveillance. *Front. Immunol.* **2017**, *8*, 1194. [CrossRef]
14. Caligiuri, M.A. Human natural killer cells. *Blood* **2008**, *112*, 461–469. [CrossRef]
15. Vivier, E.; Tomasello, E.; Baratin, M.; Walzer, T.; Ugolini, S. Functions of natural killer cells. *Nat. Immunol.* **2008**, *9*, 503–510. [CrossRef]
16. Cao, G.; Wang, J.; Zheng, X.; Wei, H.; Tian, Z.; Sun, R. Tumor Therapeutics Work as Stress Inducers to Enhance Tumor Sensitivity to Natural Killer (NK) Cell Cytolysis by Up-regulating NKp30 Ligand B7-H6*. *J. Biol. Chem.* **2015**, *290*, 29964–29973. [CrossRef]
17. Simon, T.; Hero, B.; Schulte, J.H.; Deubzer, H.; Hundsdoerfer, P.; von Schweinitz, D.; Fuchs, J.; Schmidt, M.; Prasad, V.; Krug, B.; et al. 2017 GPOH Guidelines for Diagnosis and Treatment of Patients with Neuroblastic Tumors. *Klin. Padiatr.* **2017**, *229*, 147–167. [CrossRef] [PubMed]
18. Choi, S.H.; Jung, D.; Kim, K.Y.; An, H.J.; Park, K.-S. Combined use of cisplatin plus natural killer cells overcomes immunoresistance of cisplatin resistant ovarian cancer. *Biochem. Biophys. Res. Commun.* **2021**, *563*, 40–46. [CrossRef]
19. Markasz, L.; Stuber, G.; Vanherberghen, B.; Flaberg, E.; Olah, E.; Carbone, E.; Eksborg, S.; Klein, E.; Skribek, H.; Szekely, L. Effect of frequently used chemotherapeutic drugs on the cytotoxic activity of human natural killer cells. *Mol. Cancer Ther.* **2007**, *6*, 644–654. [CrossRef]
20. Siebert, N.; Zumpe, M.; Jüttner, M.; Troschke-Meurer, S.; Lode, H.N. PD-1 blockade augments anti-neuroblastoma immune response induced by anti-GD(2) antibody ch14.18/CHO. *Oncoimmunology* **2017**, *6*, e1343775. [CrossRef]
21. Ng, H.Y.; Li, J.; Tao, L.; Lam, A.K.; Chan, K.W.; Ko, J.M.Y.; Yu, V.Z.; Wong, M.; Li, B.; Lung, M.L. Chemotherapeutic Treatments Increase PD-L1 Expression in Esophageal Squamous Cell Carcinoma through EGFR/ERK Activation. *Transl. Oncol.* **2018**, *11*, 1323–1333. [CrossRef] [PubMed]
22. Eastman, A. Improving anticancer drug development begins with cell culture: Misinformation perpetrated by the misuse of cytotoxicity assays. *Oncotarget* **2017**, *8*, 8854–8866. [CrossRef] [PubMed]
23. Mehta, G.; Hsiao, A.Y.; Ingram, M.; Luker, G.D.; Takayama, S. Opportunities and challenges for use of tumor spheroids as models to test drug delivery and efficacy. *J. Control. Release* **2012**, *164*, 192–204. [CrossRef]
24. Nath, S.; Devi, G. Three-dimensional culture systems in cancer research: Focus on tumor spheroid model. *Pharmacol. Ther.* **2016**, *163*, 94–108. [CrossRef] [PubMed]
25. Hoffmann, O.I.; Ilmberger, C.; Magosch, S.; Joka, M.; Jauch, K.-W.; Mayer, B. Impact of the spheroid model complexity on drug response. *J. Biotechnol.* **2015**, *205*, 14–23. [CrossRef]
26. Torisawa, Y.-S.; Takagi, A.; Shiku, H.; Yasukawa, T.; Matsue, T. A multicellular spheroid-based drug sensitivity test by scanning electrochemical microscopy. *Oncol. Rep.* **2005**, *13*, 1107–1112. [CrossRef]
27. Lin, R.-Z.; Chang, H.-Y. Recent advances in three-dimensional multicellular spheroid culture for biomedical research. *Biotechnol. J.* **2008**, *3*, 1172–1184. [CrossRef]
28. Mozhi, A.; Sunil, V.; Zhan, W.; Ghode, P.B.; Thakor, N.V.; Wang, C.-H. Enhanced penetration of pro-apoptotic and anti-angiogenic micellar nanoprobe in 3D multicellular spheroids for chemophototherapy. *J. Control. Release* **2020**, *323*, 502–518. [CrossRef]
29. Azharuddin, M.; Roberg, K.; Dhara, A.K.; Jain, M.V.; Darcy, P.; Hinkula, J.; Slater, N.K.H.; Patra, H.K. Dissecting multi drug resistance in head and neck cancer cells using multicellular tumor spheroids. *Sci. Rep.* **2019**, *9*, 20066. [CrossRef]
30. Nii, T.; Makino, K.; Tabata, Y. A Cancer Invasion Model Combined with Cancer-Associated Fibroblasts Aggregates Incorporating Gelatin Hydrogel Microspheres Containing a p53 Inhibitor. *Tissue Eng. Part C Methods* **2019**, *25*, 711–720. [CrossRef]
31. Joy, M.S.; La, M.; Wang, J.; Bridges, A.S.; Hu, Y.; Hogan, S.L.; Frye, R.F.; Blaisdell, J.; Goldstein, J.A.; Dooley, M.A.; et al. Cyclophosphamide and 4-hydroxycyclophosphamide pharmacokinetics in patients with glomerulonephritis secondary to lupus and small vessel vasculitis. *Br. J. Clin. Pharmacol.* **2012**, *74*, 445–455. [CrossRef]
32. Lowis, S.P.; Pearson, A.D.; Newell, D.R.; Cole, M. Etoposide pharmacokinetics in children: The development and prospective validation of a dosing equation. *Cancer Res.* **1993**, *53*, 4881–4889. [PubMed]
33. Veal, G.J.; Cole, M.; Errington, J.; Pearson, A.D.J.; Gerrard, M.; Whyman, G.; Ellershaw, C.; Boddy, A.V. Pharmacokinetics of carboplatin and etoposide in infant neuroblastoma patients. *Cancer Chemother. Pharmacol.* **2010**, *65*, 1057–1066. [CrossRef] [PubMed]
34. Peng, B.; English, M.; Boddy, A.; Price, L.; Wyllie, R.; Pearson, A.; Tilby, M.; Newell, D. Cisplatin pharmacokinetics in children with cancer. *Eur. J. Cancer* **1997**, *33*, 1823–1828. [CrossRef] [PubMed]
35. Crom, W.R.; de Graaf, S.S.; Synold, T.; Uges, D.R.; Bloemhof, H.; Rivera, G.; Christensen, M.L.; Mahmoud, H.; Evans, W.E. Pharmacokinetics of vincristine in children and adolescents with acute lymphocytic leukemia. *J. Pediatr.* **1994**, *125*, 642–649. [CrossRef]
36. Siebert, N.; Eger, C.; Seidel, D.; Jüttner, M.; Zumpe, M.; Wegner, D.; Kietz, S.; Ehlert, K.; Veal, G.J.; Siegmund, W.; et al. Pharmacokinetics and pharmacodynamics of ch14.18/CHO in relapsed/refractory high-risk neuroblastoma patients treated by long-term infusion in combination with IL-2. *MAbs* **2016**, *8*, 604–616. [CrossRef]
37. Bresciani, G.; Hofland, L.J.; Dogan, F.; Giamas, G.; Gagliano, T.; Zatelli, M.C. Evaluation of Spheroid 3D Culture Methods to Study a Pancreatic Neuroendocrine Neoplasm Cell Line. *Front. Endocrinol.* **2019**, *10*, 682. [CrossRef]

38. Matlashov, M.E.; Shcherbakova, D.M.; Alvelid, J.; Baloban, M.; Pennacchietti, F.; Shemetov, A.A.; Testa, I.; Verkhusha, V.V. A set of monomeric near-infrared fluorescent proteins for multicolor imaging across scales. *Nat. Commun.* **2020**, *11*, 239. [CrossRef]
39. Osawa, T.; Shibuya, M. Targeting cancer cells resistant to hypoxia and nutrient starvation to improve anti-angiogeneic therapy. *Cell Cycle* **2013**, *12*, 2519–2520. [CrossRef]
40. Nashimoto, Y.; Okada, R.; Hanada, S.; Arima, Y.; Nishiyama, K.; Miura, T.; Yokokawa, R. Vascularized cancer on a chip: The effect of perfusion on growth and drug delivery of tumor spheroid. *Biomaterials* **2020**, *229*, 119547. [CrossRef]
41. Huang, Q.; Hu, X.; He, W.; Zhao, Y.; Hao, S.; Wu, Q.; Li, S.; Zhang, S.; Shi, M. Fluid shear stress and tumor metastasis. *Am. J. Cancer Res.* **2018**, *8*, 763–777. [PubMed]
42. Zeng, Y.; Fest, S.; Kunert, R.; Katinger, H.; Pistoia, V.; Michon, J.; Lewis, G.; Ladenstein, R.; Lode, H.N. Anti-neuroblastoma effect of ch14.18 antibody produced in CHO cells is mediated by NK-cells in mice. *Mol. Immunol.* **2005**, *42*, 1311–1319. [CrossRef] [PubMed]
43. Pogge von Strandmann, E.; Shatnyeva, O.; Hansen, H. NKp30 and its ligands: Emerging players in tumor immune evasion from natural killer cells. *Ann. Transl. Med.* **2015**, *3*, 314. [PubMed]
44. Han, Y.; Liu, D.; Li, L. PD-1/PD-L1 pathway: Current researches in cancer. *Am. J. Cancer Res.* **2020**, *10*, 727–742. [PubMed]
45. Williams, A.P.; Bate, J.; Brooks, R.; Chisholm, J.; Clarke, S.C.; Dixon, E.; Faust, S.N.; Galanopoulou, A.; Heath, P.T.; Maishman, T.; et al. Immune reconstitution in children following chemotherapy for acute leukemia. *eJHaem* **2020**, *1*, 142–151. [CrossRef] [PubMed]
46. Baychelier, F.; Sennepin, A.; Ermonval, M.; Dorgham, K.; Debré, P.; Vieillard, V. Identification of a cellular ligand for the natural cytotoxicity receptor NKp44. *Blood* **2013**, *122*, 2935–2942. [CrossRef]
47. Cantoni, C.; Bottino, C.; Vitale, M.; Pessino, A.; Augugliaro, R.; Malaspina, A.; Parolini, S.; Moretta, L.; Moretta, A.; Biassoni, R. NKp44, A Triggering Receptor Involved in Tumor Cell Lysis by Activated Human Natural Killer Cells, Is a Novel Member of the Immunoglobulin Superfamily. *J. Exp. Med.* **1999**, *189*, 787–796. [CrossRef]
48. Furman, W.L.; McCarville, B.; Shulkin, B.L.; Davidoff, A.; Krasin, M.; Hsu, C.-W.; Pan, H.; Wu, J.; Brennan, R.; Bishop, M.W.; et al. Improved Outcome in Children With Newly Diagnosed High-Risk Neuroblastoma Treated With Chemoimmunotherapy: Updated Results of a Phase II Study Using hu14.18K322A. *J. Clin. Oncol.* **2022**, *40*, 335–344. [CrossRef]
49. Doi, T.; Ishikawa, T.; Okayama, T.; Oka, K.; Mizushima, K.; Yasuda, T.; Sakamoto, N.; Katada, K.; Uchiyama, K.; Handa, O.; et al. The JAK/STAT pathway is involved in the upregulation of PD-L1 expression in pancreatic cancer cell lines. *Oncol. Rep.* **2017**, *37*, 1545–1554. [CrossRef]
50. Kim, S.B.; Kim, J.S.; Lee, J.H.; Yoon, W.J.; Lee, D.S.; Ko, M.S.; Kwon, B.S.; Choi, D.H.; Cho, H.R.; Lee, B.J.; et al. NF-kappaB activation is required for cisplatin-induced apoptosis in head and neck squamous carcinoma cells. *FEBS Lett.* **2006**, *580*, 311–318. [CrossRef]
51. Antonangeli, F.; Natalini, A.; Garassino, M.C.; Sica, A.; Santoni, A.; Di Rosa, F. Regulation of PD-L1 Expression by NF-κB in Cancer. *Front. Immunol.* **2020**, *11*, 584626. [CrossRef] [PubMed]
52. Battula, V.L.; Nguyen, K.; Sun, J.; Pitner, M.K.; Yuan, B.; Bartholomeusz, C.; Hail, N.; Andreeff, M. IKK inhibition by BMS-345541 suppresses breast tumorigenesis and metastases by targeting GD2+ cancer stem cells. *Oncotarget* **2017**, *8*, 36936–36949. [CrossRef] [PubMed]

Disclaimer/Publisher's Note: The statements, opinions and data contained in all publications are solely those of the individual author(s) and contributor(s) and not of MDPI and/or the editor(s). MDPI and/or the editor(s) disclaim responsibility for any injury to people or property resulting from any ideas, methods, instructions or products referred to in the content.

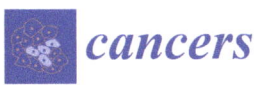

Article

Characterization of Estrogen Receptors in Pancreatic Adenocarcinoma with Tertiary Lymphoid Structures

Xuan Zou [1,2,3,4,†], Yu Liu [1,2,3,4,†], Xuan Lin [1,2,3,4], Ruijie Wang [1,2,3,4], Zhengjie Dai [1,2,3,4], Yusheng Chen [1,2,3,4], Mingjian Ma [1,2,3,4], Yesiboli Tasiheng [1,2,3,4], Yu Yan [1,2,3,4], Xu Wang [1,2,3,4,5], Xianjun Yu [1,2,3,4], He Cheng [1,2,3,4,*] and Chen Liu [1,2,3,4,*]

[1] Department of Pancreatic Surgery, Fudan University Shanghai Cancer Center, Shanghai 200032, China
[2] Department of Oncology, Shanghai Medical College, Fudan University, Shanghai 200032, China
[3] Shanghai Pancreatic Cancer Institute, Shanghai 200032, China
[4] Pancreatic Cancer Institute, Fudan University, Shanghai 200032, China
[5] Cancer Institute, Shanghai Key Laboratory of Radiation Oncology, Fudan University Shanghai Cancer Center, Shanghai 200032, China
* Correspondence: chenghe@fudanpci.org (H.C.); liuchen@fudanpci.org (C.L.)
† These authors contributed equally to this work.

Simple Summary: The role of estrogen signaling in pancreatic adenocarcinoma (PAAD) was unclear. Here we investigated the expression patterns of three estrogen receptors (ERα, ERβ, and GPER) in 174 PAAD samples via immunohistochemistry staining. Positive expression of all three estrogen receptors was significantly correlated with better clinicopathological characteristics and prognosis, as well as more tertiary lymphoid structure (TLS) presence in PAAD. Upregulated expression of ERα and ERβ in PAAD was also significantly associated with increased CD8$^+$ T-cell infiltration in vitro. In-silico analyses also revealed that the expression of estrogen receptors affects multiple pathways relevant to T-cell and B-cell behaviors. In summary, estrogen receptors may remodel the immune microenvironment and regulate the development of TLS in PAAD.

Abstract: The role of estrogen signaling in antitumor immunology remains unknown for non-traditional sex-biased cancer types such as pancreatic adenocarcinoma (PAAD). Tertiary lymphoid structures (TLS) are active zones composed of multiple types of immune cells, whose presence indicates anti-tumor immune responses. In this study, we employed a 12-chemokine signature to characterize potential gene categories associated with TLS development and identified seventeen major gene categories including estrogen receptors (ERs). Immunohistochemistry staining revealed the expression patterns of three ERs (ERα, ERβ, and GPER) in 174 PAAD samples, and their correlation with clinicopathological characteristics, immune cell infiltration levels, and intratumoral TLS presence was analyzed. The results indicated that ERα (+) and ERβ (+) were correlated with high tumor grade, and ERβ (+) and GPER (+) were correlated with lower TNM stage, and both ERα (+) and GPER (+) displayed a beneficial effect on prognosis in this cohort. Interestingly, positive staining of all three ERs was significantly correlated with the presence of intratumoral TLSs and infiltration of more active immune cells into the microenvironment. Moreover, the chemotaxis of CD8$^+$ T-cells to PAAD cells was significantly increased in vitro with upregulated expression of ERα or ERβ on PAAD cells. To conclude, our study showed a novel correlation between ER expression and TLS development, suggesting that ERs may play a protective role by enhancing anti-tumor immune responses in PAAD.

Keywords: pancreatic adenocarcinoma; estrogen receptor; tertiary lymphoid structure; tumor microenvironment

Citation: Zou, X.; Liu, Y.; Lin, X.; Wang, R.; Dai, Z.; Chen, Y.; Ma, M.; Tasiheng, Y.; Yan, Y.; Wang, X.; et al. Characterization of Estrogen Receptors in Pancreatic Adenocarcinoma with Tertiary Lymphoid Structures. *Cancers* **2023**, *15*, 828. https://doi.org/10.3390/cancers15030828

Academic Editors: Xianda Zhao, Timothy K. Starr and Subbaya Subramanian

Received: 11 January 2023
Accepted: 20 January 2023
Published: 29 January 2023

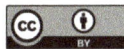

Copyright: © 2023 by the authors. Licensee MDPI, Basel, Switzerland. This article is an open access article distributed under the terms and conditions of the Creative Commons Attribution (CC BY) license (https://creativecommons.org/licenses/by/4.0/).

1. Introduction

Pancreatic adenocarcinoma (PAAD) is one of the most common cancers with poor survival worldwide [1]. Although PAAD is not a traditional gender-biased cancer like breast cancer and prostate cancer, the incidence rate and mortality of male patients are still higher than that of female patients [2]. Gender differences are attributed to enormous factors including genetic, physiological, and environmental factors such as cigarette smoking, obesity, and alcohol intake. At the physiological level, sex hormone pathways undoubtedly have a dominant impact [1].

Estrogens are typical sex hormones that play regulatory roles in multiple physiological processes from reproduction to neuronal development [3]. Emerging evidence indicated that estrogen signaling was extensively involved in regulating cancer cell proliferation, angiogenesis, epithelial-mesenchymal transition, and anti-tumor immunity in multiple tumor types [4–6]. Estrogens exert biological effects via two nuclear receptors, estrogen receptor α (ERα) and estrogen receptor β (ERβ) [7], but recent reports have suggested that G-protein coupled ER (GPER) is also involved in the regulation of tumor metabolism and the immune microenvironment [8]. In PAAD, the potential role of ERs has long been debated, and even the expression characteristics of ERs in PAAD are still controversial. The lack of large-sample studies evaluating the expression of different ER isoforms using isoform-specific antibodies (ERα, ERβ, and GPER) likely contributes to the inconsistency of published results concerning ERs expression in PAAD [9]. For example, in a retrospective study of 10 PAAD patients [10], only nuclear ERα expression was detected and found to be expressed in intralobular stromal and islet cells rather than tumor cells in PAAD. Another recently published study identified the broad expression of several ERβ isoforms in 18 PAAD patients [11]. These studies still had rather limited sample sizes and lacked comprehensive analyses of different ERs including both nuclear and membrane ERs.

PAAD is characterized by a complex immune microenvironment, and recent studies have revealed that the successful establishment of adaptive anti-tumor immune responses may be represented by the presence of tertiary lymphoid structures (TLSs) [12,13]. Tertiary lymphoid structures (TLSs) are ectopic lymphoid organs developing in non-lymphoid tissues at sites of chronic inflammation [14]. Intratumoral TLSs are active sites for the generation and activation of innate and adaptive anti-tumor immune responses, and their presence has been shown to be associated with superior prognosis in many cancers [13]. In this study, we first performed bioinformatic analyses to characterize potential regulatory signaling categories for TLS development in PAAD, and the results interestingly revealed a potential link between ER signaling and TLS expression in PAAD. The regulatory roles of estrogen and its receptors in anti-tumor immunity have been gradually revealed [5]. For example, in PAAD, ectopic GPER expression suppressed tumor cell proliferation and normalized the immune microenvironment, indicating the translational value of ERs manipulation for PAAD immunotherapy [15–17]. However, few studies have investigated the potential role of ER signaling in the development of tumor-associated TLS structures.

In this study, we focused on the expression patterns of ERα, ERβ, and GPER, and revealed their correlation with immune status including tumor-infiltrated immune cells and TLS presence in PAAD. For the first time, our study investigated the role of ERs in PAAD prognosis and revealed their potential roles in TLS development.

2. Methods

2.1. Data Source

Transcriptome data of the Cancer Genome Atlas Program (TCGA)-PAAD and the Clinical Proteomic Tumor Analysis Consortium (CPTAC)-PDAC datasets [18] were analyzed in this study. For TCGA-PAAD, fragments per kilobase per million (FPKM) normalized RNA-sequencing (RNA-seq) gene expression data were downloaded and converted to transcripts per million (TPM) format. The Genome Reference Consortium Human Build 38 (GRCh38) assembly was referenced for gene symbol annotation. Gene expression and clinical information matrices of 178 pancreatic adenocarcinoma samples from TCGA-PAAD and 141 from CPTAC-PDAC were analyzed as follows.

2.2. Bioinformatic Analysis Methods

TLS score was calculated using a 12-chemokine (CCL2, CCL3, CCL4, CCL5, CCL8, CCL18, CCL19, CCL21, CXCL9, CXCL10, CXCL11, and CXCL13) TLS signature, which was reported as a predictor of TLS expression [19,20], using the single-sample gene set enrichment analysis (ssGSEA) method. For each sample, the TLS expression level was represented by the normalized enrichment score (NES) of ssGSEA result. GSEA analysis was conducted to compare the differentially enriched pathways between two distinct groups, using the classical gene sets from the Kyoto Encyclopedia of Genes and Genomes (KEGG), Gene Oncology (GO), Reactome, and BioCarta databases (https://www.gsea-msigdb.org accessed on 1 June 2022). Spearman correlation analyses were performed to screen the TLS score-correlated genes. The DAVID gene functional classification tool [21] was applied to group functionally related genes from the identified gene list. The abundance of 22 tumor-infiltrated immune cells was inferred from bulk-tissue transcriptome profiles using the CIBERSORTx tool [22].

2.3. Patients and Samples

Tumor tissue specimens were collected from PAAD patients receiving upfront surgery between 2012 and 2020 at the Department of Pancreatic Surgery, Fudan University Shanghai Cancer Center. Written informed consent was obtained from each participant. Tissue samples were preserved in formalin-fixed, paraffin-embedded (FFPE) tissue blocks for long-term storage. Hematoxylin and eosin (H&E) staining slides from 348 PAAD patients were first analyzed to investigate the general association between gender, intratumoral TLS presence, and prognosis. The final cohort of 174 samples with complete clinicopathological information and immunohistochemistry staining results was further analyzed to explore the association between ERs expression and clinicopathological features as well as tumor immunity characteristics.

2.4. Immunohistochemistry (IHC)

The protein expression level and localization of three ERs and the infiltration level of several immune cells were detected by IHC staining. The primary antibodies used in this study included anti-ERα antibody (1/200, pH 6.0, No. ab79413, Abcam, Waltham, MA, USA), anti-ERβ antibody (1/200, pH 9.0, No. ab288, Abcam, Waltham, MA, USA), anti-GPER antibody (1/200, pH 9.0, No. ab260033, Abcam, Waltham, MA, USA), anti-CD4 antibody (1/200, pH 9.0, No. ab133616, Abcam, Waltham, MA, USA), anti-CD8 antibody (1/100, pH 9.0, No. ab178089, Abcam, Waltham, MA, USA), anti-CD20 antibody (1/100, pH 6.0, No. ab64088, Abcam, Waltham, MA, USA), anti-HLA-DR-antibody (1/200, pH 6.0, No. ab20181, Abcam, Waltham, MA, USA), and anti-FOXP3 antibody (1/100, pH 9.0, No. ab20034, Abcam, Waltham, MA, USA). The accuracy of the anti-ERα, ERβ, and GPER antibodies has been verified in previous studies [23–25]. IHC staining was performed following standard procedures of sample dewaxing and hydration, endogenous enzyme removal and antigen repair, blocking, antibody incubation, and DAB staining. Samples with positive staining in more than 10% of tumor cells were regarded as positive for ERs expression. Intratumoral TLS was identified as the regional aggregation of immune cells (mainly T-cells and B-cells) that lacked integrated capsules within tumors on hematoxylin and Eosin (H&E) stained pathology slides, followed by sequential sections stained with T-cell and B-cell markers (CD4, CD8, and CD20) to determine the characteristic cellular compositions and concentric distribution patterns. The relative infiltration level of each immune cell type was calculated as the mean density in more than 3 random sites under a 20-fold microscope magnification.

2.5. Immune Cell Chemotaxis Assay

Peripheral blood samples of PAAD patients were diluted in phosphate-buffered saline and added to Ficoll (GE Healthcare, Chicago, IL, USA) for gradient centrifugation to obtain peripheral blood mononuclear cells (PBMCs). $CD8^+$T-cells were purified from PBMCs using the Human T-Cell Isolation Kit (STEMCELL Technologies, Vancouver, BC, Canada) according to the manufacturer's protocol. Human PAAD cell lines BxPC-3 and Capan-2 were cultured respectively in RPMI-1640 medium (Gibco, Waltham, MA, USA) and McCoy's 5a medium (ATCC) supplemented with 10% fetal calf serum (Sigma, Burlington, NJ, USA) and 10 nM 17 β-estradiol (Sigma, Burlington, NJ, USA) in a humidified atmosphere containing 5% CO_2 at 37 °C. ESR1 or ESR2 was overexpressed in human PAAD cell lines via the transfection of pLVX-ESR1(ESR2)-GFP plasmids. The overexpression efficiency was assessed by quantitative reverse transcription-polymerase chain reaction (qRT-PCR) and flow cytometry.

Chemotactic assays were performed to measure the chemotaxis of ERs expressed in PAAD cells on $CD8^+$T-cells. $CD8^+$T-cells (1×10^6) and human PAAD cells with or without ESR overexpression (1×10^6) were separately seeded in transwell chambers (3 μm, Corning, New York, NY, USA) or at the bottom of chambers. After 24 h of co-culture, the culture supernatant of PAAD cells was collected and the number of $CD8^+$T-cells was counted.

2.6. Statistical Methods and Software

The correlation between gene expression level and TLS score was measured by spearman correlation analysis. Chi-squared testing was conducted to evaluate the association between ERs expression and intratumoral TLS presence or other clinicopathological features. The survival distribution of samples from two groups was compared by Kaplan-Meier survival analysis. TLS scores and immune cell infiltration levels were compared between two independent groups using Wilcoxon test. "GSVA", "limma", and "GSEABase" R packages were used for ssGSEA analysis [26,27]. Statistical analyses were performed on SPSS (version 25.0), Prism (version 7.0), and R (version 4.1.1) software. A two-tailed *p-value* < 0.05 was considered statistically significant.

3. Results

3.1. Characterization of Regulatory Factors of TLS Development in PAAD

As previously reported, a 12-chemokine signature served as a pan-cancer marker of TLS expression and immunophenotype, and its predictive value had been validated in various types of cancer [19,20,28]. To investigate the potential regulatory signaling of TLS development in PAAD, we first employed the signatures to calculate the TLS scores of samples from two PAAD datasets (TCGA and CPTAC). After that, GSEA analyses were performed to compare groups with high and low TLS scores (the median value as a cutoff) to identify pathways significantly associated with TLS phenotype (Table S1). A total of 1056 genes whose expression levels were significantly correlated with TLS scores in both datasets were identified and analyzed for gene functional classification (Table S2). The genes were classified into seventeen groups with distinct biological categories such as cytokine receptors, C-type lectins, and toll-like receptors (Table S3). In addition, TLS scores were also significantly correlated with the expression of some genes in RAS oncogene family, APOBEC family, and nuclear hormone receptors (including nuclear ER-encoded genes ESR1 and ESR2), etc. (Figure 1A).

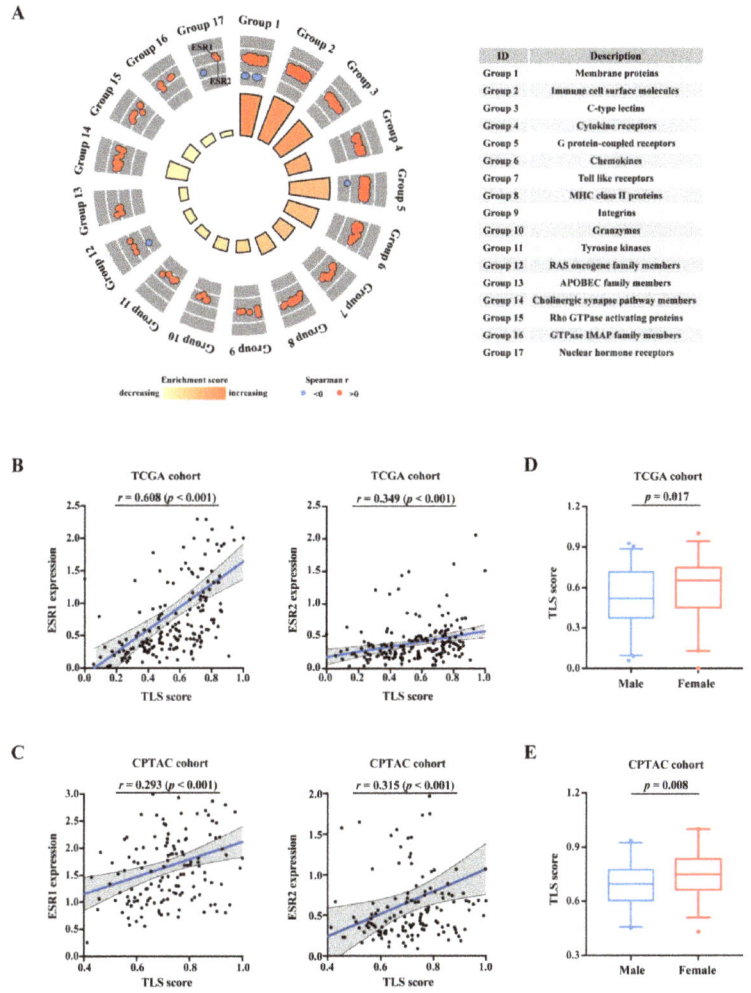

Figure 1. Association between estrogen signaling and TLS scores in two public databases. (**A**) Circular plot showing gene categories significantly correlated with TLS score; the inner circle displays the gene number and enrichment score in each group; the outer circle displays the scatter plots of spearman's r-values of gene members. (**B**) Scatter plots of the positive correlation between TLS score and ESR1 and ESR2 expression in the TCGA cohort ($n = 178$). (**C**) Scatter plots of the positive correlation between TLS score and ESR1 and ESR2 expression in the CPTAC cohort ($n = 141$). (**D**) Comparison of TLS scores between males and females in the TCGA cohort ($n = 178$). (**E**) Comparison of TLS scores between males and females in the TCGA cohort ($n = 141$).

3.2. Correlation of Estrogen Receptors with TLS Development

Interestingly, several pathways associated with estrogen signaling (e.g., "extra-nuclear estrogen signaling", "estrogen-dependent nuclear events downstream of ESR-membrane signaling", "ESR mediated signaling", "steroid hormone biosynthesis") were found to be enriched in the differentially expressed genes between the groups with high and low TLS scores (Table S1). Particularly, ESR1 and ESR2 (Figure 1B,C) were significantly and positively correlated with TLS scores in both datasets. Meanwhile, female patients displayed significantly higher TLS scores than male patients (Figure 1D,E), suggesting that the presence of TLS may be gender-biased and relevant to the expression of estrogen receptors.

3.3. Gender Bias in PAAD Prognosis and TLS Expression

The influence of sex on patient prognosis and TLS expression was first investigated by H&E staining analysis in a large cohort of 348 PAAD patients from Fudan University Shanghai Cancer Center. As shown in Figure 2, the female patients displayed a better overall survival than the male patients (Figure 2A). In this cohort, intratumoral TLS structures were found in 22.1% (77/348) patients, and TLS presence may indicate a more favorable prognosis (Figure 2B). Female patients were found to have a marginally higher proportion of TLS (+) samples (24.4% vs. 20.3%), although no statistically significant difference was found ($p > 0.05$, chi-square test; Figure 2C). Notably, female PAAD patients with positive intratumoral TLS and male patients without TLS represented the best and the worst survival (Figure 2D). The result indicated a marginal trend that the ER signaling played a protective role in PAAD.

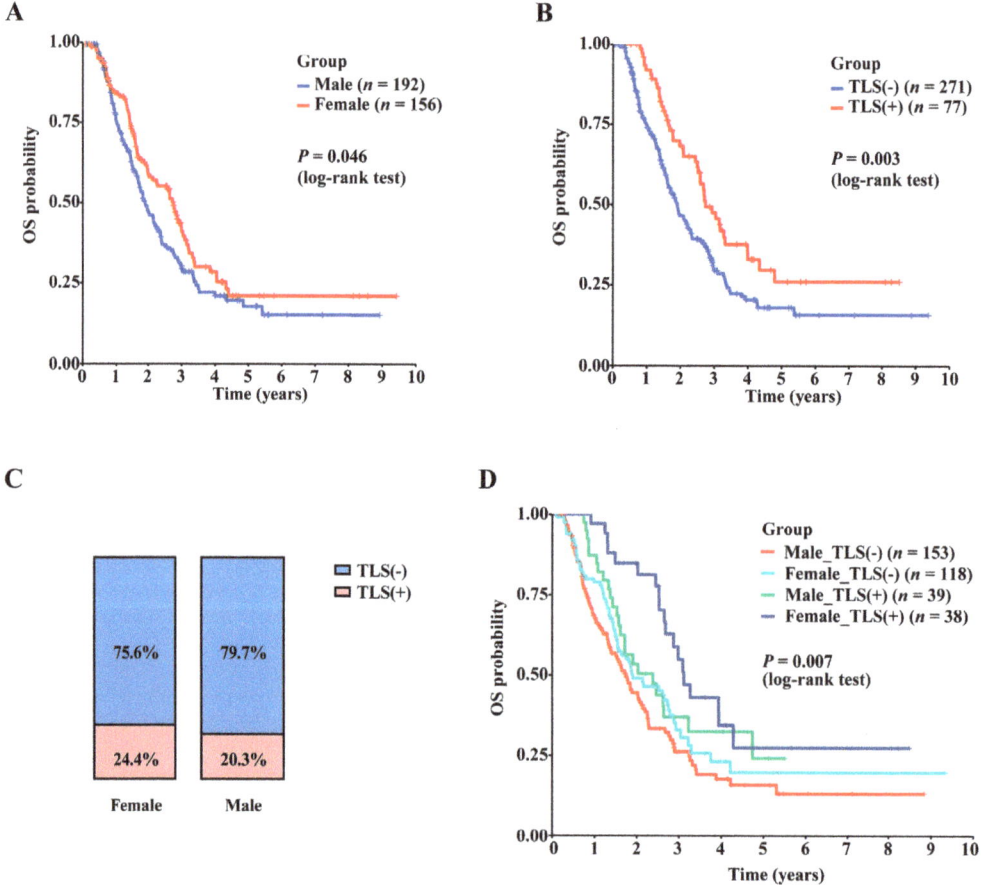

Figure 2. Gender difference of TLS incidences and prognosis in PAAD patients. (**A**) The overall survival curves of male and female PAAD patients. (**B**) The overall survival curves of intratumoral TLS (+) and TLS (−) PAAD patients. (**C**) Proportion distribution of TLS (+) and TLS (−) samples in different gender groups; $p > 0.05$, chi-square test. (**D**) Survival curve analysis based on gender and TLS classification.

3.4. Expression Patterns of ERs in PAAD

The expression of three major estrogen receptors, classical nuclear ERs (ERα and ERβ) and transmembrane GPER, were investigated in 174 PAAD samples via IHC analysis. The positive rates of ERβ and GPER expression were 73.0% and 77.0% respectively, while ERα was positively detected in 41.4% of all PAAD samples. Interestingly, although the ERs' expression in individuals displayed distinct patterns, there were no statistical differences in their positive rates between males and females (Table 1). ERα (Figure 3A) and ERβ (Figure 3B) were expressed in the nucleus and cytoplasm of tumor cells, while GPER (Figure 3C) was mainly located in the cell membrane and cytoplasm. In addition to tumor cells, ERs were also expressed in stromal cells, immune cells, and islets in PAAD tumor tissue.

Table 1. Expression of ERs in PAAD and its association with patients' clinicopathological features.

Variables	ERα Expression			ERβ Expression			GPER Expression		
	ERα(+)	ERα(−)	Chi-Square Test	ERβ(+)	ERβ(−)	Chi-Square Test	GPER(+)	GPER(−)	Chi-Square Test
Total	72(41.4%)	102(58.6%)		127(73.0%)	47(27.0%)		134(77.0%)	40(23.0%)	
Gender			0.475			0.821			0.954
Male	37(21.3%)	58(33.3%)		70(40.2%)	25(14.4%)		73(42.0%)	22(12.6%)	
Female	35(20.1)	44(25.3%)		57(32.8%)	22(12.6%)		61(35.1%)	18(10.3%)	
Age			0.413			0.628			0.453
≤60	35(20.1%)	56(32.2%)		65(37.4%)	26(14.9%)		68(39.1%)	23(13.2%)	
>60	37(21.3%)	46(26.4%)		62(35.6%)	21(12.1%)		66(37.9%)	17(9.8%)	
TNM Stage			0.153			0.017			0.006
I/II	50(28.7%)	60(34.5%)		87(50.0%)	23(13.2%)		92(52.9%)	18(10.3%)	
III/IV	22(12.6%)	42(24.1%)		40(23.0%)	24(13.8%)		42(24.1%)	22(12.6%)	
T			0.470			0.002			0.024
T1/T2	49(28.2%)	64(36.8%)		91(52.3%)	22(12.6%)		93(53.4%)	20(11.5%)	
T3/T4	23(13.2%)	38(21.8%)		36(20.7%)	25(14.4%)		41(23.6%)	20(11.5%)	
N			0.733			0.245			0.826
N0	40(23.0%)	54(31.0%)		72(41.4%)	22(12.6%)		73(42.0%)	21(12.1%)	
N1/N2	32	48(27.6%)		55(31.6%)	25(14.4%)		61(35.1%)	19(10.9%)	
M			0.216			0.938			0.090
M0	67(38.5%)	89(51.1%)		114(65.5%)	42(24.1%)		123(70.7%)	33(19.0%)	
M1	5(2.9%)	13(7.5%)		13(7.5%)	5(2.9%)		11(6.3%)	7(4.0%)	
Grade			0.011			0.023			0.200
G1/2	23(13.2%)	16(9.2%)		34(19.5%)	5(2.9%)		33(19.0%)	6(3.4%)	
G3	49(28.2%)	86(49.4%)		93(53.4%)	42(24.1%)		101(58.0%)	34(19.5%)	
Nerve Invasion			0.975			0.453			0.439
No	10(5.7%)	14(8.0%)		16(9.2%)	8(4.6%)		17(9.8%)	7(4.0%)	
Yes	62(35.6%)	88(50.6%)		111(63.8%)	39(22.4%)		117(67.2%)	33(19.0%)	
Vascular Invasion			0.256			0.221			0.107
No	57(32.8%)	73(42.0%)		98(56.3%)	32(18.4%)		104(59.8%)	26(14.9%)	
Yes	15(8.6%)	29(16.7%)		29(16.7%)	15(8.6%)		30(17.2%)	14(8.0%)	

The association between ERs expression and clinicopathological characteristics was further analyzed. ERα (+) (Figure 3D) and GPER (+) (Figure 3H) patients had better survival than the negative groups, but no significant difference was found for ERβ (Figure 3F). In addition, patients with positive ERs expression displayed more protective clinicopathological features (Table 1). ERα (Figure 3E) and ERβ (Figure 3G) expression were significantly correlated with lower tumor grades. Meanwhile, patients in the early stages had higher rates of positive ERβ (Figure 3G) and GPER (Figure 3I) expression. Together, the results revealed the potential beneficial effects of ERs and ER signaling in PAAD.

3.5. Association between Positive Ers Expression and TLS Presence in PAAD

Bioinformatic analyses demonstrated a potential correlation between ER signaling and PAAD-associated TLS development. Here we performed IHC on 174 PAAD samples from the local center to perform further investigation. The concurrence of positive ER expression and intratumoral TLS presence in PAAD could be frequently observed for ERα (Figure 4A), ERβ (Figure 4D), and GPER (Figure 4G). For ERα, 58.3% of ERα (+) samples were TLS-positive simultaneously, significantly higher than that of ERα (−) samples ($p = 0.0000007$, Figure 4B). Compared to the ER (−) group, ERα (+) samples also had significantly higher levels of CD8[+] T-cell infiltration and higher levels of HLA-DR expression in tumor tissues (Figure 4C). The positive expression of ERβ in tumor cells was also significantly correlated with a higher incidence of TLS presence ($p = 0.003$, Figure 4E) and more CD8[+]T-cells infiltration (Figure 4F) in PAAD. The positive correlation between TLS presence and GPER expression in tumor cells was consistently identified ($p = 0.001$, Figure 4H), although CD8+T-cell levels and HLA-DR expression were only marginally higher in the GPER (+) group (Figure 4I). Taken together, ERs expression in tumor cells was statistically associated with an immune-active tumor microenvironment in PAAD.

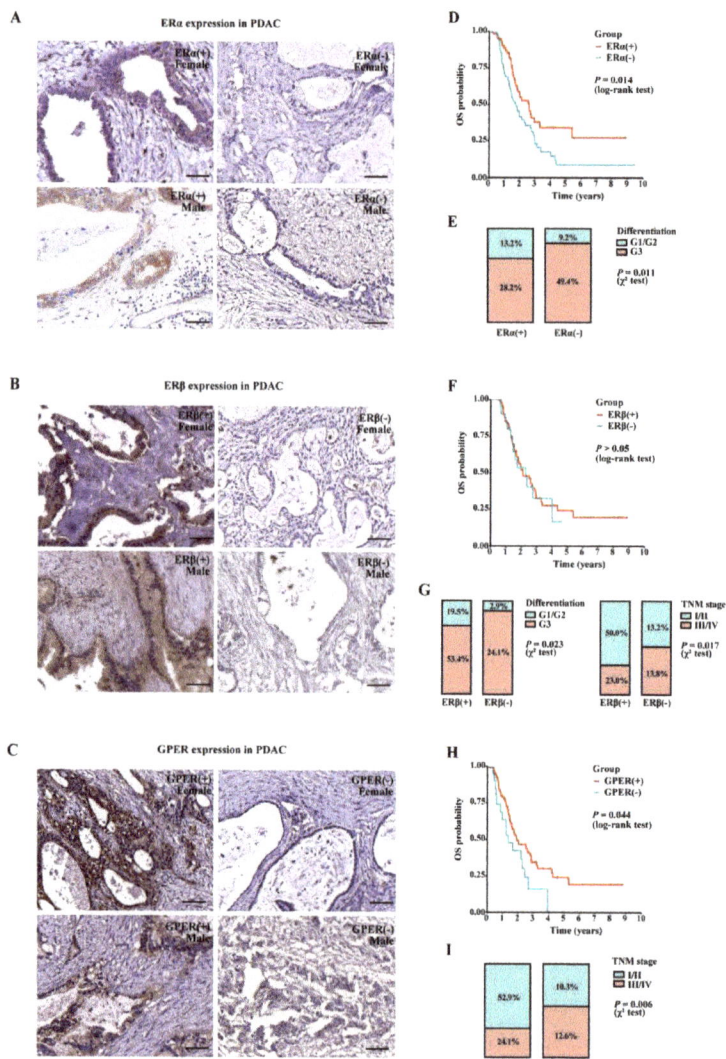

Figure 3. Expression patterns of ERα/β and GPER in PAAD tumor tissues. (**A**) Representative images of ERα staining in PAAD samples from male and female patients; scale bar: 50 μm. (**B**) Representative images of ERβ staining in PAAD samples from male and female patients; scale bar: 50 μm. (**C**) Representative images of GPER staining in PAAD samples from male and female patients; scale bar: 50 μm. (**D**) The overall survival curves of ERα (+) and ERα (−) patients. (**E**) Association between ERα expression and tumor grade in 174 patients. (**F**) The overall survival curves of ERβ (+) and ERβ (−) patients. (**G**) Association between ERβ expression and tumor grade, TNM stage in 174 patients. (**H**) The overall survival curves of GPER (+) and GPER (−) patients. (**I**) Association between GPER expression and tumor grade in 174 patients.

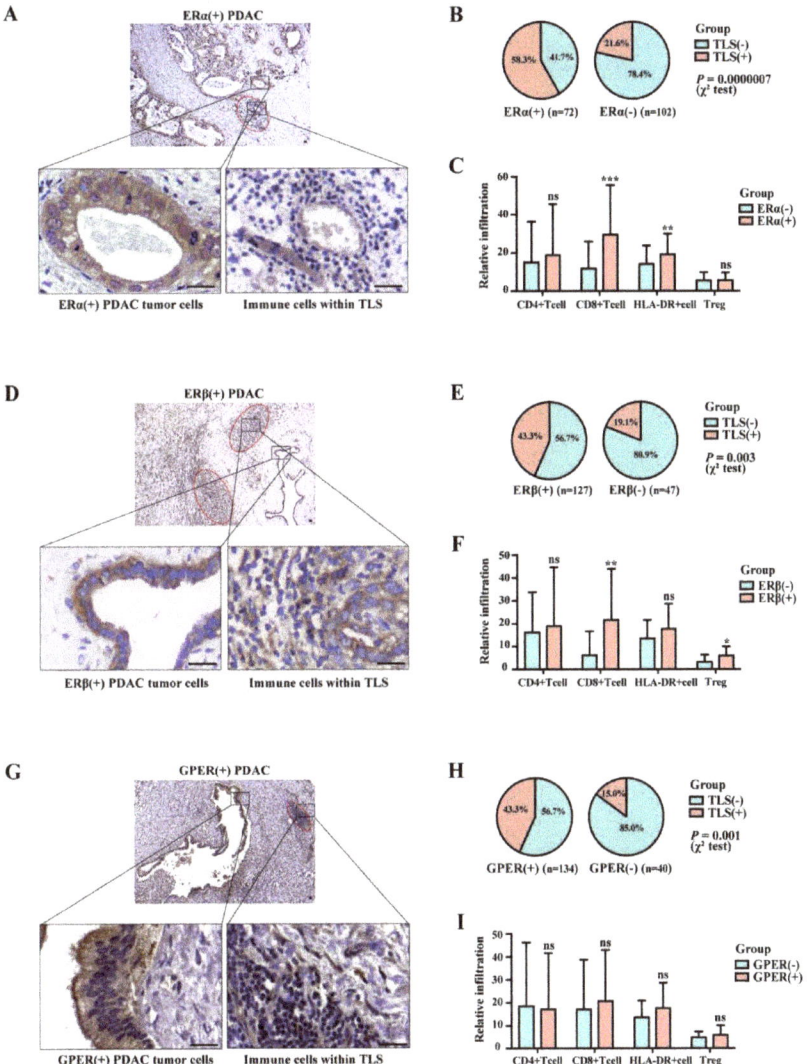

Figure 4. Correlation between ERs expression and tumor-infiltrating immune cells in PAAD. (**A**) Representative IHC images of ERα (+) PAAD tumor tissues with concurrent intratumoral TLS structures; TLS was circled in red line; scale bar: 20 μm. (**B**) Pie plots of the proportion of TLS (+) samples in ERα (+) and ERα (−) groups. (**C**) Histograms of relative infiltration levels of CD4+T-cells, CD8+T-cells, HLA-DR+ activated immune cells, and FOXP3+ Tregs in ERα (+) and ERα (−) groups; Treg: regulatory T-cell; ** $p < 0.01$, *** $p < 0.001$, ns: non-significant. (**D**) Representative IHC images of ERβ (+) PAAD tumor tissues with concurrent intratumoral TLS structures; TLS was circled in red line; scale bar: 20 μm. (**E**) Pie plots of the proportion of TLS (+) samples in ERβ (+) and ERβ (−) groups. (**F**) Histograms of relative infiltration levels of CD4+T-cells, CD8+T-cells, HLA-DR+ activated immune cells, and FOXP3+ Tregs in ERα (+) and ERα (−) groups; * $p < 0.05$, ** $p < 0.01$, ns: non-significant. (**G**) Representative IHC images of GPER (+) PAAD tumor tissues with concurrent intratumoral TLS structures; TLS was circled in red line; scale bar: 20 μm. (**H**) Pie plots of the proportion of TLS (+) samples in GPER (+) and GPER (−) groups. (**I**) Histograms comparing relative infiltration levels of CD4+T-cells, CD8+T-cells, HLA-DR+ activated immune cells and FOXP3+ Tregs in ERα (+) and ERα (−) groups; ns: non-significant.

3.6. In Vitro Verification of the Influence of Ers Expression on Immune Cell Chemotaxis

By analyzing the IHC staining from 174 PAAD samples, we found that both the positive expression of ERα and ERβ on PAAD tumor cells were significantly associated with high infiltration of CD8$^+$T-cells in the tumor microenvironment. To validate the finding in vitro, we constructed ESR1 or ESR2-overexpressed PAAD cell lines and then used chemotaxis assays to evaluate the influence of ERs expression on CD8$^+$T-cell migration. After transfected with ESR1 or ESR2, both the mRNA (Figure 5A) and protein (Figure 5B) expression levels of ESR1 or ESR2 in tumor cells were significantly upregulated. CD8$^+$T-cells in the transwell chamber were co-cultured with or without ESR1 or ESR2-overexpressed PAAD cells seeded at the bottom (Figure 5C). After 24 h, the numbers of CD8$^+$T-cells migrating to the bottom were counted (Figure 5D). Notably, the chemotaxis of CD8$^+$T-cells was significantly increased with upregulated expression of ERα or ERβ on PAAD cells, further demonstrating the significant roles of ERs in anti-tumor immunity in PAAD.

Significant roles of ERs in anti-tumor immunity in PAAD.

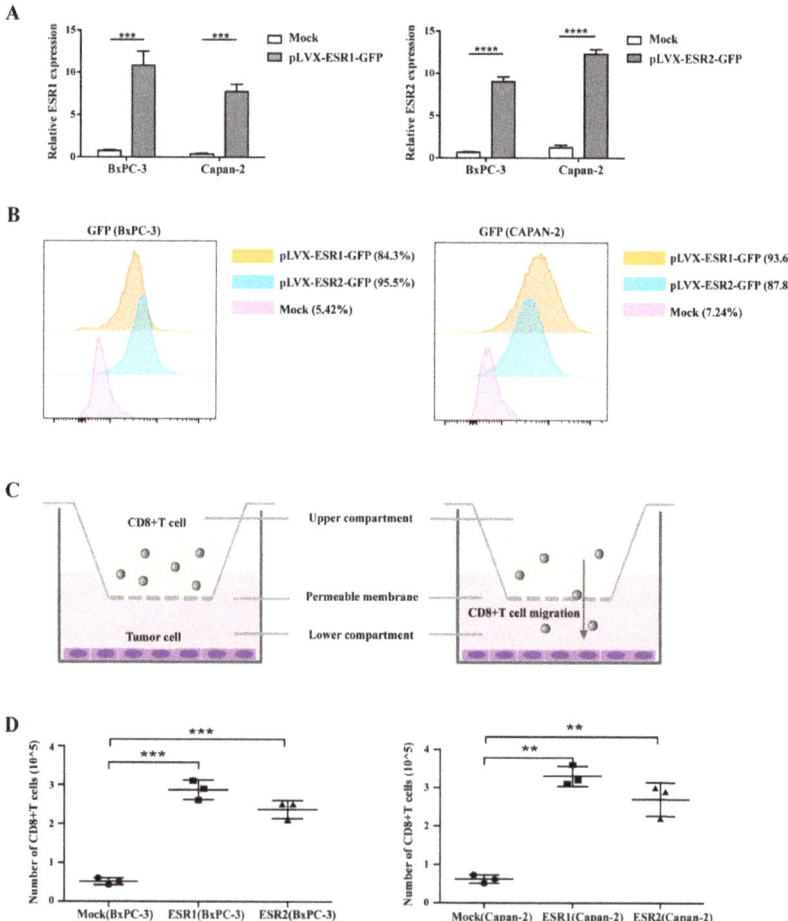

Figure 5. Immune cell chemotaxis assay. (**A**) Expression efficiency of ESR1 and ESR2 in PAAD tumor cells detected by qRT-PCR; *** $p < 0.001$, **** $p < 0.0001$. (**B**) Efficiency of ESR1 or ESR2 (GFP) overexpression in BxPC-3 or Capan-2 cells detected by flow cytometry. (**C**) The schematic diagram of chemotaxis assay. (**D**) The number of CD8$^+$T-cells in the supernatant of BxPC-3 or Capan-2 cells in chemotaxis assay; ** $p < 0.01$, *** $p < 0.001$.

3.7. In-Silico Analyses of the Influence of Estrogen Receptors on Tumor Immune Microenvironment

The potential immune stimulator function of ERs was further explored in the TCGA-PAAD dataset via immune-cell abundance estimation using CIBERSORTx and functional enrichment analysis using GSEA. CIBERSORTx analysis helped interpret transcriptome data into proportions of 22 tumor-infiltrated immune cells. With this tool, we could verify the findings of IHC experiments from a different perspective through bioinformatic analysis. Spearman correlation analysis was then conducted to assess the potential correlation between ERs-encoded gene expression and immune cell infiltration levels. Consistent with IHC findings, the expression levels of ESR1 and ESR2 were positively and significantly correlated with CD4/CD8$^+$T-cell infiltration in PAAD (Figure 6A).

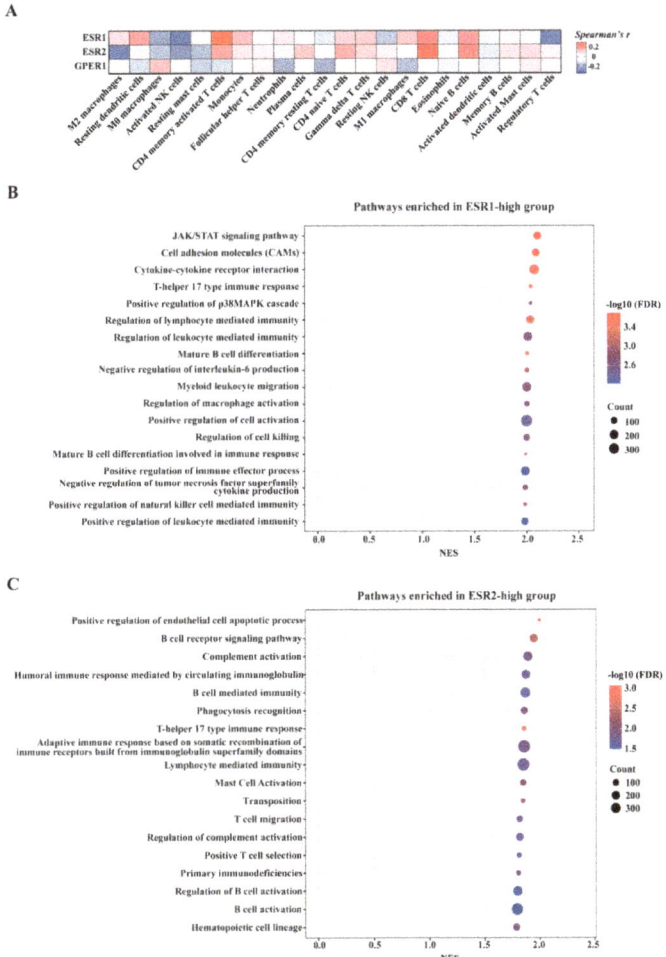

Figure 6. In silico functional exploration of ERs in PAAD. (**A**) Heatmap showing the association between ERs gene expression levels and proportions of 22 immune cell types in tumor microenvironment. (**B**) Diagram of the pathways enriched in the ESR1-high group; the median of gene expression was used as a cutoff value for sample classification. (**C**) Diagram of the pathways enriched in the ESR2-high group.

To gain insights into the biological mechanisms of ESR1 and ESR2 in PAAD, samples from the TCGA-PAAD dataset were divided into ESR1(ESR2)-high and low groups based on the median value of ESR1(ESR2) mRNA expression, and GSEA analyses were performed between the two groups. Figure 6B,C show the most significantly enriched pathways in ESR1-high and ESR2-high groups, including the B-cell receptor signaling pathway, mature B-cell differentiation, T-cell migration, positive T-cell selection, T-helper 17 type immune response, etc. Since B-cells and T-cells were the predominant cell types in TLS structures, the results identified significantly up-regulated T/B-cell-related pathways in PAAD with high ERs expression, which further demonstrated the potential stimulatory role of ER signaling in PAAD-associated TLS formation and function.

4. Discussion

4.1. Prognostic Value of ERs in Non-Traditional Sex-Biased Cancer

Recent studies revealed gender disparities in the incidence and mortality rates of multiple cancers. For most cancers, including PAAD, males have a higher incidence and worse prognosis than females of all ages and races [29]. In addition, there was growing evidence of sex differences in responses to chemotherapy or immunotherapy in certain cancer types [30]. Sex bias in cancers may involve multidimensional mechanisms, including gender-related genetic or epigenetic regulation, and environmental factors. Sex hormones (estrogen in particular) and their receptors were reported to play important roles in cancer biology by affecting cancer stem cell self-renewal, cancer metabolism, and the immune microenvironment [31].

Estrogen, acting through estrogen receptors (nuclear receptors ERα and ERβ and membrane receptors GPER), was extensively deregulated during the development and progression of esophageal cancer [32], gastric cancer [33], and colon cancer [34]. Both elevated estrogen levels and ectopic ERs expression affected the carcinogenesis of certain cancer types, with a variety of outcomes [35,36]. In PAAD, ER signaling was generally reported to be a repressive factor in tumor development, but expression patterns and potential mechanisms of ER signaling are still poorly understood [37,38].

In this study, the influence of gender and TLS expression on patient prognosis was first investigated by H&E staining analysis in a large cohort of 348 PAAD patients from our institute. Through the large sample study, we confirmed the prognostic value of intratumoral TLS in PAAD. In addition, we found that female patients had a slightly better prognosis and a relatively higher proportion of TLS (+) samples than male patients. Together, the result indicated a potential protective role of ER signaling in PAAD.

We then attempted to investigate the expression patterns and assess the prognostic values for all three ERs in PAAD. Positive staining can be detected for ERα, ERβ, and GPER in 41.4%, 73.0%, and 77.0% of PAAD tumor tissues, respectively. In particular, ERα (+) and ERβ (+) were correlated with high tumor grade, ERβ (+) and GPER (+) were correlated with lower TNM stage, and both ERα and GPER showed a beneficial effect in this cohort. These findings revealed that the positive expression of ERs in tumor cells might serve novel beneficial prognostic factors for PAAD.

4.2. Estrogen Signaling as a Target to Remodel PAAD Microenvironment

PAAD is featured by a "desmoplasia, inflammation, and immune suppression" microenvironment and recent studies suggested that GPER may harbor the capacity to remodel the microenvironment [15–17]. Our study reported that the expression of ERs (including GPER) in PAAD was strongly correlated with the presence of intratumoral TLSs and more infiltration of active immune cells in the tumor microenvironment. In vitro analyses further revealed that the chemotaxis of CD8$^+$T-cells was significantly increased under the influence of upregulated ERα or ERβ on PAAD cells, demonstrating the role of ERs in anti-tumor immunity in PAAD.

However, whether ER signaling can serve as a therapeutic target to induce TLSs in PAAD and to remodel the immune microenvironment remains unclear. Recently, the rapid development of molecular dynamics and other computational approaches has greatly facilitated the understanding of dynamic receptor–ligand interactions [39,40]. These tools may become an appropriate complement to understanding the roles of ER signaling in PAAD and identifying potential therapeutics targeting ERs to improve PAAD prognosis.

Nevertheless, the functions of estrogen signaling in regulating immune response were well-understood in both autoimmune diseases and other cancers [41]. Previous evidence demonstrated that ER signaling could contribute to the maturation, activation, or proliferation of a diversity of immune cells (e.g., effector T-cells and B-cells) [42–44]. Since intratumoral TLS formation was based on crosstalk among immune cells, further study will focus on the TLS-inducing mechanism of estrogen signaling.

To conclude, our study provided an overview of ERα, ERβ, and GPER expression patterns in PAAD. The expression of all three ERs was correlated with the formation and development of PAAD-associated TLSs, and the manipulation of ER signaling may contribute to the remodeling of the PAAD immune microenvironment.

Supplementary Materials: The following supporting information can be downloaded at: https://www.mdpi.com/article/10.3390/cancers15030828/s1, Table S1; Table S2; Table S3.

Author Contributions: Conceptualization, C.L. and X.Y.; methodology, Y.L.; software, X.L.; validation, R.W.; formal analysis, Z.D.; resources, Y.C.; data curation, M.M.; writing—original draft preparation, X.Z.; writing—review and editing, H.C. and X.W.; visualization, Y.Y.; supervision, Y.T. All authors have read and agreed to the published version of the manuscript.

Funding: This work was supported by the National Natural Science Foundation of China (grant numbers 82072693, 81902417, 82172884, U21A20374), the Scientific Innovation Project of Shanghai Education Committee (2019-01-07-00-07-E00057), Shanghai Municipal Science and Technology Major Project (21JC1401500), Clinical and Scientific Innovation Project of Shanghai Hospital Development Center (SHDC12018109), Clinical Research Plan of Shanghai Hospital Development Center (SHDC2020CR1006A), National Key Research and Development Program of China (2020YFA0803202), and Xuhui District Artificial Intelligence Medical Hospital Cooperation Project (2021-011).

Institutional Review Board Statement: The study was approved by the Medical Ethics Committee of Fudan University Shanghai Cancer Center (ID: 050432-4-2108*).

Informed Consent Statement: Informed consent was obtained from all subjects involved in the study.

Data Availability Statement: All the transcriptome data generated or analyzed during the present study was downloaded from the TCGA (https://portal.gdc.cancer.gov accessed on 10 January 2023) and CPTAC (https://cptac-data-portal.georgetown.edu accessed on 10 January 2023) databases that could be available with open access.

Conflicts of Interest: The authors declare no conflict of interest.

References

1. Klein, A.P. Pancreatic cancer epidemiology: Understanding the role of lifestyle and inherited risk factors. *Nat. Rev. Gastroenterol. Hepatol.* **2021**, *18*, 493–502. [CrossRef] [PubMed]
2. Siegel, R.L.; Miller, K.D.; Fuchs, H.E.; Jemal, A. Cancer Statistics, 2021. *CA Cancer J. Clin.* **2021**, *71*, 7–33. [CrossRef] [PubMed]
3. Mauvais-Jarvis, F.; Clegg, D.; Hevener, A. The role of estrogens in control of energy balance and glucose homeostasis. *Endocr. Rev.* **2013**, *34*, 309–338. [CrossRef] [PubMed]
4. Miyamoto, H. Sex Hormone Receptor Signals in Human Malignancies. *Int. J. Mol. Sci.* **2019**, *20*, 2677. [CrossRef]
5. Wang, T.; Jin, J.; Qian, C.; Lou, J.; Lin, J.; Xu, A.; Xia, K.; Jin, L.; Liu, B.; Tao, H.; et al. Estrogen/ER in anti-tumor immunity regulation to tumor cell and tumor microenvironment. *Cancer Cell Int.* **2021**, *21*, 295. [CrossRef]
6. Rothenberger, N.J.; Somasundaram, A.; Stabile, L. The Role of the Estrogen Pathway in the Tumor Microenvironment. *Int. J. Mol. Sci.* **2018**, *19*, 611. [CrossRef]
7. Delaunay, F.; Pettersson, K.; Tujague, M.; Gustafsson, J.Å. Functional differences between the amino-terminal domains of estrogen receptors alpha and beta. *Mol. Pharmacol.* **2000**, *58*, 584–590. [CrossRef]
8. Liu, Q.; Chen, Z.; Jiang, G.; Zhou, Y.; Yang, X.; Huang, H.; Liu, H.; Du, J.; Wang, H. Epigenetic down regulation of G protein-coupled estrogen receptor (GPER) functions as a tumor suppressor in colorectal cancer. *Mol. Cancer* **2017**, *16*, 87. [CrossRef]
9. Satake, M.; Sawai, H.; Go, V.L.W.; Satake, K.; Reber, H.A.; Hines, O.J.; Eibl, G. Estrogen receptors in pancreatic tumors. *Pancreas* **2006**, *33*, 119–127. [CrossRef]
10. Chan, K.S.; Ho, B.C.S.; Shelat, V.G. A pilot study of estrogen receptor (ER) expression in pancreatic ductal adenocarcinoma (PDAC). *Transl. Gastroenterol. Hepatol.* **2021**, *6*, 9. [CrossRef] [PubMed]

11. Younes, M.; Ly, C.J.; Singh, K.; Ertan, A.; Younes, P.S.; Bailey, J.M. Expression of estrogen receptor beta isoforms in pancreatic adenocarcinoma. *Oncotarget* **2018**, *9*, 37715–37720. [CrossRef] [PubMed]
12. Gunderson, A.J.; Rajamanickam, V.; Bui, C.; Bernard, B.; Pucilowska, J.; Ballesteros-Merino, C.; Schmidt, M.; McCarty, K.; Philips, M.; Piening, B.; et al. Germinal center reactions in tertiary lymphoid structures associate with neoantigen burden, humoral immunity and long-term survivorship in pancreatic cancer. *Oncoimmunology* **2021**, *10*, 1900635. [CrossRef] [PubMed]
13. Schumacher, T.N.; Thommen, D. Tertiary lymphoid structures in cancer. *Science* **2022**, *375*, eabf9419. [CrossRef] [PubMed]
14. Sautès-Fridman, C.; Petitprez, F.; Calderaro, J.; Fridman, W.H. Tertiary lymphoid structures in the era of cancer immunotherapy. *Nat. Rev. Cancer* **2019**, *19*, 307–325. [CrossRef] [PubMed]
15. Natale, C.A.; Li, J.; Pitarresi, J.R.; Norgard, R.J.; Dentchev, T.; Capell, B.C.; Seykora, J.T.; Stanger, B.Z.; Ridky, T.W. Pharmacologic Activation of the G Protein-Coupled Estrogen Receptor Inhibits Pancreatic Ductal Adenocarcinoma. *Cell. Mol. Gastroenterol. Hepatol.* **2020**, *10*, 868–880.e1. [CrossRef]
16. Cortes, E.; Sarper, M.; Robinson, B.; Lachowski, D.; Chronopoulos, A.; Thorpe, S.D.; Lee, D.A.; Hernández, A.E.D.R. GPER is a mechanoregulator of pancreatic stellate cells and the tumor microenvironment. *EMBO Rep.* **2019**, *20*, e46556. [CrossRef] [PubMed]
17. Cortes, E.; Lachowski, D.; Robinson, B.; Sarper, M.; Teppo, J.S.; Thorpe, S.D.; Lieberthal, T.J.; Iwamoto, K.; Lee, D.A.; Okada-Hatakeyama, M.; et al. Tamoxifen mechanically reprograms the tumor microenvironment via HIF-1A and reduces cancer cell survival. *EMBO Rep.* **2019**, *20*, e46557. [CrossRef]
18. Cao, L.; Huang, C.; Cui Zhou, D.; Hu, Y.; Lih, T.M.; Savage, S.R.; Krug, K.; Clark, D.J.; Schnaubelt, M.; Chen, L.; et al. Proteogenomic characterization of pancreatic ductal adenocarcinoma. *Cell* **2021**, *184*, 5031–5052.e26. [CrossRef]
19. Li, X.; Wan, Z.; Liu, X.; Ou, K.; Yang, L. A 12-chemokine gene signature is associated with the enhanced immunogram scores and is relevant for precision immunotherapy. *Med. Oncol.* **2022**, *39*, 43. [CrossRef]
20. Tokunaga, R.; Nakagawa, S.; Sakamoto, Y.; Nakamura, K.; Naseem, M.; Izumi, D.; Kosumi, K.; Taki, K.; Higashi, T.; Miyata, T.; et al. 12-Chemokine signature, a predictor of tumor recurrence in colorectal cancer. *Int. J. Cancer* **2020**, *147*, 532–541. [CrossRef]
21. Huang, D.W.; Sherman, B.T.; Tan, Q.; Collins, J.R.; Alvord, W.G.; Roayaei, J.; Stephens, R.; Baseler, M.W.; Lane, H.C.; Lempicki, R.A. The DAVID Gene Functional Classification Tool: A novel biological module-centric algorithm to functionally analyze large gene lists. *Genome Biol.* **2007**, *8*, R183. [CrossRef] [PubMed]
22. Steen, C.B.; Liu, C.L.; Alizadeh, A.A.; Newman, A.M. Profiling Cell Type Abundance and Expression in Bulk Tissues with CIBERSORTx. *Methods Mol. Biol.* **2020**, *2117*, 135–157. [PubMed]
23. Liu, Y.; Xu, Z.; Zhang, Z.; Wen, G.; Sun, J.; Han, F. Efficacy and safety of TE/TEC/intensive paclitaxel neoadjuvant chemotherapy for the treatment of breast cancer. *Oncol. Lett.* **2019**, *17*, 907–912. [CrossRef] [PubMed]
24. Warfvinge, K.; Krause, D.N.; Maddahi, A.; Edvinsson, J.C.; Edvinsson, L.; Haanes, K.A. Estrogen receptors alpha, beta and GPER in the CNS and trigeminal system—Molecular and functional aspects. *J. Headache Pain* **2020**, *21*, 131. [CrossRef]
25. Carmeci, C.; Thompson, D.A.; Ring, H.Z.; Francke, U.; Weigel, R. Identification of a gene (GPR30) with homology to the G-protein-coupled receptor superfamily associated with estrogen receptor expression in breast cancer. *Genomics* **1997**, *45*, 607–617. [CrossRef]
26. Ritchie, M.E.; Belinda, P.; Wu, D.; Hu, Y.; Law, C.W.; Shi, W.; Smyth, G.K. limma powers differential expression analyses for RNA-sequencing and microarray studies. *Nucleic Acids Res.* **2015**, *43*, e47. [CrossRef]
27. Subramanian, A.; Tamayo, P.; Mootha, V.K.; Mukherjee, S.; Ebert, B.L.; Gillette, M.A.; Paulovich, A.; Pomeroy, S.L.; Golub, T.R.; Lander, E.S.; et al. Gene set enrichment analysis: A knowledge-based approach for interpreting genome-wide expression profiles. *Proc. Natl. Acad. Sci. USA* **2005**, *102*, 15545–15550. [CrossRef]
28. Prabhakaran, S.; Rizk, V.T.; Ma, Z.; Cheng, C.-H.; Berglund, A.E.; Coppola, D.; Khalil, F.; Mulé, J.J.; Soliman, H.H. Evaluation of invasive breast cancer samples using a 12-chemokine gene expression score: Correlation with clinical outcomes. *Breast Cancer Res.* **2017**, *19*, 71. [CrossRef]
29. Lopes-Ramos, C.M.; Quackenbush, J.; DeMeo, D.L. Genome-Wide Sex and Gender Differences in Cancer. *Front. Oncol.* **2020**, *10*, 597788. [CrossRef]
30. Conforti, F.; Pala, L.; Bagnardi, V.; De Pas, T.; Martinetti, M.; Viale, G.; Gelber, R.D.; Goldhirsch, A. Cancer immunotherapy efficacy and patients' sex: A systematic review and meta-analysis. *Lancet Oncol.* **2018**, *19*, 737–746. [CrossRef]
31. Clocchiatti, A.; Cora, E.; Zhang, Y.; Dotto, G.P. Sexual dimorphism in cancer. *Nat. Rev. Cancer* **2016**, *16*, 330–339. [CrossRef] [PubMed]
32. Chen, C.; Gong, X.; Yang, X.; Shang, X.; Du, Q.; Liao, Q.; Xie, R.; Chen, Y.; Xu, J. The roles of estrogen and estrogen receptors in gastrointestinal disease. *Oncol. Lett.* **2019**, *18*, 5673–5680. [CrossRef] [PubMed]
33. Qin, J.; Liu, M.; Ding, Q.; Ji, X.; Hao, Y.; Wu, X.; Xiong, J. The direct effect of estrogen on cell viability and apoptosis in human gastric cancer cells. *Mol. Cell. Biochem.* **2014**, *395*, 99–107. [CrossRef] [PubMed]
34. Wilkins, H.R.; Doucet, K.; Duke, V.; Morra, A.; Johnson, N. Estrogen prevents sustained COLO-205 human colon cancer cell growth by inducing apoptosis, decreasing c-myb protein, and decreasing transcription of the anti-apoptotic protein bcl-2. *Tumour Biol.* **2010**, *31*, 16–22. [CrossRef]
35. Al-Khyatt, W.; Tufarelli, C.; Khan, R.; Iftikhar, S.Y. Selective oestrogen receptor antagonists inhibit oesophageal cancer cell proliferation in vitro. *BMC Cancer* **2018**, *18*, 121. [CrossRef]

36. Yue, W.; Yager, J.D.; Wang, J.-P.; Jupe, E.R.; Santen, R.J. Estrogen receptor-dependent and independent mechanisms of breast cancer carcinogenesis. *Steroids* **2013**, *78*, 161–170. [CrossRef]
37. Rawla, P.; Sunkara, T.; Gaduputi, V. Epidemiology of Pancreatic Cancer: Global Trends, Etiology and Risk Factors. *World J. Oncol.* **2019**, *10*, 10–27. [CrossRef]
38. Andersson, G.; Borgquist, S.; Jirström, K. Hormonal factors and pancreatic cancer risk in women: The Malmö Diet and Cancer Study. *Int. J. Cancer* **2018**, *143*, 52–62. [CrossRef]
39. Celik, L.; Lund, J.D.D.; Schiøtt, B. Conformational dynamics of the estrogen receptor alpha: Molecular dynamics simulations of the influence of binding site structure on protein dynamics. *Biochemistry* **2007**, *46*, 1743–1758. [CrossRef]
40. Allec, S.I.; Sun, Y.; Sun, J.; Chang CE, A.; Wong, B.M. Heterogeneous CPU+GPU-Enabled Simulations for DFTB Molecular Dynamics of Large Chemical and Biological Systems. *J. Chem. Theory Comput.* **2019**, *15*, 2807–2815. [CrossRef]
41. Chakraborty, B.; Byemerwa, J.; Krebs, T.; Lim, F.; Chang, C.-Y.; McDonnell, D.P. Estrogen receptor signaling in the immune system. *Endocr. Rev.* **2022**, *44*, 117–141. [CrossRef] [PubMed]
42. Hill, L.; Jeganathan, V.; Chinnasamy, P.; Grimaldi, C.; Diamond, B. Differential roles of estrogen receptors α and β in control of B-cell maturation and selection. *Mol. Med.* **2011**, *17*, 211–220. [CrossRef] [PubMed]
43. Fu, Y.; Li, L.; Liu, X.; Ma, C.; Zhang, J.; Jiao, Y.; You, L.; Chen, Z.J.; Zhao, Y. Estrogen promotes B cell activation in vitro through down-regulating CD80 molecule expression. *Gynecol. Endocrinol.* **2011**, *27*, 593–596. [CrossRef]
44. Mohammad, I.; Starskaia, I.; Nagy, T.; Guo, J.; Yatkin, E.; Väänänen, K.; Watford, W.T.; Chen, Z. Estrogen receptor α contributes to T cell-mediated autoimmune inflammation by promoting T cell activation and proliferation. *Sci. Signal.* **2018**, *11*, eaap9415. [CrossRef]

Disclaimer/Publisher's Note: The statements, opinions and data contained in all publications are solely those of the individual author(s) and contributor(s) and not of MDPI and/or the editor(s). MDPI and/or the editor(s) disclaim responsibility for any injury to people or property resulting from any ideas, methods, instructions or products referred to in the content.

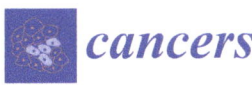

Article

The Immunocytokine FAP-IL-2v Enhances Anti-Neuroblastoma Efficacy of the Anti-GD$_2$ Antibody Dinutuximab Beta

Nikolai Siebert *,†, Justus Leopold †, Maxi Zumpe, Sascha Troschke-Meurer, Simon Biskupski, Alexander Zikoridse and Holger N. Lode *

Department of Pediatric Oncology and Hematology, University Medicine Greifswald, 17475 Greifswald, Germany
* Correspondence: nikolai.siebert@med.uni-greifswald.de (N.S.); holger.lode@uni-greifswald.de (H.N.L.);
  Tel.: +49-3834-86-6329 (N.S.); +49-3834-86-6300 (H.N.L.)
† These authors contributed equally to this work.

Simple Summary: Since IL-2 co-treatment did not show any therapeutic benefit in the GD$_2$-directed treatment of high-risk neuroblastoma (NB) but strongly induced regulatory T cells (Treg), we investigated here the immunocytokine FAP-IL-2v stimulating NK and cytotoxic T cells without induction of Treg. We first detected FAP on NB- and myeloid-derived suppressor cells (MDCS) in tumor tissue and showed a tumor-cell-dependent enhancement in FAP expression by fibroblasts. Treatment of leukocytes with FAP-IL-2v increased ADCC mediated by the anti-GD$_2$ antibody dinutuximab beta (DB) against NB cells. We next evaluated the antitumor efficacy of a combinatorial immunotherapy by applying DB and FAP-IL-2v and observed strongly reduced tumor growth and improved survival in experimental mice. Analysis of tumor tissue revealed increased NK and cytotoxic T cell numbers and reduced Treg compared to controls. Our data show that FAP-IL-2v is a potent immunocytokine that augments the efficacy of DB against NB, providing a promising alternative to IL-2.

Citation: Siebert, N.; Leopold, J.; Zumpe, M.; Troschke-Meurer, S.; Biskupski, S.; Zikoridse, A.; Lode, H.N. The Immunocytokine FAP-IL-2v Enhances Anti-Neuroblastoma Efficacy of the Anti-GD$_2$ Antibody Dinutuximab Beta. *Cancers* **2022**, *14*, 4842. https://doi.org/10.3390/cancers14194842

Academic Editor: David Wong

Received: 8 September 2022
Accepted: 29 September 2022
Published: 4 October 2022

Publisher's Note: MDPI stays neutral with regard to jurisdictional claims in published maps and institutional affiliations.

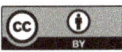

Copyright: © 2022 by the authors. Licensee MDPI, Basel, Switzerland. This article is an open access article distributed under the terms and conditions of the Creative Commons Attribution (CC BY) license (https://creativecommons.org/licenses/by/4.0/).

Abstract: Treatment of high-risk neuroblastoma (NB) patients with the anti-GD$_2$ antibody (Ab) dinutuximab beta (DB) improves survival by 15%. Ab-dependent cellular cytotoxicity (ADCC) is the major mechanism of action and is primarily mediated by NK cells. Since IL-2 co-treatment did not show a therapeutic benefit but strongly induced Treg, we investigated here a DB-based immunotherapy combined with the immunocytokine FAP-IL-2v, which comprises a fibroblast activation protein α (FAP)-specific Ab linked to a mutated IL-2 variant (IL-2v) with abolished binding to the high-affinity IL-2 receptor, thus stimulating NK cells without induction of Treg. Effects of FAP-IL-2v on NK cells, Treg and ADCC mediated by DB, as well as FAP expression in NB, were investigated by flow cytometry, calcein-AM-based cytotoxicity assay and RT-PCR analysis. Moreover, the impact of soluble factors released from tumor cells on FAP expression by primary fibroblasts was assessed. Finally, a combined immunotherapy with DB and FAP-IL-2v was evaluated using a resistant syngeneic murine NB model. Incubation of leukocytes with FAP-IL-2v enhanced DB-specific ADCC without induction of Treg. FAP expression on NB cells and myeloid-derived suppressor cells (MDCS) in tumor tissue was identified. A tumor-cell-dependent enhancement in FAP expression by primary fibroblasts was demonstrated. Combination with DB and FAP-IL-2v resulted in reduced tumor growth and improved survival. Analysis of tumor tissue revealed increased NK and cytotoxic T cell numbers and reduced Treg compared to controls. Our data show that FAP-IL-2v is a potent immunocytokine that augments the efficacy of DB against NB, providing a promising alternative to IL-2.

Keywords: neuroblastoma; immunotherapy; dinutuximab beta; fibroblast activation protein α; FAP-IL-2v; myeloid-derived suppressor cells

1. Introduction

Neuroblastoma (NB) is a malignant disease of childhood with a poor prognosis in the high-risk group [1]. In Europe, treatment of high-risk NB patients with the chimeric anti-GD$_2$

antibody (Ab) dinutuximab beta (DB) in combination with the immune stimulating cytokine interleukin-2 (IL-2) resulted in a 15% improvement in 5-year survival compared to the standard treatment [2]. Therapeutic Ab directed against tumor antigens mediates antitumor effects primarily through the induction of antibody-dependent cellular cytotoxicity (ADCC), whereby natural killer (NK) cells are the major effector cells. Indeed, it was shown that the depletion of NK cells resulted in the complete abrogation of the antitumor effects mediated by DB [3]. The rationale of combining DB with IL-2 for NB treatment was based on the stimulating effects of IL-2 on NK cells. However, evaluation of the progression-free (PFS) and overall survival (OS) probabilities in high-risk NB patients treated with or without IL-2 did not reveal any additional treatment benefit of IL-2, while higher treatment-related toxicity was observed in the patients who additionally received IL-2 [4]. Although administration of IL-2 resulted in an approximately three-fold increase in cytotoxic NK cells [5], thus confirming the rationale of using IL-2 in combination with DB, the undesired strong expansion of regulatory T cells (Treg) with increased levels over 20-fold compared to the baseline was also detected in the patients of the combinatorial cohort [5]. These results explain in part the unexpected absence of the clinical benefit of IL-2.

The use of alternative immune-stimulating agents that do not preferentially induce immune-inhibiting cells may provide an alternative. One promising molecule in this context is the mutated variant of IL-2 (IL-2v), with reduced binding to the IL-2RA subunit of the high-affinity trimeric IL-2 receptor (IL-2RABG; A, B and G for α (CD25), β (CD122) and γ receptor chain (CD132)) [6] expressed by Treg but with efficient binding to the intermediate-affinity dimeric IL-2RBG [6] expressed by NK and resting T cells. Recently, the proliferation of NK cells and effective activation of cytotoxic T cells without preferential activation of Treg has been shown in vitro after incubation of peripheral blood mononuclear cells with IL-2v conjugated with an Ab against the fibroblast activation protein α (FAP) [7]. Due to abolished Fcγ receptor binding (P329G LALA mutations), FAP-IL-2v does not induce ADCC against FAP-positive cells and serves as a vehicle for IL-2v, transporting it into the tumor microenvironment. Importantly, the activating effects of FAP-IL-2v on effector cells by IL-2v has been shown to be translated into the considerably enhanced antitumor activity of these effector cells against tumor cells mediated by the therapeutic Ab [7], thus clearly showing advantageous therapeutic effects compared to the non-modified IL-2.

Moreover, as the administration of cytokines is known to be associated with systemic side effects, the usage of immunocytokines (tumor-specific Ab genetically linked to cytokines) transporting cytokines directly into the site of tumor could overcome this obstacle. A common tumor-associated antigen is the fibroblast-activating protein (FAP), which is detectable in tumor tissue of different malignancies. FAP is a dimeric protease localized primarily on the cell surfaces of cancer-associated fibroblasts (CAFs), which have been shown to play a protumoral role [8]. Generally, CAFs are known to increase tumor cell invasion, angiogenesis and tumor growth and their presence correlates with a poor prognosis [8]. Importantly, CAFs have been detected in NB [9], thus suggesting FAP targeting as a promising therapeutic strategy against this aggressive tumor. Based on these observations, we hypothesized that a combinatorial treatment of NB with DB and the immunocytokine FAP-IL-2v can further augment the antitumor efficacy of DB.

In the present study, we first investigated the effects of FAP-IL-2v on Treg and ADCC mediated by DB against NB cells. Next, we assessed FAP expression by primary and well-known NB cells, as well as in a murine NB tumor tissue. We then investigated the impact of soluble factors released from tumor cells on FAP expression by primary fibroblasts isolated from murine skin tissue. Finally, we evaluated the antitumor efficacy of the combinatorial treatment with DB and FAP-IL-2v in vivo using our syngeneic murine-resistant NB model, followed by the analysis of tumor-infiltrating effector cells.

2. Materials and Methods

2.1. Ethics Statement

All procedures involving human participants were in accordance with the ethical standards of the institutional and national research committee and with the 1964 Helsinki declaration and its later amendments or comparable ethical standards. Informed consent was obtained from all individual participants (Ethics Board of the Medical Faculty of the University Greifswald, approval code number: BB 014/14, 24 January 2014). All procedures involving animal experiments were approved by the animal welfare committee (Landesamt für Landwirtschaft, Lebensmittelsicherheit und Fischerei Mecklenburg-Vorpommern, approval code number: LALLF M-V/7221.3-1-011/20, 7 September 2020) and approved and supervised by the commissioner for animal welfare at the University Medicine Greifswald representing the Institutional Animal Care and Use Committee (IACUC).

2.2. Cell Cultivation

The human NB cell lines CHLA-20, CHLA-90, CHLA-136 and CHLA-172, as well as in-house-established cell lines from tumor samples derived from high-risk NB patients (HGW-1, HGW-3, HGW-5) [10] and the newly established cell line HGW-B, were cultivated in IMDM (PAN-Biotech GmbH, Aidenbach, Germany) supplemented with 4 mM stable glutamine (Fisher Scientific, Waltham, MA, USA), 30 U/mL penicillin and 0.03 mg/mL streptomycin (0.3× P/S; PAN-Biotech GmbH, Aidenbach, Germany) and 20% FBS Good (PAN-Biotech GmbH, Aidenbach, Germany). The primary cell line HGW-B was established as described for the cell lines HGW-1, HGW-3, HGW-5 [10]. The human NB cells Kelly, SMS-KCN and LAN-1 were cultivated in RPMI 1640 (Capricorn Scientific GmbH, Ebsdorfergrund, Germany) supplemented with 2 mM stable glutamine, 0.3× P/S and 10% Sera Plus (PAN-Biotech GmbH, Aidenbach, Germany). The human FAP-positive cell line Wi-38 served as a positive control was cultivated in DMEM (Capricorn Scientific GmbH, Ebsdorfergrund, Germany) supplemented with 2 mM stable glutamine, 0.3× P/S, 15% FBS Good and 1× NEAA (Capricorn Scientific GmbH, Ebsdorfergrund, Germany). The murine NB cells NXS2-HGW [11,12] used for the tumor cell implantation in vivo were cultivated in DMEM supplemented with 2 mM stable glutamine, 0.3× P/S and 10% FBS Good. Primary adult murine fibroblasts (PAMF) isolated from skin tissue of A/J mice were cultivated in DMEM supplemented with 4 mM stable glutamine, 0.3× P/S, 1× ITS (Capricorn Scientific GmbH, Ebsdorfergrund, Germany) and 15% FBS Good. Prior to cultivation, mycoplasma contamination analysis was performed for every cell line using the MYCOALERT Detection Kit (Lonza Cologne GmbH, Cologne, Germany). Only mycoplasma-negative cell lines were used for experiments. All cell lines were passaged no more than 30 times.

2.3. ADCC

To analyze effects of FAP-IL-2v on the cellular cytotoxic activity of effector cells (ADCC) mediated by DB, a non-radioactive calcein-AM-based cytotoxicity assay was used, as previously described [10]. Briefly, leukocytes of healthy donors were cultivated for five days using RPMI 1640 (Capricorn Scientific GmbH, Ebsdorfergrund, Germany) supplemented with 2 mM stable glutamine, 0.3× P/S and 10% Sera Plus (PAN-Biotech GmbH, Aidenbach, Germany). To show the effects of FAP-IL-2v on ADCC, culture medium was supplemented with 1 µg/mL/day of FAP-IL-2v. Untreated leukocytes and leukocytes incubated with IL-2 (3000 IU/mL/day) served as controls. To induce ADCC against NB cells, DB (10 µg/mL) and an effector-to-target cell ratio of 40:1 were used. The GD_2-positive human NB cells LAN-1 (5000 cells/well) served as targets cells. The GD_2 specificity of ADCC was confirmed using the anti-idiotype Ab ganglidiomab [13]. The DB-independent cytotoxicity of leukocytes (AICC, antibody-independent cellular cytotoxicity) was evaluated by incubation of leukocytes with tumor cells with rituximab.

2.4. Isolation of PAMF

To assess FAP expression by primary fibroblasts and address whether the injection of syngeneic NB cells in combination with primary fibroblasts results in the development of CAF-positive tumors, we first isolated fibroblasts from the skin tissue of female adult A/J mice. After mice were sacrificed, the fur was removed with hair removal cream. Following disinfection (70% ethanol), skin samples were extracted and cut into small pieces of around 2×2 mm size using a scalpel. Tissue samples were then enzymatically digested using a Tumor Dissociation Kit (Miltenyi Biotech, Bergisch Gladbach, Germany) for 90 min at 37 °C. To remove debris, the samples were then filtered using a 70 μm cell strainer. The obtained single-cell solution was finally cultivated in PAMF-specific medium, as described above.

2.5. Analysis of Tumor-Cell-Dependent Impact of FAP Expression by PAMF

To evaluate the effects of soluble factors released by NB cells on the FAP expression on primary fibroblasts, PAMF were cultivated with tumor-conditioned medium (TCM) followed by flow cytometry analysis of FAP. For this, 1×10^4 PAMF of the first or second passage was seeded and cultivated for 24 h. Thereafter, 50% of the culture medium was replaced with the tumor-conditioned medium harvested after 48 h cultivation of the murine NB cells NXS2-HGW.

Finally, the treated cells were harvested and used for flow cytometry analysis.

2.6. Establishment of a Resistant Version of the NB Model In Vivo

Since the immunotherapy with DB (i.p., five consecutive days, 3 mg/kg bw/day, start of treatment: four days after tumor cell implantation) showed strong antitumor efficacy against NB in our syngeneic tumor model, resulting in constant tumor regression [12,14], we aimed to establish a more resistant version of this model allowing the evaluation of different therapeutic agents in combination with DB. For this, we started DB treatments in a later tumor growth phase. The new treatment protocol was established by the comparison of the following three time points at which the DB immunotherapy was started: day 11, 12 and 14. Briefly, for all in vivo experiments, mice were randomized prior to tumor cell injection. Female 11-week-old A/J mice (Charles River Laboratories, Sulzfeld, Germany) were granted a two-week acclimatization time, accommodated in groups of maximum 6 animals in standard animal laboratories (12 h light/dark cycle, 20 °C ± 2 °C room temperature, 60% ± 20% humidity) with ad libitum access to water and standard laboratory chow. Mice of all experimental groups were subcutaneously injected with 2×10^6 tumor cells on the left ventral flank, followed by the DB immunotherapy (i.p., five consecutive days, 3 mg/kg/day bw). Untreated controls received an equivalent volume of 0.9% NaCl. The treatments were started either on day 8 or day 11 or day 14 after tumor cell implantation. Tumor and/or treatment burden parameters [12] were assessed every two days after tumor cell injection and daily starting on day 8. Tumors were measured using a caliper, followed by tumor volume calculation according to the formula (length $\times$ width $\times$ height)/2. Mice were sacrificed when tumors exceeded 750 mm³. For those mice killed ahead of schedule, the tumor volume data of the last measurement were included into the calculation of the group-specific average volumes at the subsequent time points.

After a more resistant version of our syngeneic tumor model was established, the new treatment protocol was used in the following in vivo experiments for the evaluation of the antitumor efficacy of the combinatorial therapy with FAP-IL-2v and DB.

2.7. Induction of CAF Development in Tumor Tissue In Vivo

Prior to the evaluation of the antitumor efficacy of the combinatorial treatment, we investigated whether injection of the tumor cells NXS2-HGW in combination with the syngeneic PAMF led to the development of CAFs in tumor tissue. For this, mice of an additional experimental group were subcutaneously injected in the left ventral flank with 2×10^6 tumor cells in combination with 1×10^6 PAMF ($\geq$95% viability). Prior to this, PAMF were isolated from murine skin tissue and cultivated for one week, as described above.

2.8. Evaluation of Antitumor Effects of Combinatorial Immunotherapy with DB and FAP-IL-2v

To evaluate the treatment efficacy of DB in combination with FAP-IL-2v, a lethal syngeneic murine NB model in a more resistant version was used, as described above. Mice were treated i.p. with DB (five consecutive days, 3 mg/kg/day bw) or FAP-IL-2v Ab (twice a week, 1 mg/kg bw) or with a combination of both. Untreated controls received the equivalent volumes of 0.9% NaCl. Moreover, to show IL-2-dependent effects, mice of an additional control group were treated with IL-2 (twice a week, 3×10^6 IU/kg bw/day).

2.9. Flow Cytometry

To identify different populations of tumor-infiltrating leukocytes or fibroblasts or to determine the surface abundance of FAP in different cell types, flow cytometry analysis was performed. For this, PE-labeled anti-human anti-FAP Ab (R&D Systems, Minneapolis, MN, USA) or rabbit anti human/mouse anti-FAP (Abcam plc, Cambridge, UK) and respective PE-labeled Fc-specific secondary Ab (Abcam plc, Cambridge, UK) were used. NB cells were detected using the Alexa Fluor647-labeled anti-GD_2 chimeric Ab DB. Fibroblasts were identified using FITC-labeled anti-mouse anti-CD140a REAfinity Ab (Miltenyi Biotec, Teterow, Germany). For detection of different tumor-infiltrating leukocyte populations described below, the following Ab were utilized: APC-Vio® 770-labeled anti-mouse CD3 REAfinity™ Ab, VioGreen™-labeled anti-mouse CD4 Antibody REAfinity™, PerCP-labeled anti-mouse CD8a REAfinity™ Ab, Vio® Bright FITC-labeled anti-mouse CD11b REAfinity™ Ab, PE-Vio® 770-labeled anti-mouse CD25 REAfinity™ Ab, PE-labeled anti-mouse CD335 REAfinity™ Ab, APC-labeled anti-mouse FoxP3 REAfinity™ Ab (all Miltenyi Biotec, Teterow, Germany), APC/Cy-7-labeled anti-mouse Ly6C Ab and PerCP-labeled anti-mouse Ly6G Ab (BioLegend, San Diego, CA, USA). For every primary Ab, respective ITC were used to determine the potential background caused by nonspecific Ab binding.

First, primary tumors were resected from the experimental mice, followed by the preparation of tumor tissue single-cell suspensions using a Tumor Dissociation Kit (Miltenyi Biotech, Teterow, Germany), according to the manufacturer's protocol. After assessment of cell numbers and viability, $1 \mp 2 \times 10^6$ cells were used for the analysis.

The following leukocyte populations were detected in murine tumor tissue using antigen-specific Ab: T cells (CD45+/CD3+), cytotoxic T cells (CD45+/CD3+/CD8+), NK cells (CD45+/CD3−/CD335+), Treg (CD3+/CD4+/CD25+/FoxP3+), CD11b-positive immune cells (CD45+/CD11b+), M-MDSC (CD45+/CD11b+/Ly6C^{high}/Ly6G−), PMN-MDSC (CD45+/CD11b+/Ly6C^{low}/Ly6G+) and Ly6C− and Ly6G-negative immune cells expressing CD11b (CD45+/CD11b+/Ly6C−/Ly6G−). Respective human leukocyte populations were identified as follows: NK cells (CD3−/CD56+), Treg (CD3+/CD4+/CD25+/CD127−).

To exclude unspecific binding of the detection Ab to Fc receptor-expressing cells, samples were first incubated with the FcR Blocking Reagent (Miltenyi Biotech, Teterow, Germany). For intracellular staining, the FoxP3 Staining Buffer Set (Miltenyi Biotech, Teterow, Germany) was used according to the manufacturer's protocol. To exclude dead cells in the samples prepared for the detection of the cell surface antigens, 4 µL of a 0.1 mg/mL 4′,6-diamino-2-phenylindole (DAPI) solution was added 5 min prior to acquisition using a BD CANTO II cytometer and FACS Diva software (BD Biosciences, Heidelberg, Germany). For the intracellular staining, Viobility™ 405/452 Fixable Dye (Miltenyi Biotec, Teterow, Germany) was used according to manufacturer's protocol. Data were analyzed with FlowJo V10 software (Ashland, OR, USA). Moreover, based on the flow cytometry results, the numbers of NK and cytotoxic T cells as well as Treg were calculated as a percentage of all viable tumor-infiltrating leukocytes and T cells, respectively. Additionally, the ratio of cytotoxic T cells to Treg was assessed.

2.10. Statistics

For statistical analysis, SigmaPlot software (Version 13.0, Jandel Scientific Software, San Rafael, CA, USA) was used. First, the acquired data sets were tested for normal distribution. Based on the outcome, either the Mann–Whitney-U-test or Student *t*-test, if the assumption of normality was met, and analysis of variance (ANOVA) to compare more than two samples regarding the significance of a metric trait, were applied. All data are presented as mean ± SEM (standard error of the mean). Survival probabilities (event-free survival (EFS)) were estimated using the LogRank test, and multiple comparison was done with the Holm–Sidak method for post-hoc testing. A tumor volume of 300 mm^3 was defined as an event. A p value of <0.05 (* p or # p) was considered significant, <0.01 (** p) very significant and <0.001 highly significant (*** p).

3. Results

3.1. FAP-IL-2v Effects on ADCC Mediated by DB against NB Cells

To investigate whether the immunocytokine FAP-IL-2v augments ADCC mediated by DB against NB cells, we used a calcein-AM-based cytotoxicity assay. Untreated leukocytes and leukocytes incubated with IL-2 instead of FAP-IL-2v served as controls.

As expected, IL-2 treatment enhanced the cytotoxic activity of leukocytes against the GD$_2$-positive NB cells LAN-1 (Figure 1A) compared to the untreated controls. This effect was GD$_2$-specific, as incubation with the anti-idiotype Ab ganglidiomab completely abrogated ADCC, resulting in similar cytotoxicity levels compared to the negative control (AICC). Similar to the effects observed for IL-2, treatment of leukocytes with the immunocytokine FAP-IL-2v significantly increased ADCC mediated by DB (Figure 1A). An additional incubation with ganglidiomab confirmed the GD$_2$ specificity of the observed effects.

These data clearly show a positive effect of FAP-IL-2v on ADCC against NB cells mediated by DB.

3.2. FAP-IL-2v and IL-2 Effects on Treg

Next, we investigated effects of FAP-IL-2v on Treg. Leukocytes incubated with IL-2 served as controls. Additionally, the effects of both agents on NK cells and cytotoxic T cells (CD8+) were evaluated.

As expected, incubation of leukocytes with IL-2 resulted in a strong increase in Treg numbers compared to the untreated controls (Figure 1B). In contrast, we found similar numbers of Treg after the treatment of leukocytes with FAP-IL-2 compared to the negative control, clearly confirming the fact that IL-2v does not stimulate this cell population. Interestingly, we did not observe any change in the CD8+- and NK cell numbers compared to the untreated controls (Figure 1B).

In summary, incubation of leukocytes with FAP-IL-2v did not stimulate Treg, in contrast to the strong effects of IL-2, leading to an almost two-fold increase in their numbers. These data suggest the rationale of using FAP-IL-2v in combination with DB instead of IL-2.

3.3. FAP Expression by Neuroblastoma Cells

To investigate FAP expression by human NB cells, both well-known (CHLA-15, CHLA-20, CHLA-90, CHLA-136, CHLA-172, LAN-1, Kelly and SMS-KCN) and primary cell lines established from tumor samples derived from high-risk NB patients (HGW-1, HGW-3, HGW-5 and HGW-B) were analyzed by RT-PCR.

While most of the human cell lines analyzed were found to be FAP-negative, FAP mRNA was detected in the cell lines HGW-B, CHLA-90 and CHLA-172 (Figure 2A). Additional analysis of FAP surface abundance using flow cytometry confirmed our RT-PCR results, showing different levels of FAP for these three cell lines (Figure 2B).

These results show both FAP-positive and FAP-negative NB cells, suggesting FAP's role in NB.

3.4. Impact of Tumor Cells on FAP Expression by Primary Fibroblasts (PAMF)

Since soluble factors released by tumor cells can induce CAF development in tumor tissue [15,16], we investigated whether the expression of FAP by primary fibroblasts can be affected by the soluble factors released by the murine NB cells NXS2-HGW used in our in vivo experiments. We first isolated primary adult murine fibroblasts (PAMF) from the skin of adult A/J mice, followed by the flow cytometry analysis of the basal FAP abundance (Figure 3A), as described in the Materials and Methods Section. Additionally, a fibroblast marker, CD140a, was used to identify fibroblasts by flow cytometry.

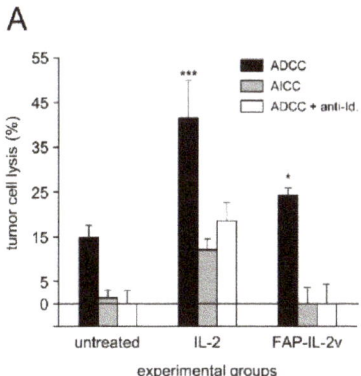

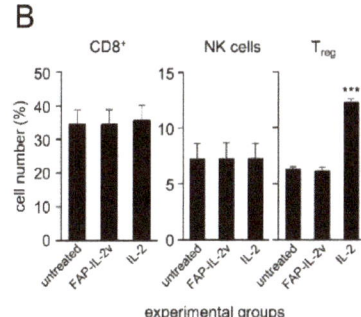

Figure 1. Analysis of FAP-IL-2v effects on GD_2-directed ADCC mediated by dinutuximab beta and on the number of cytotoxic T cells, NK cells and Treg. Leukocytes of healthy donors were treated with either FAP-IL-2v or IL-2 for five days, followed by the analysis of the DB ADCC against the GD_2-positive NB cells LAN-1 and flow cytometry analysis of different effector cell populations. Leukocytes cultivated without FAP-IL-2 and IL-2 served as negative controls (untreated). (**A**) ADCC (black columns) against tumor cells using DB and leukocytes treated with either FAP-IL-2 or IL-2 was assessed using a calcein-AM-based cytotoxicity assay. To show DB-independent tumor cells' lysis (AICC; grey columns) and the GD_2 specificity of the ADCC (white columns), additional samples were incubated with rituximab instead of DB and the anti-idiotype Ab of DB ganglidiomab, respectively. t-test. *** $p < 0.001$ vs. untreated ADCC; * $p < 0.05$ vs. untreated ADCC. (**B**) The effects of FAP-IL-2v and IL-2 on the number of cytotoxic T cells (CD8+), NK cells and Treg were analyzed using flow cytometry. Data are presented as % of the cells relative to all CD3+, lymphocytes and CD4+ cells for cytotoxic T cells, NK cells and Treg, respectively. ANOVA followed by appropriate post-hoc comparison test. *** $p < 0.001$ vs. untreated and FAP-IL-2v.

As expected, PAMF showed a clear signal for CD140a (Figure 3A). Similarly, flow cytometry analysis revealed a basal level of FAP (Figure 3A), thus confirming the suitability of both markers for fibroblast detection. Importantly, incubation of PAMF with tumor-conditioned medium (TCM) for 48 h resulted in a significant, approximately two-fold increase in FAP expression compared to the untreated control (Figure 3B). Interestingly, a TCM-dependent increase in CD140a was also observed (Figure 3C); however, the difference was not statistically significant.

These results clearly show a tumor-cell-dependent enhancement in FAP levels by primary fibroblasts, suggesting the NB-dependent induction of CAFs in tumor tissue.

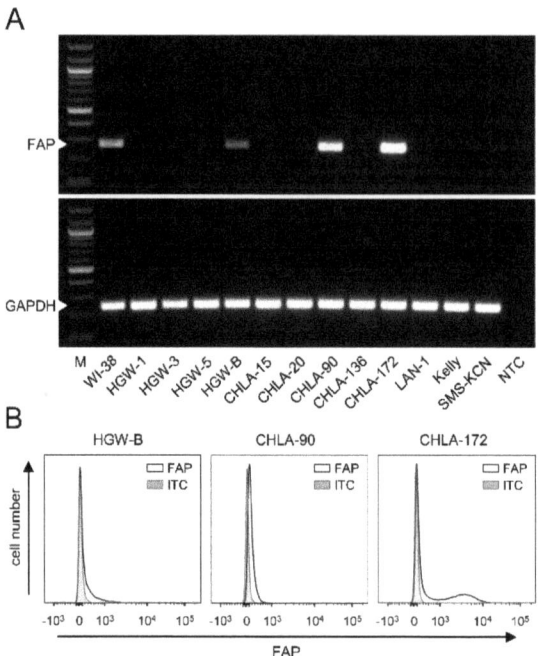

Figure 2. Analysis of FAP expression by human NB cells. (**A**) Representative images of the RT-PCR analysis of FAP mRNA levels (PCR product size: 268 bp) in NB cells derived from tumors of high-risk NB patients (HGW-1, HGW-3, HGW-5, HGW-B) and well-known NB cell lines (CHLA-15, CHLA-20, CHLA-90, CHLA-136, CHLA-172, LAN-1, Kelly, SMS-KCN). Human fibroblasts WI-38 were used as a positive and GAPDH (PCR product size: 238 bp) as an internal control. M: marker, NTC: no template control. (**B**) Representative histograms of the flow cytometry analysis of FAP abundance in human NB cells (HGW-B, CHLA-90, CHLA-172). Cells were stained with anti-human FAP-PE Ab (black curve) or appropriate ITC (grey-filled curve). Full gel images can be found at Supplementary Materials.

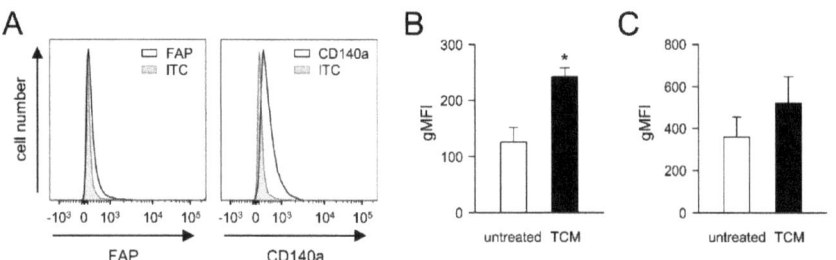

Figure 3. Analysis of tumor-cell-dependent effects on FAP abundance in PAMF. (**A**) Representative histograms of flow cytometry analysis of baseline levels of FAP and CD140a by PAMF. Primary fibroblasts were isolated from skin of female adult A/J mice and cultivated for up to two passages prior to analysis. Cells were then stained with mouse anti-FAP IgG and PE-labeled anti-murine IgG Ab, which served as primary and secondary Ab, respectively (black curve), and with FITC-labeled anti-mouse CD140a Ab or appropriate ITC (grey-filled curve). (**B**,**C**) Impact of soluble factors secreted by the tumor cells NXS2-HGW on FAP (**B**) and CD140a expression by PAMF (**C**). PAMF were incubated with either TCM (TCM, black columns) or control medium for 48 h (untreated, open columns). Expression levels are presented as gMFI quantified according to the following formula: gMFI of sample—gMFI of ITC. *t*-test. * $p < 0.05$.

3.5. FAP Expression in Primary Murine Tumor Tissue

Next, we analyzed FAP mRNA levels in primary tumors collected from the experimental mice three weeks after s.c. injection of the syngeneic NB cells NXS2-HGW. RT-PCR analysis revealed a clear FAP signal in all tumor tissue samples analyzed (Figure 4A).

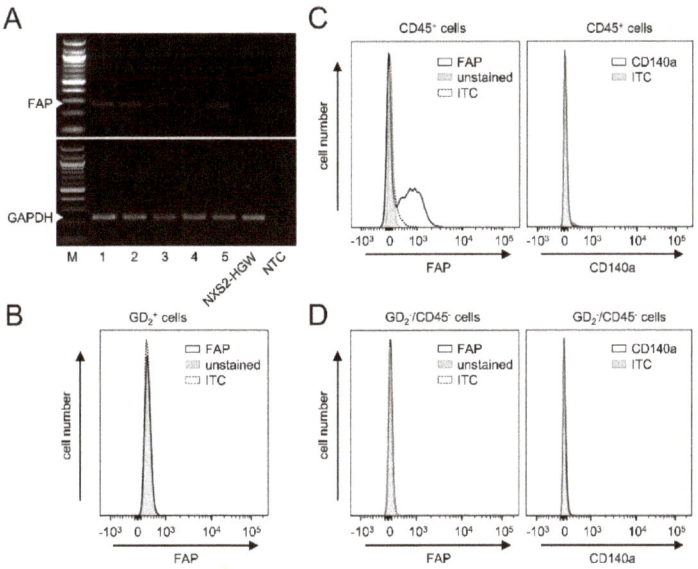

Figure 4. Analysis of FAP and CD140a expression in murine tumor tissue. (**A**) Representative images of the RT-PCR analysis of FAP mRNA levels (PCR product size: 268 bp) in five tumor tissue samples (1–5) and by the murine tumor cells NXS2-HGW that were used for tumor cell implantation. GAPDH (PCR product size: 238 bp) served as an internal control. M: marker, NTC: no template control. (**B**) A representative histogram of the flow cytometry analysis of FAP and CD140a abundance in the GD_2- and CD45 double-negative cells within primary tumor tissue. Samples were collected when tumors reached a size of 750 mm^3, followed by enzymatic digestion to obtain a single-cell solution. Samples were then stained with rabbit anti-mouse anti-FAP IgG and PE-labeled anti-rabbit IgG Ab, which served as primary and secondary Ab and FITC-labeled anti-mouse CD140a Ab, respectively (black curve), or appropriate ITC (black dashed curve). Unstained cells served as negative control (unstained; grey-filled curve). (**C**) A representative histogram of the flow cytometry analysis of FAP and CD140a abundance in the CD45-positive cells detected in tumor tissue. (**D**) A representative histogram of the flow cytometry analysis of FAP levels in NXS2-HGW cells that served for induction of primary tumors. Full gel images can be found at Supplementary Materials.

Interestingly, in contrast to the tumor tissue, we could not detect any FAP mRNA by the GD_2-positive murine NB cells NXS2-HGW that served for tumor establishment in vivo (Figure 4A). These results could be confirmed by flow cytometry, showing a lack of FAP by NXS2-HGW (Figure 4D).

Next, we analyzed which cell populations within the tumor tissue express FAP. We defined CAFs as double-positive cells for FAP and CD140a and double-negative cells for GD_2 (NB-specific marker) and CD45 (leukocyte-specific marker). Surprisingly, we could not detect CAFs in tumor tissue (Figure 4B), thus suggesting a lack of these cells in our model. Interestingly, FAP could be clearly detected by the CD45 cell population (Figure 4C), suggesting a role for FAP as a target in the tumor microenvironment expressed by tumor-infiltrating leukocytes.

In summary, our results show clear FAP expression in primary tumor tissue, thus showing the suitability of our syngeneic tumor model to test a combinatorial treatment with DB and the immunocytokine FAP-IL-2v. Since the NB cells that were used for tumor implantation were found to be FAP-negative and we could not detect CAFs in the primary tumor tissue, we hypothesized FAP's role by tumor-infiltrating leukocytes.

Next, we investigated in more detail which cell populations of the tumor-infiltrating leukocytes express FAP. Since we previously showed a tumor-promoting role of CD11b-positive cells in NB [14], we assessed first FAP expression by this cell population (GD$_2$-/CD45+/CD11b+). In contrast to the CD11b-negative cells (GD$_2$−/CD45+/CD11b−) (Figure 5D), CD11b-positive cells showed a clear signal for FAP (Figure 5A), suggesting an additional role of CD11b-positive cells in FAP-mediated effects in NB.

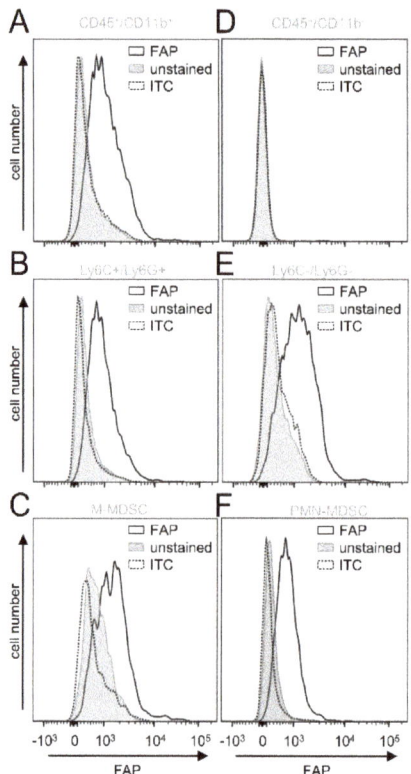

Figure 5. Analysis of FAP expression by tumor-infiltrating leukocytes. (**A–F**) Representative histograms of the flow cytometry analysis of FAP expression by leukocytes (CD45+) found within primary tumor tissue. Samples were collected when tumors reached a size of 750 mm^3, followed by enzymatic digestion to obtain a single-cell solution. Samples were then analyzed to show FAP expression (black solid line) using mouse anti-FAP IgG and PE-labeled anti-murine IgG Ab as primary and secondary Ab by CD11b-positive (**A**; CD45+/CD11b+) and CD11b-negative leukocytes (**D**; CD45+/CD11b−), MDCS (**B**; CD45+/CD11+/Ly6C+/Ly6G+), CD11b+ leukocytes excepting MDSC (**E**; CD45+/CD11b+/Ly6C−/Ly6G−), as well as two MDCS populations, M-MDSC (**C**; CD45+/CD11b+/Ly6C^{high}/Ly6G−) and PMN-MDCS (**F**; CD45+/CD11b+/Ly6C^{low}/Ly6G+). Unstained cells (unstained; grey-filled curve) and cells incubated with appropriate isotype control (ITC, grey dashed line) served as negative controls.

To further characterize the FAP-positive CD11b cell fraction, we included additional cell markers to determine the immune-suppressive cells of the myeloid lineage MDSC, namely monocytic (M)- (CD11b+/Ly6C^{high}/Ly6G−) and polymorphonuclear (PMN)-MDSC CD11b+/Ly6C^{low}/Ly6G+). Interestingly, both MDSC populations (Figure 5C,F) and the CD11b+ cells that did not express Ly6C and Ly6G showed a clear FAP signal (Figure 5B,E).

In summary, analysis of tumor tissue revealed a lack of CAFs in our in vivo model. Importantly, we detected FAP on tumor-infiltrating CD11b+ cells, especially by M- and PMN-MDSC, as well as CD11b+ cells that did not express Ly6C and -G, probably tumor-associated macrophages (TAM), as has been shown in tumors of Lewis lung carcinoma [17].

3.6. Impact of Fibroblasts Injected in Combination with Tumor Cells on Tumor Growth

Based on our data showing the tumor-cell-dependent induction of FAP on primary fibroblasts and on the fact that CAFs were found in human NB [9,15], but not in our murine tumor model, we addressed the question of whether the injection of murine tumor cells in combination with PAMF results in the development of CAF-positive tumors. Tumor development was evaluated daily after the implantation of tumor cells in combination with PAMF in a ratio of 2:1 in comparison to the growth of tumor cells injected without PAMF.

Although the analysis of tumor growth revealed significantly higher tumor volumes in mice injected with tumor cells in combination with PAMF between days 16 and 18 compared to the controls (tumor cells only), tumor growth in both groups was found to be very similar on most days (Figure 6A). Unexpectedly, flow cytometry analysis of tumor tissue collected three weeks after the injection of tumor cells in combination with PAMF did not show any FAP- or CD140a-positive cells in the $GD_2-/CD45-$ cell population (Figure 6B).

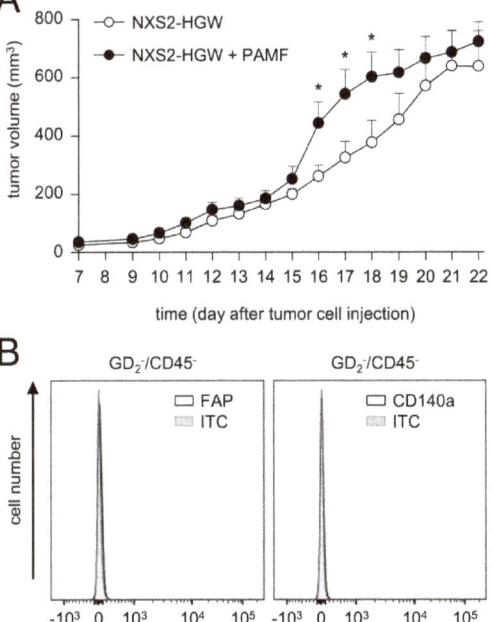

Figure 6. Impact of PAMF on tumor growth. (**A**) Analysis of tumor growth in mice injected with either NXS2-HGW (open circles) or NXS2-HGW in combination with PAMF (closed circles). Tumors were surgically resected on day 22 after tumor cell injection. Co-injection was performed at the tumor-cell-to-PAMF ratio of 2:1. When mice were sacrificed ahead of schedule due to tumor burden, the last measurement was included into the calculation of tumor growth at subsequent time points. Data are given as mean + SEM. * $p < 0.05$, t-test (**B**) Representative histograms of flow cytometry analysis of FAP and CD140a levels in tumor tissue of mice injected with NXS2-HGW in combination with PAMF. To detect CAFs (FAP+/CD140a+), leukocytes and tumor cells were excluded from the analysis using CD45 and GD_2 expression, respectively.

These results indicate that the development of CAFs in our model could not be effectively induced by the co-injection of syngeneic primary fibroblasts and tumor cells. Based on these observations, we injected NB cells without PAMF for tumor induction in further in vivo experiments.

3.7. Establishment of a More Resistant In Vivo Tumor Model

Since the immunotherapy with DB (i.p., five consecutive days, 3 mg/kg bw/day, start of treatment: four days after tumor cell implantation) showed, in our syngeneic tumor model, strong antitumor efficacy against NB, resulting in constant tumor regression [12,14], we aimed to establish a more resistant version of this tumor model allowing the evaluation of the combinatorial immunotherapy with DB and FAP-IL-2v. For this, we started DB treatments in a later tumor growth phase (day 11, 12 and 14), after the development of measurable tumors.

As expected, starting the DB immunotherapy on days 11, 12 and 14 resulted in a steady decrease in the antitumor effects compared to starting on day 4 (Figure 7A). Untreated mice showed the strongest tumor growth compared to every experimental group receiving DB; however, the differences between the tumor volumes of the untreated mice and the mice of the two groups "day 12" and "day 14" were statistically not significant, thus indicating the development of a more resistant tumor against DB treatment compared with the mice of the "day 11" and "day 4" groups.

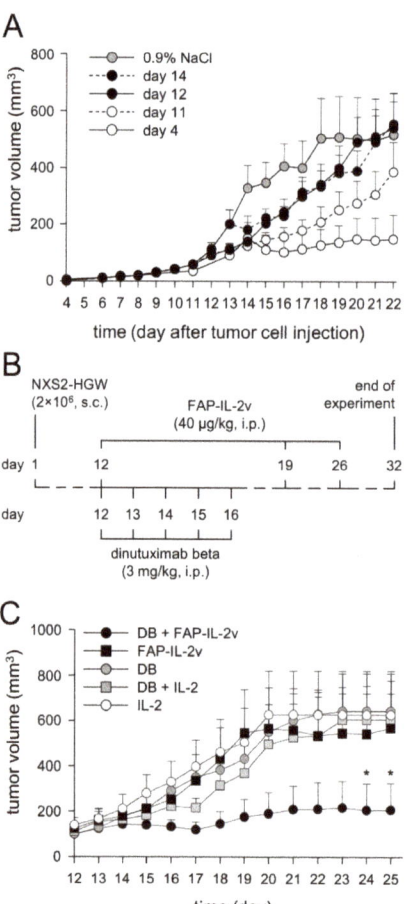

Figure 7. Cont.

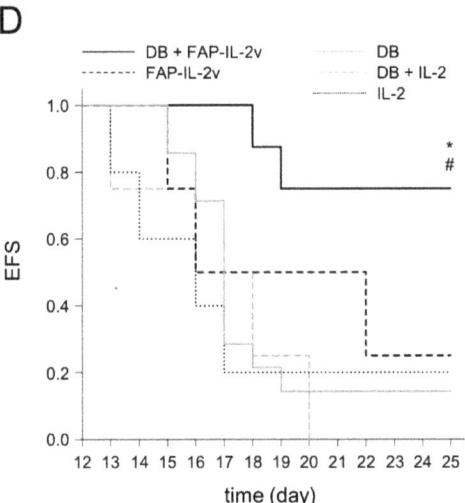

Figure 7. Establishment of a more resistant in vivo tumor model (**A**) and effects of the combinatorial immunotherapy with DB and FAP-IL-2v in vivo (**B–D**). (**A**) To establish a more resistant version of the murine syngeneic NB tumor model, DB treatment was started in a later tumor growth phase. After establishment of primary tumors, three later time points at which DB treatment was started (day 11 (open circles, dashed line), 12 (closed circles, solid line) and 14 (closed circles, dashed line)) were compared with day 4, representing the DB treatment starting time point of the previous NB model (open circles, solid line). Mice receiving equivalent doses of 0.9% NaCl served as controls (grey circles, solid line). When mice were sacrificed ahead of schedule due to tumor burden, the last measurement was included into the calculation of tumor growth at subsequent time points. Data are given as mean + SEM. (**B**) Schematic overview of the treatment protocol. The murine syngeneic GD_2-expressing NB cells NXS2-HGW were injected on day 1, followed by establishment of primary tumors. When tumor size of 100 mm³ was reached (indicated as day 12), treatment was started. Mice received either DB or FAP-IL-2v or a combination of both. To investigate IL-2-dependent effects, mice of two additional control groups were treated with IL-2 and DB in combination with IL-2. Tumor growth was determined daily. (**C**) Analysis of tumor growth in mice treated with DB in combination with FAP-IL-2v (DB + FAP-IL-2v, black solid line, closed circles), FAP-IL-2v (black solid line, closed squares), DB (black solid line, grey circles), DB in combination with IL-2 (DB+ IL-2, black solid line, grey squares) and IL-2 (black solid line, open circles). When mice were sacrificed ahead of schedule due to tumor burden, the last measurement was included into the calculation of tumor growth at subsequent time points. Data are given as mean + SEM. * $p < 0.05$ vs. DB + IL-2, t-test. (**D**) Analysis of event-free survival (EFS) probabilities in mice treated with DB in combination with FAP-IL-2v (DB + FAP-IL-2v, black solid line), FAP-IL-2v (black dashed line), DB (grey solid line), DB in combination with IL-2 (DB+ IL-2, grey dashed line) and IL-2 (black dotted line). A tumor volume of 300 mm³ was defined as an event. Statistical analysis was performed using LogRank test; multiple comparison was done with Holm–Sidak method. * $p < 0.05$ vs. DB; # $p < 0.05$ vs. DB + IL-2.

For further experiments, we used the treatment schedule of the first group of the treated mice that showed similar tumor growth to the untreated controls, namely the "day 12" group. In this group, tumors achieved a volume of approximately 100 mm3 at the start of treatment.

3.8. Evaluation of Antitumor Effects of Combinatorial Immunotherapy with DB and FAP-IL-2v

After the successful establishment of a more resistant version of our syngeneic tumor model allowing the evaluation of the antitumor efficacy of combinatorial therapeutic strategies, we treated mice showing tumors of approximately 100 mm³ volume with DB in combination with the immunocytokine FAP-IL-2v (Figure 7B). Additionally, mice treated with IL-2 instead of FAP-IL-2v, as well as mice receiving IL-2 only, served as controls.

As expected, the immunotherapy with DB showed, in the resistant tumor model, similar tumor growth compared to the monotherapy controls with FAP-IL-2 or IL-2 (Figure 7C). Interestingly, additional treatment of mice that received DB with IL-2 did not show any beneficial effects of IL-2 on tumor growth compared with the mice that were treated with DB without IL-2 (Figure 7C). In contrast, the combinatorial immunotherapy with DB and FAP-IL-2v resulted in superior antitumor effects, showing the strongest tumor growth inhibition compared to every control group (Figure 7C). These results clearly show that an additional treatment with FAP-IL-2v Ab augments the efficacy of the immunotherapy with DB against NB.

Further analysis of EFS confirmed our results of tumor growth evaluation. The superior effects on EFS could be observed in the mice treated with DB in combination with FAP-IL-2v (Figure 7D), further underlining the improvement in anti-GD$_2$ Ab immunotherapies by the immunocytokine FAP-IL-2v against NB.

Together, our results show an FAP-IL-2v-dependent improvement in the DB-mediated antitumor effects against resistant NB, resulting in delayed tumor growth and an increase in survival compared to the respective monotherapy. Moreover, IL-2 did not show any benefit in combination with DB, confirming data reported in high-risk NB patients [4].

3.9. Assessment of Therapy-Dependent Effects on Tumor-Infiltrating Lymphocytes

Finally, we investigated the effects of the combinatorial treatment on different leukocyte populations infiltrating tumor tissue. We focused our analysis on the antitumoral effector NK and cytotoxic T cells (CD8+) as well as immune-suppressive Treg. Although the flow cytometry analysis was performed using tumors showing a volume of around 750 mm^3, i.e., in a late growth phase, we still could observe clear therapy-dependent effects.

Compared to the control mice treated with IL-2 only, mice of the DB immunotherapy group showed higher numbers of NK and CD8+ T cells (Figure 8A,B), indicating the induction of antitumoral effector cells. However, the difference between the groups was statistically not significant, probably due to the low number of tumors available for the analysis. Furthermore, we observed, in the mice treated with DB, reduced Treg numbers (Figure 8C), thus further indicating the antitumor efficacy of the anti-GD$_2$ Ab DB even in a more resistant model. As hypothesized, an additional treatment with the immunocytokine FAP-IL-2v augmented the antitumor effects of DB, resulting in a further increase in NK and CD8+ T cells as well as a reduction in Treg (Figure 8A–C). However, a single-agent treatment of mice with FAP-IL-2 Ab also led to elevated numbers of NK and CD8+ T cells as well as a reduction in Treg (Figure 8A–C), suggesting the immune-stimulating effects of IL-2v.

These results could be clearly confirmed by the analysis of the CD8+/Treg ratio, showing the highest levels in the mice receiving either DB in combination with FAP-IL-2v or FAP-IL-2v as a single-agent treatment (Figure 8D).

Together, the single-agent treatment of resistant NB with the anti-GD$_2$ Ab DB resulted in an increase in antitumoral NK and CD8+ T cells as well as a reduction in immune-suppressive Treg-infiltrating primary tumors. The combinatorial treatment of mice with DB and FAP-IL-2v further increased the infiltration of tumors by NK and CD8+ T cells and resulted in a further reduction in Treg, probably due to the preferential stimulation of antitumoral effector cells by IL-2v. These results show an improvement in the DB immunotherapeutic efficacy by the immunocytokine FAP-IL-2, thus suggesting this combinatorial treatment as a promising strategy against resistant NB.

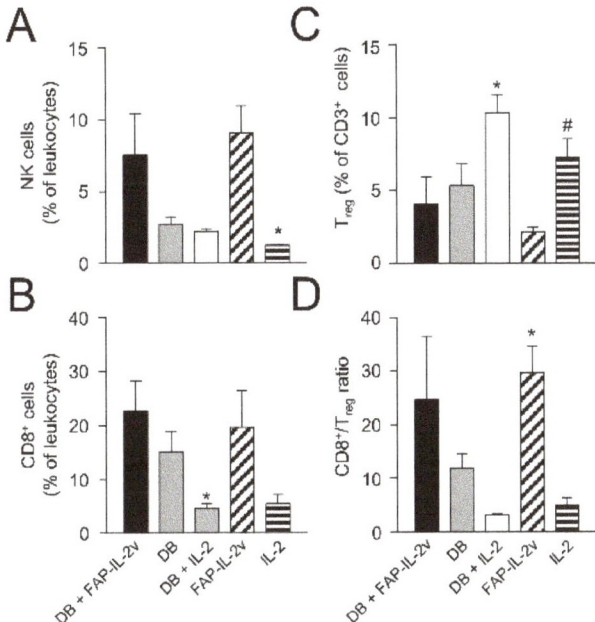

Figure 8. Flow cytometry analysis of tumor-infiltrating lymphocytes. To investigate effects of the combinatorial DB + FAP-IL-2v treatment on tumor-infiltrating lymphocytes, primary tumor tissue was analyzed using flow cytometry. After resection, primary tumor tissue samples were enzymatically digested to obtain a single-cell solution. To assess NK (**A**) and cytotoxic T cells (**B**) as well as Treg (**C**), the effector-cell-population-specific antigens CD335 and CD8 as well as CD25 and FocP3 were marked, respectively. Additionally, the ratio of cytotoxic T cells to Treg (**D**) was calculated. Results are presented as a percentage of the respective effector cell population cells relative to all viable CD45- or CD3-positive leukocytes for NK and cytotoxic T cells or Treg, respectively. ANOVA followed by appropriate post-hoc comparison test and t-test. (**A**) * $p < 0.05$ vs. FAP-IL-2v, (**B**) * $p < 0.05$ vs. DB + FAP-IL-2v, (**C**) * $p < 0.05$ vs. DB + FAP-IL-2v, # $p < 0.05$ vs. FAP-IL-2v, (**D**) * $p < 0.05$ vs. IL-2.

4. Discussion

The successful treatment of high-risk NB remains a major challenge in pediatric oncology. Although immunotherapeutic approaches, especially with monoclonal anti-GD$_2$ Ab, have shown promising results, around one third of NB patients still die [18]. To improve the antitumor efficacy of anti-GD$_2$ Ab, different cytokines were additionally included into the treatment protocols. The most prominent are IL-2 and GM-CSF, which activate two cell populations primarily mediating ADCC, namely NK cells and granulocytes, respectively. In Europe, an effective increase in NK cells could be shown in high-risk NB patients after the application of DB in combination with IL-2 compared to the patients of the IL-2-free treatment arm [5]. We here additionally confirmed in vitro a stimulating effect of IL-2 on the antitumor cytotoxicity of effector cells, showing an almost two-fold increase in ADCC mediated by DB after treatment of leukocytes with IL-2. However, the positive effects of IL-2 on NK cells and ADCC did not result in the improved survival of the high-risk NB patients compared to those patients who received immunotherapy without IL-2 [4]. A detailed comparison of the immune cells in the patients of both cohorts revealed a strong (21-fold) induction of Treg after application of IL-2 and almost unchanged Treg levels in the patients of the IL-2-free treatment arm [5]. Such a preferential induction of the immune-inhibiting cells by IL-2 can partly explain the missing survival benefit of the additional usage of IL-2 against NB, thus underlining a need for alternative strategies to activate antitumor effector cells only.

One promising alternative cytokine that showed the effective activation of NK cells, increasing the GD_2-specific ADCC against NB cells in vitro, as well anti-NB efficacy in vivo, is IL-15 [19]. Importantly, recombinant human IL-15 has been already evaluated in cancer patients [20]. However, the systemic application of cytokines is associated with strong side effects. To overcome this problem, tumor-specific Ab conjugated with immune-stimulating cytokines, called immunocytokines, were developed and showed promising results in the treatment of cancer patients. In melanoma patients, treatment with the GD_2-specitifc Ab hu14.18-IL-2 resulted in immune activation and showed reversible clinical toxicity with no grade 4 adverse events [21,22]. This immunocytokine was also used in clinical trials against refractory or recurrent NB, demonstrating safety profiles and antitumor efficacy [23,24]. Despite these promising results, the application of such immunocytokines can still activate Treg, thus hampering the antitumor effects of the immunotherapy.

Here, we investigated the anti-NB effects of the immunocytokine FAP-IL-2v in combination with DB. The rationale of using FAP-IL-2v was based on the fact that the mutated IL-2 (IL-2v) is able to preferentially stimulate antitumor effector cells such as NK cells without activating effects on the immune-inhibiting Treg [7]. Moreover, it was shown that the incubation of effector cells with FAP-IL-2v enhanced ADCC against colon and gastric cancer cells by the therapeutic Ab directed against tumor antigens [7]. In the present study, we could clearly confirm these results in NB, showing a strong FAP-IL-2-dependent increase in ADCC against tumor cells mediated by DB. Moreover, flow cytometry analysis of Treg did not show any induction compared to the untreated controls. In contrast, IL-2 treatment resulted in a strong increase in Treg, confirming the results in NB patients treated with DB in combination with IL-2 [5].

The observed increase in DB-specific ADCC by FAP-IL-2 in our in vitro experiments was clearly translated into an FAP-IL-2v-dependent improvement in the antitumor effects of DB against aggressively growing GD_2-positive NB tumors in vivo. In contrast to our previously established tumor model [12], whereby treatments were started four days after tumor cell implantation, in the present study, we used a more resistant model of NB allowing the evaluation of combinatorial treatments. We changed the start of treatment to a later time point, at least 12 days after tumor cell implantation, after primary tumors were established at a size of 100 mm^3, thus showing more resistant characteristics. Our in vivo data are in line with the data of Klein and colleagues, showing, in murine models of human cancers, such as leukemia, breast or lung cancer, FAP-IL-2v efficacy when combined with therapeutic Ab directed against tumor antigens [6]. Moreover, in the present study, the comparison of the antitumor efficacy of DB given as a monotherapy and DB in combination with IL-2 did not show any benefit regarding the additional treatment with IL-2, thus further confirming the results from the clinical study published by Ladenstein and colleagues showing a lack of superior effects of IL-2 [4].

Although the application of FAP-IL-2 has been reported to stimulate effector cells in the periphery [6] as well, the fusion of IL-2v to the anti-FAP Ab was performed to preferentially transport an additional stimulating agent (IL-2v) into the tumor tissue. Since FAP expression has been shown in NB and we could here confirm both FAP expression by human NB cell lines and in murine primary tumor tissue, as well as the NB-cell-dependent induction of FAP on fibroblasts, we suggest that both effects contribute to the efficacy of the immunocytokine FAP-IL-2v in the periphery and in the tumor tissue. In our tumor model, we detected FAP only by tumor-infiltrating CD11b-positive leukocytes, especially by the two MDCS populations, M- and PMN-MDSC. We found FAP also on the Ly6C and Ly6G double-negative cells, which are probably TAM, as has been reported by Arnold and colleagues [17]. To clarify the question of whether these FAP-positive cells in tumor tissue are indeed TAMs, further studies are required.

5. Conclusions

In summary, we showed a FAP-IL-2v-dependent increase in ADCC against NB cells mediated by the chimeric anti-GD_2 Ab DB. We detected FAP in tumor tissue, with major expression by tumor-infiltrating MDSC. The combinatorial treatment of resistant NB with DB and FAP-IL-2 in vivo effectively inhibited tumor growth, improved the survival of tumor-bearing mice and resulted in an increase in cytotoxic T and NK cells, as well as a reduction in Treg found in tumor tissue. These data indicate that treatment with the immunocytokine FAP-IL-2v augments the efficacy of DB against resistant NB, probably by targeting MDSC and stimulating NK cells.

Supplementary Materials: The following supporting information can be downloaded at: https://www.mdpi.com/article/10.3390/cancers14194842/s1. Full gel images can be found at Supplementary Materials.

Author Contributions: Conceptualization, N.S., S.T.-M., M.Z. and H.N.L.; methodology, N.S., S.T.-M., M.Z, J.L. and H.N.L.; data curation, S.T.-M., M.Z., J.L., S.B. and A.Z.; writing—original draft preparation, N.S.; writing—review and editing, N.S., S.T.-M., M.Z., J.L., J.L., S.B., A.Z. and H.N.L.; supervision, N.S. and H.N.L.; project administration, N.S., S.T.-M. and M.Z.; funding acquisition, N.S. and H.N.L. All authors have read and agreed to the published version of the manuscript.

Funding: This research was funded by the University Medicine Greifswald, grant number 97237000; F. Hoffmann-La Roche Ltd., Deutsche Forschungsgemeinschaft (DFG) and Hector Stiftungen, Germany, grant number M2116.

Institutional Review Board Statement: All procedures involving human participants were in accordance with the ethical standards of the institutional and national research committee and with the 1964 Helsinki declaration and its later amendments or comparable ethical standards. Informed consent was obtained from all individual participants (Ethics Board of the Medical Faculty of the University Greifswald, approval code number: BB 014/14, 24 January 2014). All procedures involving animal experiments were approved by the animal welfare committee (Landesamt für Landwirtschaft, Lebensmittelsicherheit und Fischerei Mecklenburg-Vorpommern, approval code number: LALLF M-V/7221.3-1-011/20, 7 September 2020) and approved and supervised by the commissioner for animal welfare at the University Medicine Greifswald representing the Institutional Animal Care and Use Committee (IACUC).

Informed Consent Statement: Informed consent was obtained from all subjects involved in the study.

Data Availability Statement: The data of this study are available from the corresponding author upon reasonable request.

Acknowledgments: The authors thank Theodor Koepp and Maria Asmus (University Medicine Greifswald, Pediatric Hematology and Oncology, Greifswald, Germany) for their excellent technical assistance and Ana Rodriguez (F. Hoffmann-La Roche Ltd.) for her excellent support in the coordination of the project. FAP-IL-2v was provided by the Roche Innovation Center Zurich.

Conflicts of Interest: The authors declare no conflict of interest. The funders had no role in the design of the study; in the collection, analyses, or interpretation of data; in the writing of the manuscript, or in the decision to publish the results.

References

1. Paraboschi, I.; Privitera, L.; Kramer-Marek, G.; Anderson, J.; Giuliani, S. Novel Treatments and Technologies Applied to the Cure of Neuroblastoma. *Children* **2021**, *8*, 482. [CrossRef]
2. Ladenstein, R.; Pötschger, U.; Valteau-Couanet, D.; Luksch, R.; Castel, V.; Ash, S.; Laureys, G.; Brock, P.; Michon, J.M.; Owens, C.; et al. Investigation of the Role of Dinutuximab Beta-Based Immunotherapy in the SIOPEN High-Risk Neuroblastoma 1 Trial (HR-NBL1). *Cancers* **2020**, *12*, 309. [CrossRef] [PubMed]
3. Zeng, Y.; Fest, S.; Kunert, R.; Katinger, H.; Pistoia, V.; Michon, J.; Lewis, G.; Ladenstein, R.; Lode, H.N. Anti-neuroblastoma effect of ch14.18 antibody produced in CHO cells is mediated by NK-cells in mice. *Mol. Immunol.* **2005**, *42*, 1311–1319. [CrossRef] [PubMed]
4. Ladenstein, R.; Pötschger, U.; Valteau-Couanet, D.; Luksch, R.; Castel, V.; Yaniv, I.; Laureys, G.; Brock, P.; Michon, J.M.; Owens, C.; et al. Interleukin 2 with anti-GD2 antibody ch14.18/CHO (dinutuximab beta) in patients with high-risk neuroblastoma (HR-NBL1/SIOPEN): A multicentre, randomised, phase 3 trial. *Lancet Oncol.* **2018**, *19*, 1617–1629. [CrossRef]

5. Troschke-Meurer, S.; Siebert, N.; Marx, M.; Zumpe, M.; Ehlert, K.; Mutschlechner, O.; Loibner, H.; Ladenstein, R.; Lode, H.N. Low CD4$^+$/CD25$^+$/CD127$^-$ regulatory T cell- and high INF-γ levels are associated with improved survival of neuroblastoma patients treated with long-term infusion of ch14.18/CHO combined with interleukin-2. *Oncoimmunology* **2019**, *8*, 1661194. [CrossRef] [PubMed]
6. Klein, C.; Waldhauer, I.; Nicolini, V.G.; Freimoser-Grundschober, A.; Nayak, T.; Vugts, D.J.; Dunn, C.; Bolijn, M.; Benz, J.; Stihle, M.; et al. Cergutuzumab amunaleukin (CEA-IL2v), a CEA-targeted IL-2 variant-based immunocytokine for combination cancer immunotherapy: Overcoming limitations of aldesleukin and conventional IL-2-based immunocytokines. *Oncoimmunology* **2017**, *6*, e1277306. [CrossRef]
7. Waldhauer, I.; Gonzalez-Nicolini, V.; Freimoser-Grundschober, A.; Nayak, T.K.; Fahrni, L.; Hosse, R.J.; Gerrits, D.; Geven EJ, W.; Sam, J.; Lang, S.; et al. Simlukafusp alfa (FAP-IL2v) immunocytokine is a versatile combination partner for cancer immunotherapy. *MAbs* **2021**, *13*, 1913791. [CrossRef] [PubMed]
8. Xin, L.; Gao, J.; Zheng, Z.; Chen, Y.; Lv, S.; Zhao, Z.; Yu, C.; Yang, X.; Zhang, R. Fibroblast Activation Protein-α as a Target in the Bench-to-Bedside Diagnosis and Treatment of Tumors: A Narrative Review. *Front. Oncol.* **2021**, *11*, 648187. [CrossRef] [PubMed]
9. Zeine, R.; Salwen, H.R.; Peddinti, R.; Tian, Y.; Guerrero, L.; Yang, Q.; Chlenski, A.; Cohn, S.L. Presence of cancer-associated fibroblasts inversely correlates with Schwannian stroma in neuroblastoma tumors. *Mod. Pathol.* **2009**, *22*, 950–958. [CrossRef]
10. Siebert, N.; Seidel, D.; Eger, C.; Juttner, M.; Lode, H.N. Functional bioassays for immune monitoring of high-risk neuroblastoma patients treated with ch14.18/CHO anti-GD2 antibody. *PLoS ONE* **2014**, *9*, e107692. [CrossRef]
11. Lode, H.N.; Xiang, R.; Varki, N.M.; Dolman, C.S.; Gillies, S.D.; Reisfeld, R.A. Targeted interleukin-2 therapy for spontaneous neuroblastoma metastases to bone marrow. *J. Natl. Cancer Inst.* **1997**, *89*, 1586–1594. [CrossRef]
12. Siebert, N.; Zumpe, M.; Juttner, M.; Troschke-Meurer, S.; Lode, H.N. PD-1 blockade augments anti-neuroblastoma immune response induced by anti-GD2 antibody ch14.18/CHO. *Oncoimmunology* **2017**, *6*, e1343775. [CrossRef] [PubMed]
13. Lode, H.N.; Schmidt, M.; Seidel, D.; Huebener, N.; Brackrock, D.; Bleeke, M.; Reker, D.; Brandt, S.; Mueller, H.P.; Helm, C.; et al. Vaccination with anti-idiotype antibody ganglidiomab mediates a GD(2)-specific anti-neuroblastoma immune response. *Cancer Immunol. Immunother.* **2013**, *62*, 999–1010. [CrossRef] [PubMed]
14. Siebert, N.; Zumpe, M.; von Lojewski, L.; Troschke-Meurer, S.; Marx, M.; Lode, H.N. Reduction of CD11b(+) myeloid suppressive cells augments anti-neuroblastoma immune response induced by the anti-GD(2) antibody ch14.18/CHO. *Oncoimmunology* **2020**, *9*, 1836768. [CrossRef]
15. Hashimoto, O.; Yoshida, M.; Koma, Y.; Yanai, T.; Hasegawa, D.; Kosaka, Y.; Nishimura, N.; Yokozaki, H. Collaboration of cancer-associated fibroblasts and tumour-associated macrophages for neuroblastoma development. *J. Pathol.* **2016**, *240*, 211–223. [CrossRef] [PubMed]
16. Sahai, E.; Astsaturov, I.; Cukierman, E.; DeNardo, D.G.; Egeblad, M.; Evans, R.M.; Fearon, D.; Greten, F.R.; Hingorani, S.R.; Hunter, T.; et al. A framework for advancing our understanding of cancer-associated fibroblasts. *Nat. Rev. Cancer* **2020**, *20*, 174–186. [CrossRef]
17. Arnold, J.N.; Magiera, L.; Kraman, M.; Fearon, D.T. Tumoral immune suppression by macrophages expressing fibroblast activation protein-α and heme oxygenase-1. *Cancer Immunol. Res.* **2014**, *2*, 121–126. [CrossRef]
18. Keyel, M.E.; Reynolds, C.P. Spotlight on dinutuximab in the treatment of high-risk neuroblastoma: Development and place in therapy. *Biologics* **2019**, *13*, 1–12. [CrossRef]
19. Nguyen, R.; Moustaki, A.; Norrie, J.L.; Brown, S.; Akers, W.J.; Shirinifard, A.; Dyer, M.A. Interleukin-15 Enhances Anti-GD2 Antibody-Mediated Cytotoxicity in an Orthotopic PDX Model of Neuroblastoma. *Clin. Cancer Res.* **2019**, *25*, 7554–7564. [CrossRef] [PubMed]
20. Miller, J.S.; Morishima, C.; McNeel, D.G.; Patel, M.R.; Kohrt HE, K.; Thompson, J.A.; Sondel, P.M.; Wakelee, H.A.; Disis, M.L.; Kaiser, J.C.; et al. A First-in-Human Phase I Study of Subcutaneous Outpatient Recombinant Human IL15 (rhIL15) in Adults with Advanced Solid Tumors. *Clin. Cancer Res.* **2018**, *24*, 1525–1535. [CrossRef]
21. King, D.M.; Albertini, M.R.; Schalch, H.; Hank, J.A.; Gan, J.; Surfus, J.; Mahvi, D.; Schiller, J.H.; Warner, T.; Kim, K.; et al. Phase I clinical trial of the immunocytokine EMD 273063 in melanoma patients. *J. Clin. Oncol.* **2004**, *22*, 4463–4473. [CrossRef]
22. Ribas, A.; Kirkwood, J.M.; Atkins, M.B.; Whiteside, T.L.; Gooding, W.; Kovar, A.; Gillies, S.D.; Kashala, O.; Morse, M.A. Phase I/II open-label study of the biologic effects of the interleukin-2 immunocytokine EMD 273063 (hu14.18-IL2) in patients with metastatic malignant melanoma. *J. Transl. Med.* **2009**, *7*, 68. [CrossRef] [PubMed]
23. Osenga, K.L.; Hank, J.A.; Albertini, M.R.; Gan, J.; Sternberg, A.G.; Eickhoff, J.; Seeger, R.C.; Matthay, K.K.; Reynolds, C.P.; Twist, C.; et al. A phase I clinical trial of the hu14.18-IL2 (EMD 273063) as a treatment for children with refractory or recurrent neuroblastoma and melanoma: A study of the Children's Oncology Group. *Clin. Cancer Res.* **2006**, *12*, 1750–1759. [CrossRef] [PubMed]
24. Shusterman, S.; London, W.B.; Gillies, S.D.; Hank, J.A.; Voss, S.D.; Seeger, R.C.; Reynolds, C.P.; Kimball, J.; Albertini, M.R.; Wagner, B.; et al. Antitumor activity of hu14.18-IL2 in patients with relapsed/refractory neuroblastoma: A Children's Oncology Group (COG) phase II study. *J. Clin. Oncol.* **2010**, *28*, 4969–4975. [CrossRef]

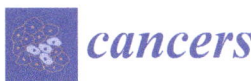

Article

Reversing PD-1 Resistance in B16F10 Cells and Recovering Tumour Immunity Using a COX2 Inhibitor

Chenyu Pi [1], Ping Jing [1], Bingyu Li [1,2], Yan Feng [1], Lijun Xu [1,2], Kun Xie [1], Tao Huang [1], Xiaoqing Xu [1], Hua Gu [1,*] and Jianmin Fang [1,3,4,*]

[1] School of Life Sciences and Technology, Tongji University, Shanghai 200092, China
[2] College of Medicine, Henan University of Science and Technology, Luoyang 471000, China
[3] Biomedical Research Center, Suzhou 230031, China
[4] Shanghai Tongji Hospital, Shanghai 200065, China
* Correspondence: gu_hua@tongji.edu.cn (H.G.); jfang@tongji.edu.cn (J.F.); Tel.: +86-021-6598-2878 (H.G. & J.F.)

Simple Summary: Some patients develop drug resistance to programmed cell death protein 1/programmed death-ligand 1(PD-1/PD-L1) therapy but the mechanism is unclear. Therefore, the study of drug resistance to PD-1 therapy is quite important. In this sense, we obtained B16F10-R tumours resistant to anti-PD-1 therapy through multiple rounds of drug resistance screening in vitro. We found that COX2 expression was significantly elevated and COX2 inhibitors in combination with anti-PD-1 monoclonal antibodies (mAbs) could reverse this resistance phenomenon. Knockout of the ptgs2 gene in B16F10-R tumours also restored tumour sensitivity to anti-PD-1 therapy. Therefore, we believe that the combination of COX2 inhibitors and anti-PD-1 mAbs may become a new choice for the drug resistance of anti-PD-1 therapy in the future.

Abstract: Immunotherapy is an effective method for tumour treatment. Anti-programmed cell death protein 1 (PD-1) and anti-programmed death-ligand 1 (PD-L1) monoclonal antibodies play a significant role in immunotherapy of most tumours; however, some patients develop drug resistance to PD-1/PD-L1 therapy. Cyclooxygenase-2 (COX2) is expressed in various solid tumours, and prostaglandin E2 (PGE2) drives the development of malignant tumours. We developed a drug-resistant B16F10 (B16F10-R) tumour mouse model through four rounds of selection in vivo. Subsequently, we investigated changes in PD-L1 expression and lymphocyte infiltration in B16F10-NR and B16F10-R tumours. Additionally, we explored the role of COX2 in acquired resistance to pembrolizumab, an anti-PD-1 treatment. Immune cell infiltration was significantly decreased in resistant tumours compared to B16F10-NR tumours; however, ptgs2 gene expression was significantly elevated in resistant tumours. Aspirin or celecoxib combined with pembrolizumab can effectively reverse tumour drug resistance. In addition, ptgs2 knockout or the use of the EP4 inhibitor E7046 abrogated drug resistance to anti-PD-1 treatment in B16F10-R tumour cells. Our study showed that inhibition of the COX2/PGE2/EP4 axis could increase the number of immune cells infiltrating the tumour microenvironment and recover drug-resistant tumour sensitivity to pembrolizumab. Thus, we highlight COX2 inhibition as a promising therapeutic target for drug-resistant tumours for future consideration.

Keywords: programmed death-ligand 1; cyclooxygenase-2; tumour resistance; immunosuppression

Citation: Pi, C.; Jing, P.; Li, B.; Feng, Y.; Xu, L.; Xie, K.; Huang, T.; Xu, X.; Gu, H.; Fang, J. Reversing PD-1 Resistance in B16F10 Cells and Recovering Tumour Immunity Using a COX2 Inhibitor. Cancers 2022, 14, 4134. https://doi.org/10.3390/cancers14174134

Academic Editor: Andrea Cavazzoni

Received: 19 July 2022
Accepted: 25 August 2022
Published: 26 August 2022

Publisher's Note: MDPI stays neutral with regard to jurisdictional claims in published maps and institutional affiliations.

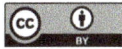

Copyright: © 2022 by the authors. Licensee MDPI, Basel, Switzerland. This article is an open access article distributed under the terms and conditions of the Creative Commons Attribution (CC BY) license (https://creativecommons.org/licenses/by/4.0/).

1. Background

In recent years, tumour immunotherapy has made major strides in cancer treatment [1]. The PD-1/PD-L1 pathway plays an important role in the immunosuppressive meshwork [2,3]. PD-1 is highly expressed on T cells and natural killer (NK) cells, whereas PD-L1/PD-L2 is expressed on antigen-presenting cells and various solid tumour cells. PD-1/PD-L1 interactions suppress T-cell immunity, leading to T-cell exhaustion, anergy, or apoptosis [4,5]. Anti-PD-1 treatment improves antitumour immune responses in patients with colorectal cancer, melanoma, renal cell carcinoma, non-small cell lung cancer, haematologic malignancies, and bladder cancer, resulting from its ability to transform anergic T cells into functional T cells [6–8]. However, the objective response rate of anti-PD-1/PD-L1 antibody therapy is approximately 10–20% for most malignancies [9,10]. Studies have shown that the tumour tissue of some tumour patients has congenital insensitivity or resistance to anti-PD-1 treatment [11]. The initial treatment showed a positive effect, but drug resistance was soon acquired in some patients [12]. However, the mechanism for primary and adaptive resistance to anti-PD-1 therapy was unclear.

Anti-PD-1 therapy can increase the expression of inflammatory cytokines, which may counteract its therapeutic effects [13,14]. Cyclooxygenase (COX) is an important rate-limiting enzyme for the conversion of arachidonic acid into various prostaglandins in the body, and it can be divided into at least two subtypes: COX1 and COX2. Unlike COX1, which is present in most tissues, COX2 expression is induced by cytokines and growth factors, and increases rapidly in response to inflammatory stimuli. COX2 activation produces prostaglandin E2 (PGE2), which is associated with enhanced tumour cell survival, migration, growth, angiogenesis, invasion, and immunosuppression [15]. COX2 is expressed in a variety of solid tumours such as colorectal cancer, nasopharyngeal carcinoma, gastrointestinal malignancies, and breast cancer [16–19]. In addition, it has been demonstrated that PGE2 could drive the development of malignant tumours [20–25]. PGE2 is significantly conserved in human cutaneous melanoma biopsies, and it is required for mutant BrafV600E mouse melanoma cell growth [20]. Inhibiting COX2 and PGE2 in colon cancer models enhanced anti-vascular endothelial growth factor therapy and suppressed angiogenesis and tumour growth [25]. In addition, blocking COX2/PGE2-mediated wound response could abrogate bladder cancer chemoresistance [22].

This study investigated the function of COX2 in anti-PD-1 acquired resistance by developing a drug-resistant B16F10 tumour mouse model. Our study showed that COX2 derived from tumours plays an essential role in adaptive tumour resistance. Inhibiting the COX2/PGE2/EP4 axis could increase the number of infiltrating T and NK cells in the tumour microenvironment (TME) and recover drug-resistant tumour sensitivity to pembrolizumab.

2. Materials and Methods
2.1. Mice and Cells

Human *Pdcd1* transgenic mice were housed in a pathogen-free environment at the Laboratory Animal Research Centre, Tongji University, as previously described [26]. All animal experiments were performed in accordance with the Animal Ethics Committee of Tongji University.

B16F10 melanoma cells were purchased from the American Type Culture Collection (Rockville, MD, USA). B16F10-NR and B16F10-R melanoma cell lines were generated by four rounds of selection for anti-PD-1 resistance. B16F10-R-knockout (KO) *ptgs2* melanoma cells were generated using the CRISPR-Cas9 system (Cas9-2hitKO). The guide RNA sequences targeting *ptgs2* were sgRNA-1, 5'-GCTTTACAGACTTAAAAGCA-3' and sgRNA-2, 5'-TTCAAGACAGATCATAAGCG-3'. All cells were maintained in Dulbecco's modified Eagle's medium (DMEM; Hyclone, Waltham, MA, USA) supplemented with 1% penicillin/streptomycin (Gibco, Waltham, MA, USA) and 10% foetal bovine serum (Gibco) at 37 °C and 5% CO_2.

2.2. Animal Experiments

B16F10, B16F10-NR, B16F10-R, and B16F10-R-knockout *ptgs2* cells (1×10^5 cells) were resuspended in phosphate-buffered saline PBS (Cytiva, Marlborough, MA, USA) and injected subcutaneously into the flanks of 6–8-week-old female human *Pdcd1* transgenic mice. Mice were randomised into groups, each comprising 6–8 mice. When tumours grew to 50 mm³, mice were administered pembrolizumab (10 mg/kg; MSD, USA) or the control isotype for ophthalmic intravenous injection twice a week, and aspirin (10 mg/kg;

Selleck, Shanghai, China), SC560 (5 mg/kg; Selleck), celecoxib (5 mg/kg; Selleck), and E7046 (10 mg/kg; Selleck) for intraperitoneal injection three times a week. The longest dimension (length) and longest perpendicular dimension (width) were measured every two days using a calliper. Tumour volume (mm^3) = (length × width × width)/2. For in vivo B16F10-R cell selection, B16F10 tumours were digested with trypsin and collagenase until reaching 1500 mm^3, which was the humane endpoint. CO_2 inhalation was used to euthanise the mice. The cells were resuspended in DMEM and cultured for two weeks. The tumour cells were re-injected subcutaneously into another mouse for subsequent rounds of in vivo selection.

2.3. Real-Time Quantitative Polymerase Chain Reaction (RT-qPCR)

Total RNA was extracted using the Animal Tissue/Cell Total RNA Extraction Kit (DAKEWE, Beijing, China) and cDNA was acquired using a reverse transcription kit (Solarbio, Beijing, China). *Ptgs1/ptgs2* transcript levels were measured using an RT-PCR SYBR Green I kit (Solarbio). RT-qPCR was performed on a ROCHE LightCycler® 96 (Roche, Basel, Switzerland) in a 96-well plate, and each sample was prepared in triplicates. The following primer pairs were used: GAPDH, forward primer 5′-TGGCCTTCCGTGTTCCTAC-3′ and reverse primer 5′-GAGTTGCTGTTGAAGTCGCA-3′; mouse COX1, forward primer 5′-TTACTATCCGTGCCAGAACCA-3′ and reverse primer 5′-CCCGTGCGAGTACAATCACA-3′; mouse COX2, forward primer 5′-AGCAAATCCTTGCTGTTCCAA-3′ and reverse primer 5′-GCAGTAATTTGATTCTTGTC-3′.

2.4. Flow Cytometry

Tumours were cut and digested with trypsin and collagenase. A 40 μm mesh filter (BioFIL, Shanghai, China) was used to filter the single-cell suspension (BioFIL, Shanghai, China). The cells were blocked with purified rat anti-mouse CD16/CD32 (553142; BD Pharmingen, San Diego, CA, USA), and dead cells were stained with BD Horizon Fixable Viability Stain 510 (564406; BD Pharmingen). Cell surface staining was performed using the following antibodies: APC-Cy™7 mouse anti-mouse CD45.2 (560694; BD Pharmingen), PE hamster anti-mouse CD3e (553063; BD Pharmingen), PerCP-Cy™5.5 rat anti-mouse CD4 (550954; BD Pharmingen), FITC rat anti-mouse CD8a (553030; BD Pharmingen), APC anti-mouse NK-1.1 antibody (108710; BioLegend, San Diego, CA, USA), FITC anti-mouse CD49b (pan-NK cells) antibody (108905; BioLegend), PE/Cyanine7 anti-mouse TCR β chain antibody (109222; BioLegend), and PE anti-mouse CD274 (B7-H1, PD-L1) antibody (124308; BioLegend). The following antibodies were used as isotype controls: APC-Cy™7 Mouse IgG2a, κ Isotype Control (557751; BD Pharmingen), PE Hamster IgG1 κ Isotype Control (553972; BD Pharmingen), PerCP-Cy™5.5 Rat IgG2a, κ Isotype Control (550765; BD Pharmingen), FITC Rat IgG2a, κ Isotype Control (553929; BD Pharmingen), APC Mouse IgG2a, κ Isotype Control (551414; BD Pharmingen), FITC Rat IgM, κ Isotype Control (555951; BD Pharmingen), PE Rat IgG2b, κ Isotype Control (553989; BD Pharmingen). All analyses were performed using a CytoFLEX LX (Beckman Coulter, Brea, CA, USA).

2.5. PGE2 Concentration Detection

Cells were plated at 0.5–1 × 10^6 cells/mL in 96-well plates at 37 °C in the absence or presence of 100 mL of conditioned medium from tumour cells plus or minus LPS (10 to 100 ng/mL) in a total volume of 200 mL. After overnight culture, PGE2 concentration in the supernatant was determined by ELISA.

2.6. Western Blotting

Cell lysis was performed with RIPA buffer (P0013D; Beyotime, Shanghai, China) supplemented with protease (Selleck, Shanghai, China) and phosphatase inhibitors (Selleck). The BCA Protein Assay Kit (PC0020; Solarbio, Beijing, China) was used to measure protein concentrations. The samples were boiled at 100 °C and centrifuged to obtain the supernatant, after which 100 μg of protein was loaded onto 10% sodium dodecyl sulphate-polyacrylamide gel electrophoresis gels (EpiZyme, Shanghai, China). The proteins were transferred to 0.45 µm polyvinylidene fluoride (PVDF) membranes (Millipore, Burlington, MA, USA), and the membranes were blocked in a Western blocking buffer (P0023B; Beyotime) for 2 h at 15 °C. The sections were then incubated with primary antibodies (1:2000) overnight at 4 °C and with the relevant secondary antibody (1:10,000) for 2 h at 15 °C. Bands were visualised using BeyoECL Plus (P0018S; Beyotime). Protein bands were quantified relative to the loading control (GAPDH). The following antibodies were used for Western blotting: anti-GAPDH (AF1186; Beyotime), anti-rabbit-IgG-HRP (A120-111P; Bethyl, Montgomery, TX, USA), and anti-COX2 (ab62331; Abcam, Cambridge, UK).

2.7. Statistical Analysis

Statistical analyses were performed using GraphPad Prism version 6.0 (GraphPad Software, San Diego, CA, USA). Statistical differences were determined using unpaired two-tailed t-tests, one-way ANOVA, or two-way ANOVA. The results are shown as the mean ± SEM, and the significance was set at $p < 0.05$. Survival analysis was based on the following criteria: tumour volume, tumour necrosis, and pathological death. Survival analysis was performed using the log-rank test.

3. Results

3.1. Development of a B16F10 Tumour Cell Line Resistant to Anti-PD-1 Therapy In Vivo

To acquire a cell line resistant to anti-PD-1 (pembrolizumab) treatment, we established an in vivo B16F10 tumour model using human *Pdcd1* transgenic mice to acquire resistance to anti-PD-1 treatment. In the human *Pdcd1* transgenic mice, the B16F10 tumour cell was sensitive to pembrolizumab treatment. We treated mice with 10 mg/kg pembrolizumab and obtained an anti-PD-1-resistant cell line (B16F10-R) after four rounds of in vivo selection (Figure 1A). Analogously, an anti-PD-1 non-resistant cell line (B16F10-NR) was acquired through four rounds of B16F10 tumour growth in vivo but treated with PBS (Figure 1A). With an increase in the number of rounds of selection, the tumour sensitivity to anti-PD-1 treatment decreased, and there was almost no difference in the fourth round (Figure 1B). Moreover, the resistance persisted through rounds five and six (Figure S1).

This B16F10-NR cell line was very sensitive to anti-PD-1 treatment, but anti-PD-1 therapy did not effectively control B16F10-R tumour growth after four selection rounds (Figure 1C). In addition, anti-PD-1 therapy effectively prolonged the mean survival time of mice in the B16F10-PD-1 group by an average of approximately 3–4 weeks compared with that in the other groups (Figure 1D).

Thus, the B16F10-R tumour model showed acquired resistance to anti-PD-1 treatment. The persistence of this phenotype in B16F10-R tumour cells after several consecutive in vitro cell cultures suggested that the acquired resistance was caused by genetic changes in the tumour cells.

3.2. The Infiltrating Immune Cells Decreased Significantly in the TME of B16F10-R Tumours

To understand the difference between drug-resistant and non-drug-resistant tumours, we hypothesised that there would be an alteration in PD-L1 expression on the tumour surface. Flow cytometry analysis showed that PD-L1 expression on the surface of B16F10-R tumour cells was slightly increased (Figure 2A). This phenomenon indicated that the tumour cells that acquired anti-PD-1 resistance were not a result of a decrease in the expression of PD-L1. Next, we determined the number of infiltrating lymphocytes in TME. A flow cytometry staining method was developed to distinguish T cells from natural killer (NK) cells (Figure 2B). We observed that infiltration of CD3+, CD4+, and CD8+ T cells was considerably lower in B16F10-R tumours than in B16F10-NR tumours (Figure 2C). In addition, NK cell infiltration significantly decreased (Figure 2C). Thus, we speculated that the acquired resistance of B16F10-R tumours was caused by the decreased infiltration of immune cells.

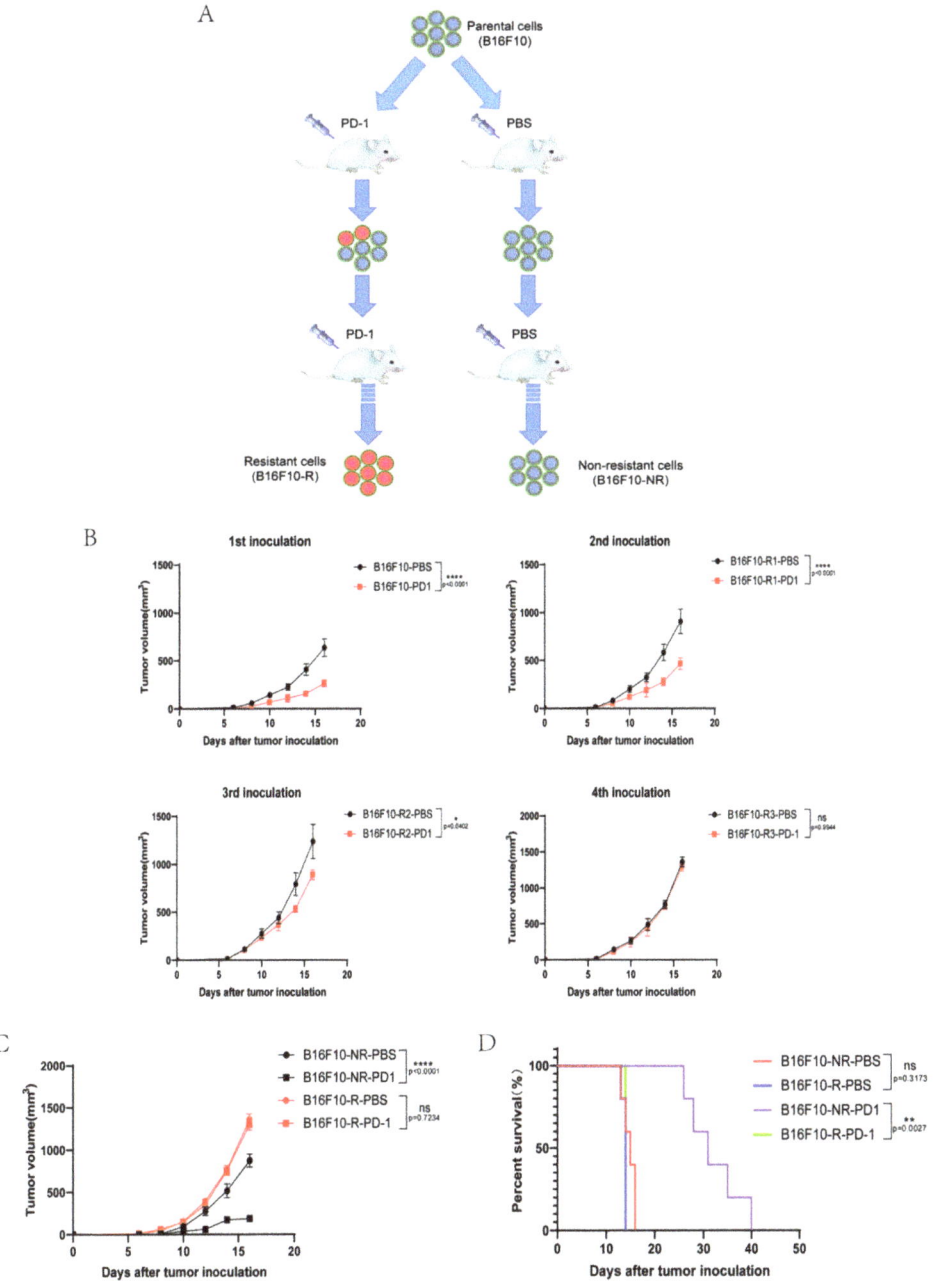

Figure 1. Construction of B16F10 tumour model resistant to anti-PD-1 therapy. (**A**) Construction method of anti-PD-1-resistant B16F10 tumour cells. (**B**) Tumour growth curves for four rounds of anti-PD-1-resistant B16F10 tumour selection ($n = 6$/group, two-way ANOVA test, Sidak). (**C**) Growth curves of B16F10-NR and B16F10-R tumours. Mice were treated with either pembrolizumab or PBS ($n = 6$–8/group, two-way ANOVA test, Tukey). (**D**) Mouse survival curves for B16F10-NR and B16F10-R tumours. Mice were treated with either pembrolizumab or PBS ($n = 6$–8/group, log-rank test of survival curve); ns, not statistically significant; * $p < 0.05$; ** $p < 0.01$; **** $p < 0.0001$.

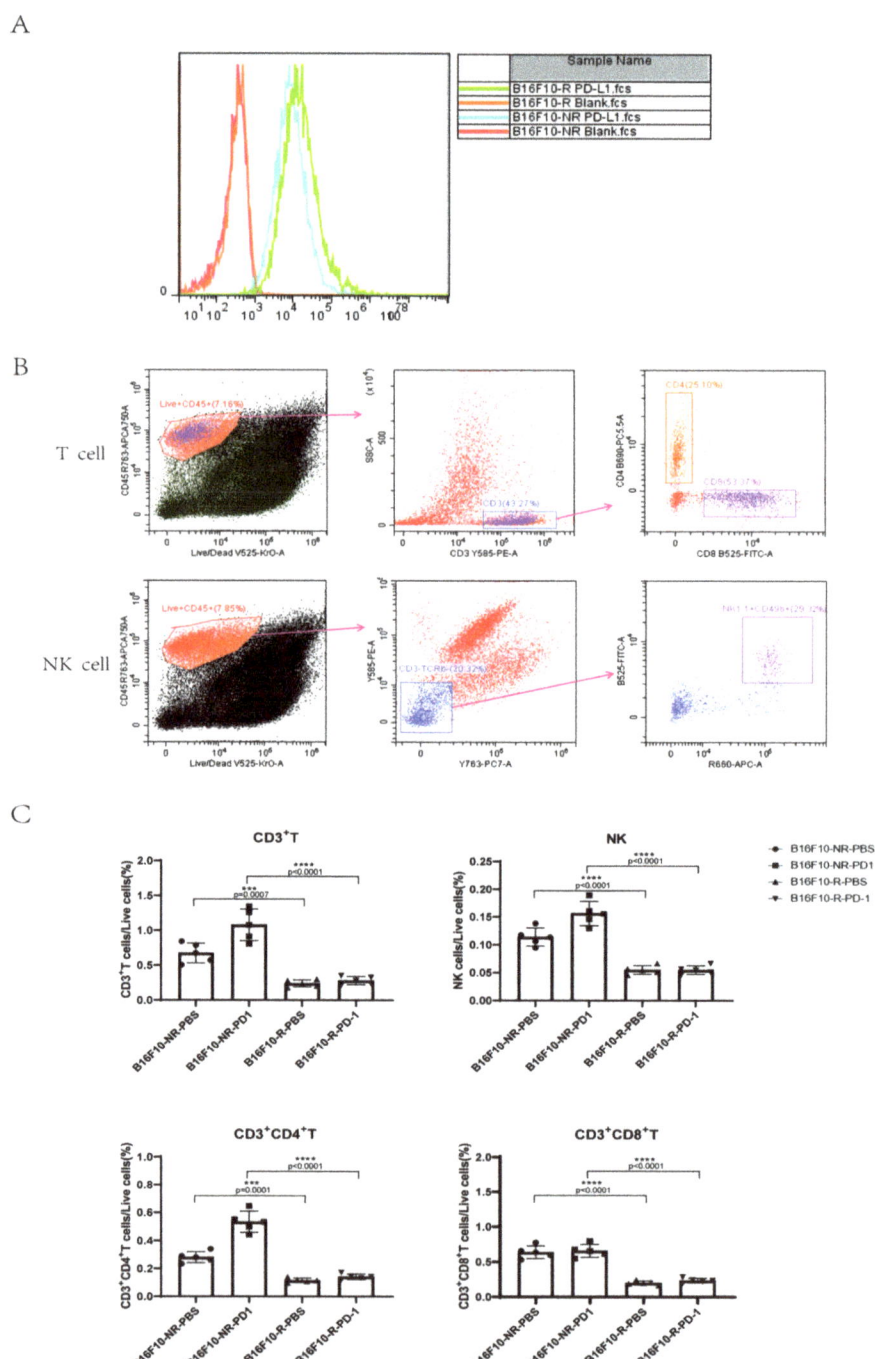

Figure 2. Differences between B16F10-NR tumour and B16F10-R tumour cells. (**A**) PD-L1 expression on the surface of B16F10-NR and B16F10-R cells. (**B**) Gating strategy to identify intratumoural T and NK cells. (**C**) Differences in the number of infiltrating lymphocytes in the TME of B16F10-NR tumours and B16F10-R tumours (one-way ANOVA test, Tukey); ns, not statistically significant; *** $p < 0.001$; **** $p < 0.0001$.

3.3. Aspirin Could Inhibit B16F10-R Tumour Growth

To further confirm whether tumour-acquired resistance to anti-PD-1 therapy was due to decreased immune cell infiltration, we investigated the effects of inhibitors that increased immune cell infiltration. Aspirin is a non-selective inhibitor of COX1/COX2 which can inhibit the expression of COX in tumour cells and then inhibit the production of PGE2, decreasing the infiltration of immune cells into tumours [27]. Next, we evaluated the tumour growth by combination therapy with aspirin and pembrolizumab in B16F10-R tumour cells. Human *Pdcd1* transgenic C57BL/6J mice were injected with aspirin, pembrolizumab, or PBS. Notably, tumour growth in the group treated with pembrolizumab alone was not affected compared to that in the PBS group. In addition, aspirin alone did not inhibit tumour growth. However, the combination of aspirin and pembrolizumab considerably inhibited tumour growth in B16F10-R tumour cells compared with that in the PBS group (Figure 3A).

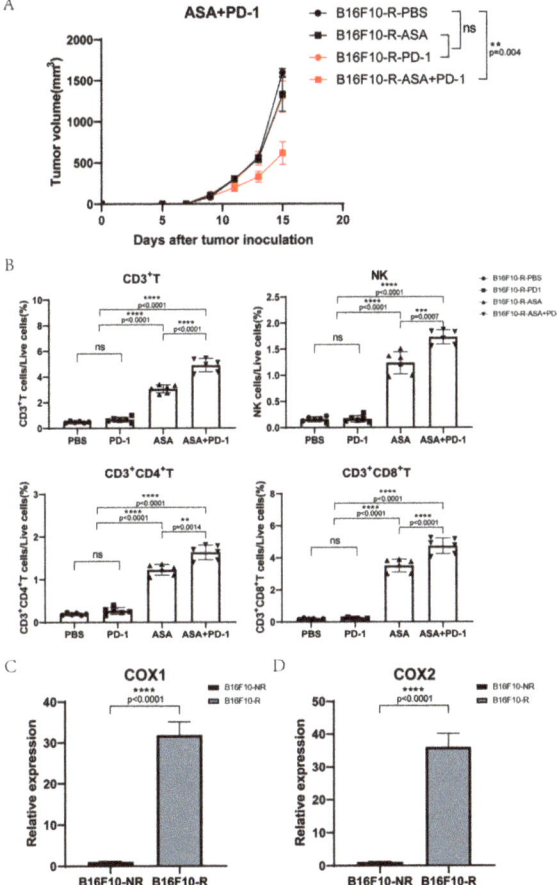

Figure 3. Effects of aspirin combined with pembrolizumab on B16F10-R tumour growth in vivo. (**A**) Growth curves of B16F10-R tumours in vivo treated with pembrolizumab, ASA, or PBS (n = 6–8/group, two-way ANOVA test, Tukey). (**B**) Differences in the number of infiltrating lymphocytes in B16F10-R tumours treated with ASA (one-way ANOVA test, Tukey). (**C,D**) RT-PCR analysis of *ptgs1* (**C**) and *ptgs2* (**D**) mRNA expression in B16F10-NR and B16F10-R tumours. GAPDH mRNA expression was used as the control (n = 8/group, unpaired, two-tailed t test); ns, not statistically significant; ** $p < 0.01$; *** $p < 0.001$; **** $p < 0.0001$.

Next, we examined the TME using flow cytometry analysis, which showed that the infiltration of CD3+, CD4+, and CD8+ T cells was markedly increased in the two aspirin groups with or without pembrolizumab (Figures 3B and S2). In addition, NK cell infiltration notably increased (Figures 3B and S2). These results suggest that aspirin can increase immune cell infiltration in tumours and overcome anti-PD-1 resistance.

3.4. COX2 Inhibitor Can Inhibit B16F10-R Tumour Growth and Recover Immune Cell Infiltration

Since aspirin is a non-selective inhibitor that inhibits both COX1 and COX2, we wanted to determine which, if any, played a more important role in tumour-acquired resistance. Thus, we verified the difference in the expression of COX1/COX2 in B16F10-R and B16F10-NR tumour tissues via RT-qPCR to estimate the relative abundance of COX1/COX2 mRNA. B16F10-R tumours exhibited significantly higher mRNA levels of both COX1 and COX2 than B16F10-NR tumours (Figure 3C,D).

To determine whether COX1 or COX2 was more vital, the selective COX1 inhibitor SC560 and selective COX2 inhibitor celecoxib were used in combination with pembrolizumab. We found that SC560 combined with pembrolizumab did not affect tumour growth (Figure 4A), whereas celecoxib effectively restricted tumour growth when combined with pembrolizumab (Figure 4B). In addition, nimesulide, another selective COX2 inhibitor, inhibited tumour growth in combination with pembrolizumab (Figure S3). Moreover, lymphocyte infiltration in the TME increased significantly after celecoxib treatment (Figures 4D and S4). However, these phenomena were not detected in the SC560 group (Figures 4C and S5). In addition, we also found that B16F10-R tumours exhibited significantly higher protein levels of COX2 than B16F10-NR tumours (Figure S6). Consistently, we also found that B16F10-R tumours secreted significantly higher levels of PGE2 than B16F10-NR tumours in vitro (Figure S7A). These results indicated that COX1 had no effect, but COX2 had a crucial effect on the development of acquired resistance in tumours. Thus, the inhibition of COX2 could effectively overcome drug resistance.

3.5. COX2 Knockout Abrogated the Acquired Resistance to Anti-PD-1 Treatment in B16F10-R Tumour Cells

To further verify the role of COX2 in the development of acquired resistance to anti-PD-1 treatment, we knocked out COX2 in B16F10-R tumour cells (Figures 5A and S6), and we found that PGE2 secretion was significantly reduced in B16F10-R-knockout tumours compared with B16F10-R tumours in vitro (Figure S7B). After COX2 knockout, anti-PD-1 therapy exhibited obvious therapeutic effects on drug-resistant tumours (Figure 5B), where lymphocyte infiltration was significantly increased in the TME (Figure 5C). Next, we compared the growth of B16F10-R tumours and B16F10-R-knockout tumours following anti-PD-1 treatment. There was no significant change in tumour growth without anti-PD-1 treatment; however, tumour growth was significantly inhibited after anti-PD-1 treatment (Figure 5D). Flow cytometry analysis showed that B16F10-R-knockout tumours had significantly more infiltrating immune cells than B16F10-R tumours did (Figures 5E and S8). This indicated that the increased infiltration of lymphocytes was caused by the knockout of COX2. However, without pembrolizumab, the tumour would have immune escape due to the PD-1/PD-L1 pathway. Moreover, the continuous blocking of the PD-1/PD-L1 pathway can have significant inhibitory effects.

3.6. EP4 Inhibitor Could Inhibit B16F10-R Tumour Growth

Most of the functions of PGE2 are mediated by four PGE2 receptors, EP1, EP2, EP3, and EP4 [28]. PGE2 inhibits the killing, cytokine production, and chemotactic activity of tumour target cells by interacting with EP4, which is expressed on NK cells [29]. EP4 is associated with drug resistance in tumours [30,31]. Therefore, we hypothesised that EP4 is related to acquired resistance to anti-PD-1 therapy in B16F10-R tumours. We used E7046, a selective EP4 inhibitor, in combination with pembrolizumab to treat B16F10-R tumours in vivo. We found that E7046 combined with pembrolizumab inhibited tumour growth;

however, the other two groups showed no significant inhibition compared to the PBS group (Figure 6A). Additionally, infiltrating immune cells were detected in the TME. We observed that the infiltrating immune cells contained CD3+, CD4+, and CD8+ T cells, as well as NK cells, and that their numbers increased significantly in the E7046 and E7046 + PD-1 groups relative to the other two groups (Figures 6B and S9). These results indicated that the EP4 receptor may be associated with the acquisition of resistance to anti-PD-1 therapy in B16F10-R cells. Thus, the inhibition of EP4 receptors can effectively address drug resistance.

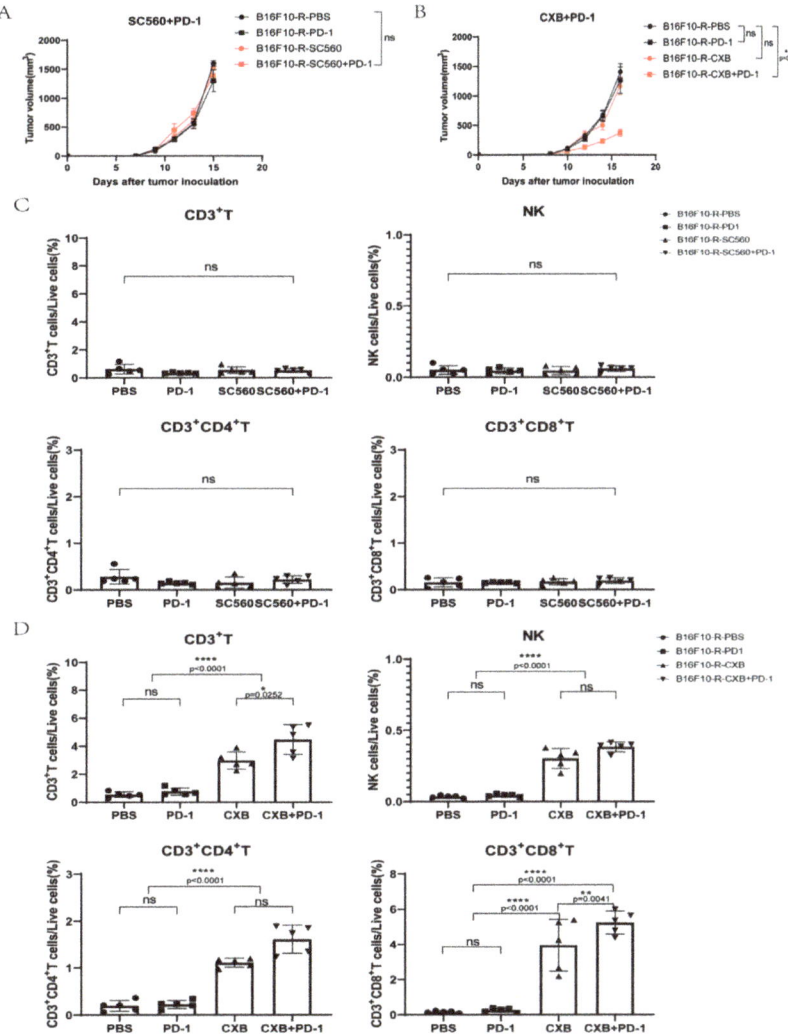

Figure 4. Effects of SC560 or celecoxib combined with pembrolizumab on B16F10-R tumour growth in vivo. (**A**) Growth curves of B16F10-R tumours in vivo treated with pembrolizumab, SC560, or PBS (*n* = 6–8/group, two-way ANOVA test, Tukey). (**B**) Growth curves of B16F10-R tumours in vivo treated with pembrolizumab, celecoxib, or PBS (*n* = 6–8/group, two-way ANOVA test, Tukey). (**C**) Differences in the number of infiltrating lymphocytes cells in B16F10-R tumours treated with celecoxib (one-way ANOVA test, Tukey). (**D**) Differences in the number of infiltrating lymphocytes in B16F10-R tumours treated with SC560 (one-way ANOVA test, Tukey); ns, not statistically significant; * $p < 0.05$; ** $p < 0.01$; **** $p < 0.0001$.

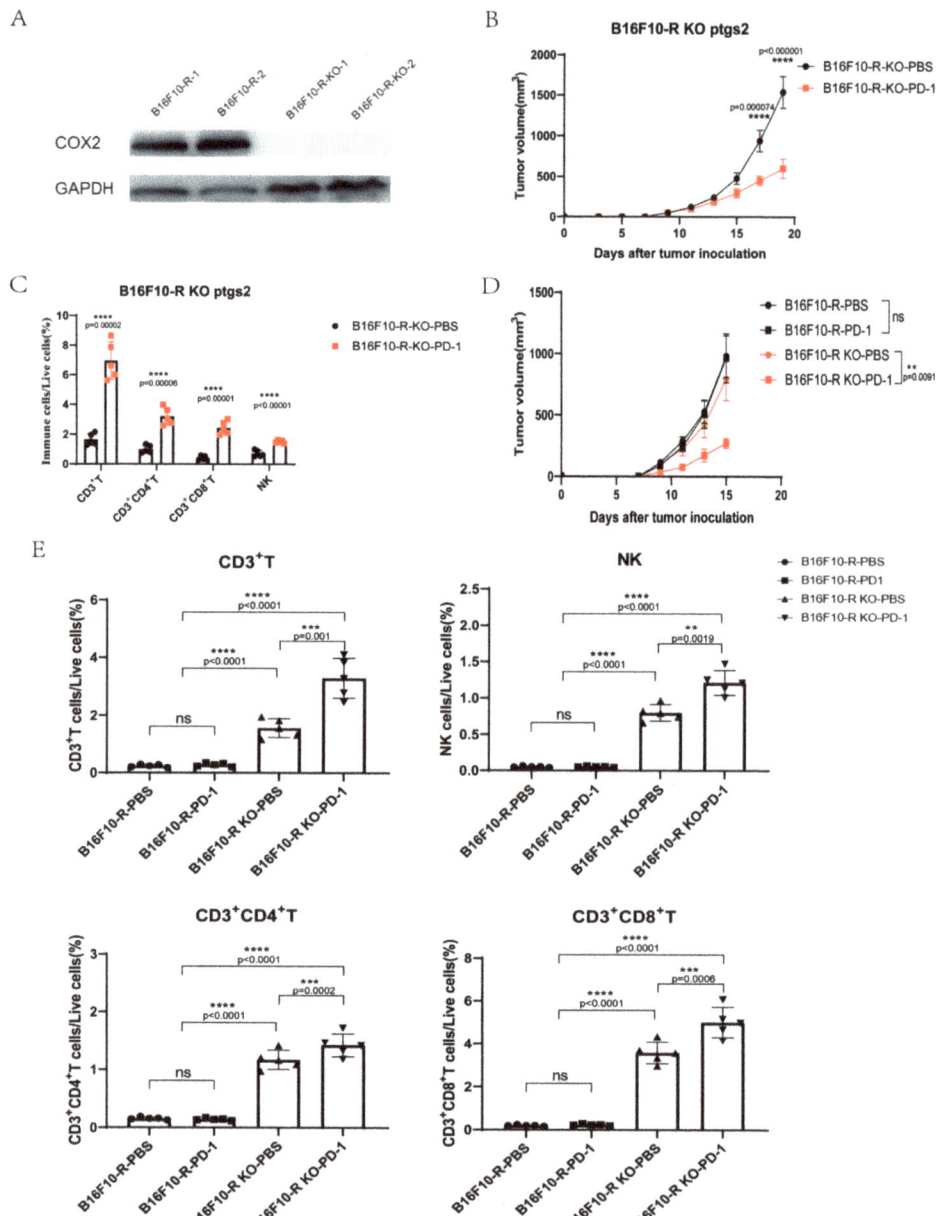

Figure 5. COX2 knockout in B16F10-R cells abrogates acquired resistance to anti-PD-1 therapy. (**A**) Western blot analysis for COX2 expression. GAPDH was the control in the two cell lines. (**B**) Tumour growth curves of B16F10-R-knockout tumours in vivo treated with pembrolizumab or PBS (n = 6–8/group, two-way ANOVA test, Tukey). (**C**) Differences in the number of infiltrating lymphocytes in B16F10-R-knockout tumours (one-way ANOVA test, Tukey). (**D**) Tumour growth curves of B16F10-R and B16F10-R-knockout tumours in vivo treated with pembrolizumab or PBS (n = 6–8/group, two-way ANOVA test, Tukey). (**E**) Differences in the number of infiltrating lymphocytes in B16F10-R-knockout tumours (one-way ANOVA test, Tukey); ns, not statistically significant; ** p < 0.01; *** p < 0.001; **** p < 0.0001.

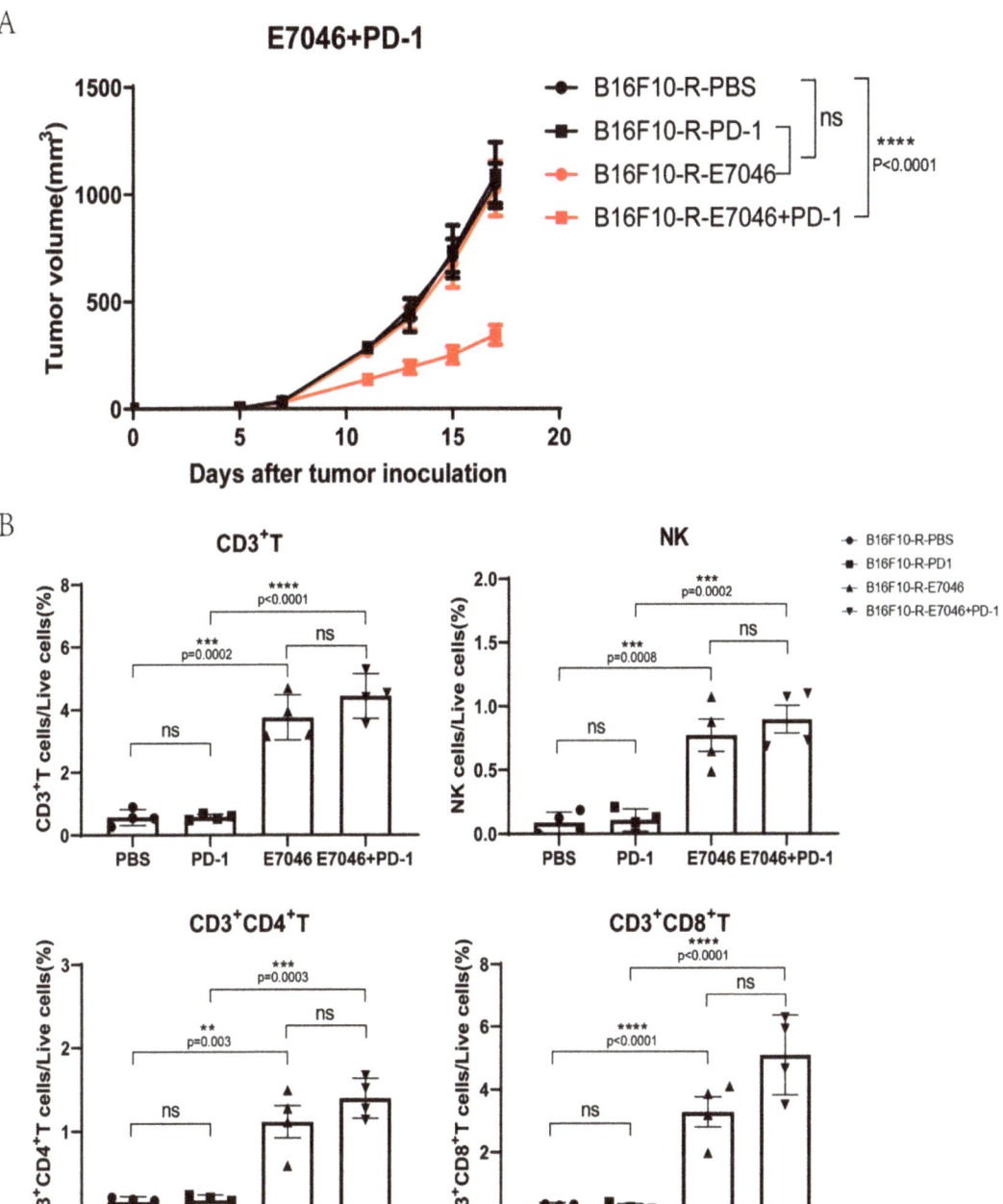

Figure 6. Effects of E7046 combined with pembrolizumab on B16F10-R tumour growth in vivo. (**A**) Growth curves of B16F10-R tumours in vivo treated with pembrolizumab, E7046, or PBS (n = 6–8/group, two-way ANOVA test, Tukey). (**B**) Differences in the number of infiltrating lymphocytes in B16F10-R tumours treated with E7046 (one-way ANOVA test, Tukey); ns, not statistically significant; ** $p < 0.01$; *** $p < 0.001$; **** $p < 0.0001$.

4. Discussion

Malignant tumours can lead to the inactivation of cytotoxic T cells after PD-1 binds to its ligand via the upregulation of PD-L1 expression. Therefore, anti-PD1 or anti-PD-L1 monoclonal antibodies can restore the immune inhibition of tumour growth by blocking the PD-1/PD-L1 pathway. In several cancer types, pembrolizumab has considerably increased patient survival through its therapeutic inhibition of PD-1 [32]. Although anti-PD-1 or anti-PD-L1 drugs are promising for cancer therapy, there are still many problems to be solved. In general, the objective response rates of anti-PD-1 or anti-PD-L1 monoclonal antibodies are nearly 10–50% in most patients [33]. In addition, patients treated with pembrolizumab for a long time are prone to drug resistance [34], thus allowing the tumour to use other signalling pathways for immune escape. Therefore, it is important to study how tumour cells develop resistance to anti-PD-1 treatment.

In this study, we established a melanoma mouse model of B16F10 tumour resistance to anti-PD-1 treatment using four rounds of pembrolizumab therapy and selection in vivo. Additionally, human Pdcd1 transgenic C57BL/6J mice were used to study secondary drug resistance. After four rounds of treatment, B16F10 tumours became resistant to pembrolizumab in vivo. This resistance persisted in cultured B16F10 cells in vitro, suggesting that the acquired resistance was caused by hereditary changes in tumour cells.

The detection of PD-L1 expression on the tumour surface ruled out the possibility that a decrease in its expression led to immune escape of the B16F10-R tumour. Flow cytometry analysis of the TME revealed that the number of infiltrating immune cells, including CD3+, CD4+, and CD8+ T cells, as well as NK cells, was considerably reduced in B16F10-R tumours compared to that in B16F10-NR tumours. We speculated whether the reduction in immune cell infiltration in B16F10-R tumours resulted in tumour immune escape against anti-PD-1 therapy.

The COX2-PGE2 pathway has been reported to be involved in the infiltration of NK and T cells in tumours [30]. In addition, it has also been reported that COX inhibitors can treat tumour patients who have been resistant to other therapies [35]. Thus, inhibiting COX2 may provide a chance to reduce immune escape in tumours [22–37]. Therefore, we used aspirin to treat drug-resistant tumours and showed that aspirin alone did not affect tumour growth, but its combination with pembrolizumab significantly inhibited tumour growth in mice.

RT-qPCR results showed that the expression of COX1/COX2 was significantly higher in drug-resistant tumours than in wild-type tumours. The combination of selective inhibitors of COX1/COX2 with pembrolizumab indicated that COX2 may be the main reason for the development of drug resistance. Therefore, we knocked out the *ptgs2* gene in drug-resistant tumour cells to verify the function of COX2 in tumour drug resistance. After knockout, the sensitivity of drug-resistant tumours to pembrolizumab changed significantly. In addition, infiltrating lymphocytes in the TME increased dozens of times. These results illustrate that COX2 expression is highly correlated with tumour drug resistance.

Subsequently, we targeted EP4 receptors, which were one of downstream receptors of PGE2, and found that EP4 was associated with drug resistance in some tumours. Moreover, we found that E7046, an inhibitor of EP4, combined with pembrolizumab, inhibited the growth of drug-resistant tumours and restored lymphocyte infiltration in the TME. This result also revealed the crucial function of the COX2/PGE2/EP4 pathway in tumour drug resistance.

In all the animal experiments related to drug-resistant tumours, we observed two common phenomena. First, the use of a single inhibitor or pembrolizumab alone did not affect tumour growth, and only a combination of therapies inhibited tumour growth. Second, as long as COX2-related inhibitors were used, the number of infiltrating immune cells in the tumours increased significantly. To explain these two phenomena, we postulated that after the tumour acquired drug resistance, the expression of PD-L1 on the tumour cell surface did not decrease, but the lymphocytes in the tumour were significantly reduced. When only pembrolizumab was used, no effect was observed, probably due to the extreme lack of immune cells. When only COX2-related inhibitors were used, the lymphocytes in the tumour recovered, but the tumour still expressed PD-L1, and immune escape was carried out through the PD-1/PD-L1 pathway; hence, there was no overall effect. Tumour growth can only be effectively inhibited by simultaneous blocking of the PD-1/PD-L1 pathway and restoration of lymphocyte infiltration in the TME with COX2 inhibitors.

In summary, upregulation of COX2 might be the reason for tumour-acquired resistance to anti-PD-1 therapy. Our work demonstrated that COX2 inhibitors could promote pembrolizumab efficacy and inhibit tumour growth in a drug-resistant model. Mechanistically, celecoxib inhibited the COX2 effect and suppressed PGE2 production, which in turn elevated the infiltration of CD3+, CD4+, and CD8+ T cells, as well as NK cells, resulting in the suppression of tumour growth.

Tumour drug resistance is a complex process caused by a range of situations. The results of our study may only reveal one of the causes of tumour-acquired resistance to anti-PD-1 therapy, and further research, including clinical tests, is needed to verify their applicability. Nonetheless, our findings further our understanding of the mechanisms underlying drug resistance in tumours. Furthermore, we identified a new role for the COX2 signalling pathway in anti-PD-1-resistant tumours. Our study suggests that elevated COX2 expression is a potential biomarker of poor immunotherapy response in anti-PD-1-resistant tumours. The dual targeting of PD-1 and COX2 in tumours may enhance the efficacy of immune checkpoint therapy and overcome drug resistance to anti-PD-1 therapy. This is an important addition to our current understanding of tumour-acquired resistance to anti-PD-1 therapy and provides research directions for developing a clinical treatment for anti-PD-1-resistant tumours and immunotherapy.

5. Conclusions

In conclusion, we developed an anti-PD-1-resistant B16F10 tumour model using human Pdcd1 transgenic mice. Lymphocyte infiltration was significantly reduced and COX2 gene expression was increased in B16F10-R tumours compared with B16F10-NR tumours. Moreover, COX2 inhibitors could restore the immune cell infiltration in tumour, and the combination with pembrolizumab could inhibit tumour growth again, lifting the limitation of drug resistance. Therefore, the combination of COX2 inhibitors and anti-PD-1 mAbs may become a new choice for the drug resistance of anti-PD-1 therapy in the future.

Supplementary Materials: The following supporting information can be downloaded at: https://www.mdpi.com/article/10.3390/cancers14174134/s1, Figure S1: Construction of B16F10 tumour model resistant to anti-PD-1 therapy. (A,B) Tumour growth curves for rounds five and rounds six of anti-PD-1 resistant B16F10 tumour selection (n = 6/group, two-way ANOVA test, Sidak); Figure S2: Flow scatter diagrams of lymphocyte infiltration in B16F10-R tumours treated with ASA. (A) Flow scatter diagram of T cell infiltration. (B) Flow scatter diagram of NK cell infiltration; Figure S3: Tumour growth curves of B16F10-R tumour in vivo treated with pembrolizumab, nimesulide or PBS (n = 6–8/group, two-way ANOVA test, Tukey); Figure S4: Flow scatter diagrams of lymphocyte infiltration in B16F10-R tumours treated with CXB. (A) Flow scatter diagram of T cell infiltration. (B) Flow scatter diagram of NK cell infiltration; Figure S5: Flow scatter diagrams of lymphocyte infiltration in B16F10-R tumours treated with SC560. (A) Flow scatter diagram of T cell infiltration. (B) Flow scatter diagram of NK cell infiltration; Figure S6: Western blot analysis for COX2 expression. GAPDH was the control in the two cell lines (one-way ANOVA test, Tukey); Figure S7: Concentration of PGE2 in the supernatant of tumour cells cultured in vitro. (A) Concentration of PGE2 of B16F10-NR or B16F10-R tumour cells cultured in vitro which was determined by ELISA (n = 6/group, unpaired, two-tailed t test). (B) Concentration of PGE2 of B16F10-R or B16F10-R-knockout tumour cells cultured in vitro which was determined by ELISA(n = 6/group, unpaired, two-tailed t test); Figure S8: Flow scatter diagrams of lymphocyte infiltration in B16F10-R or B16F10-R-knockout tumours. (A) Flow scatter diagram of T cell infiltration. (B) Flow scatter diagram of NK cell infiltration; Figure S9: Flow scatter diagrams of lymphocyte infiltration in B16F10-R tumours treated with E7046. (A) Flow scatter diagram of T cell infiltration. (B) Flow scatter diagram of NK cell infiltration.

Author Contributions: C.P.: Conceptualisation, data curation, and formal analysis. P.J.: Data curation. K.X.: Methodology. L.X.: Conceptualisation. Y.F.: Methodology. X.X.: Methodology. T.H.: Validation. B.L.: Conceptualisation and funding acquisition. H.G.: Supervision. J.F.: Conceptualisation, funding acquisition, project administration, resources, supervision, writing—review and editing. All authors have read and agreed to the published version of the manuscript.

Funding: This study was supported by grants from the National Basic Research Program of China (973 Program) (2015CB553706), the National Natural Science Foundation of China (NSFC82172604), and the Key Science and Technology Program of Henan Province (grant NO 212102310872).

Institutional Review Board Statement: All mice were housed at the Laboratory Animal Research Centre, Tongji University. The animal study protocol was approved by the Animal Research Ethics Committee of Tongji University (No. TJLAC-018-032).

Informed Consent Statement: Not applicable.

Data Availability Statement: All data relevant to the study were included in the article or uploaded as supplemental online information.

Acknowledgments: We thank all members of our laboratory for their helpful suggestions and support.

Conflicts of Interest: The authors declare no conflict of interest.

Abbreviations

PD-1	programmed cell death protein 1
PD-L1	programmed death-ligand 1
COX2	cyclooxygenase-2
PGE2	prostaglandin E2
TME	tumour microenvironment
NK cells	natural killer cells

References

1. Pardoll, D.M. The blockade of immune checkpoints in cancer immunotherapy. *Nat. Rev. Cancer* **2012**, *12*, 252–264. [CrossRef] [PubMed]
2. Zou, W. Immunosuppressive networks in the tumour environment and their therapeutic relevance. *Nat. Rev. Cancer* **2005**, *5*, 263–274. [CrossRef] [PubMed]
3. Salmaninejad, A.; Valilou, S.F.; Shabgah, A.G.; Aslani, S.; Alimardani, M.; Pasdar, A.; Sahebkar, A. PD-1/PD-L1 pathway: Basic biology and role in cancer immunotherapy. *J. Cell. Physiol.* **2019**, *234*, 16824–16837. [CrossRef]
4. Frydenlund, N.; Mahalingam, M. PD-L1 and immune escape: Insights from melanoma and other lineage-unrelated malignancies. *Hum. Pathol.* **2017**, *66*, 13–33. [CrossRef] [PubMed]
5. Zou, W.; Chen, L. Inhibitory B7-family molecules in the tumour microenvironment. *Nat. Rev. Immunol.* **2008**, *8*, 467–477. [CrossRef]
6. Tsushima, F.; Yao, S.; Shin, T.; Flies, A.; Flies, S.; Xu, H.; Tamada, K.; Pardoll, D.M.; Chen, L. Interaction between B7-H1 and PD-1 determines initiation and reversal of T-cell anergy. *Blood* **2007**, *110*, 180–185. [CrossRef]
7. Daskivich, T.J.; Belldegrun, A. Words of wisdom. Re: Safety, activity, and immune correlates of anti-PD-1 antibody in cancer. *Eur. Urol.* **2015**, *67*, 816–817. [CrossRef]
8. Brahmer, J.R.; Tykodi, S.S.; Chow, L.Q.M.; Hwu, W.J.; Topalian, S.L.; Hwu, P.; Drake, C.G.; Camacho, L.H.; Kauh, J.; Odunsi, K. Safety and activity of anti-PD-L1 antibody in patients with advanced cancer. *N. Engl. J. Med.* **2012**, *366*, 2455–2465. [CrossRef]
9. Zou, W.; Wolchok, J.D.; Chen, L. PD-L1 (B7-H1) and PD-1 pathway blockade for cancer therapy: Mechanisms, response biomarkers, and combinations. *Sci. Transl. Med.* **2016**, *8*, 328rv4. [CrossRef]
10. Balar, A.V.; Weber, J.S. PD-1 and PD-L1 antibodies in cancer: Current status and future directions. *Cancer Immunol. Immunother.* **2017**, *66*, 551–564. [CrossRef]
11. Bu, X.; Mahoney, K.M.; Freeman, G.J. Learning from PD-1 resistance: New combination strategies. *Trends Mol. Med.* **2016**, *22*, 448–451. [CrossRef] [PubMed]
12. Zaretsky, J.M.; Garcia-Diaz, A.; Shin, D.S.; Escuin-Ordinas, H.; Hugo, W.; Hu-Lieskovan, S.; Torrejon, D.Y.; Abril-Rodriguez, G.; Sandoval, S.; Barthly, L. Mutations associated with acquired resistance to PD-1 blockade in melanoma. *N. Engl. J. Med.* **2016**, *375*, 819–829. [CrossRef] [PubMed]
13. Curran, M.A.; Montalvo, W.; Yagita, H.; Allison, J.P. PD-1 and CTLA-4 combination blockade expands infiltrating T cells and reduces regulatory T and myeloid cells within B16 melanoma tumors. *Proc. Natl. Acad. Sci. USA* **2010**, *107*, 4275–4280. [CrossRef] [PubMed]

14. Dirks, J.; Egli, A.; Sester, U.; Sester, M.; Hirsch, H.H. Blockade of programmed death receptor-1 signaling restores expression of mostly proinflammatory cytokines in anergic cytomegalovirus-specific T cells. *Transpl. Infect. Dis.* **2013**, *15*, 79–89. [CrossRef]
15. Kunzmann, A.T.; Murray, L.J.; Cardwell, C.R.; McShane, C.M.; McMenamin, U.C.; Cantwell, M.M. PTGS2 (cyclooxygenase-2) expression and survival among colorectal cancer patients: A systematic review. *Cancer Epidemiol. Biomark. Prev.* **2013**, *22*, 1490–1497. [CrossRef]
16. Negi, R.R.; Rana, S.V.; Gupta, V.; Gupta, R.; Chadha, V.D.; Prasad, K.K.; Dhawan, D.K. Over-expression of cyclooxygenase-2 in Colorectal Cancer Patients. *Asian Pac. J. Cancer Prev.* **2019**, *20*, 1675–1681. [CrossRef]
17. Xie, X.Q.; Luo, Y.; Ma, X.L.; Li, S.S.; Liu, L.; Zhang, H.; Li, P.; Wang, F. Clinical significance of circulating tumor cells and their expression of cyclooxygenase-2 in patients with nasopharyngeal carcinoma. *Eur. Rev. Med. Pharmacol. Sci.* **2019**, *23*, 6951–6961. [CrossRef]
18. Nagaraju, G.P.; El-Rayes, B.F. Cyclooxygenase-2 in gastrointestinal malignancies. *Cancer* **2019**, *125*, 1221–1227. [CrossRef]
19. Harris, R.E.; Casto, B.C.; Harris, Z.M. Cyclooxygenase-2 and the inflammogenesis of breast cancer. *World J. Clin. Oncol.* **2014**, *5*, 677–692. [CrossRef]
20. Zelenay, S.; van der Veen, A.G.; Böttcher, J.P.; Snelgrove, K.J.; Rogers, N.; Acton, S.E.; Chakravarty, P.; Girotti, M.R.; Marais, R.; Quezada, S.A. Cyclooxygenase-dependent tumor growth through evasion of immunity. *Cell* **2015**, *162*, 1257–1270. [CrossRef]
21. Chen, J.H.; Perry, C.J.; Tsui, Y.C.; Staron, M.M.; Parish, I.A.; Dominguez, C.X.; Rosenberg, D.W.; Kaech, S.M. Prostaglandin E2 and programmed cell death 1 signaling coordinately impair CTL function and survival during chronic viral infection. *Nat. Med.* **2015**, *21*, 327–334. [CrossRef] [PubMed]
22. Kurtova, A.V.; Xiao, J.; Mo, Q.; Pazhanisamy, S.; Krasnow, R.; Lerner, S.P.; Chen, F.; Roh, T.T.; Lay, E.; Ho, P.L. Blocking PGE2-induced tumour repopulation abrogates bladder cancer chemoresistance. *Nature* **2015**, *517*, 209–213. [CrossRef] [PubMed]
23. Hangai, S.; Ao, T.; Kimura, Y.; Matsuki, K.; Kawamura, T.; Negishi, H.; Nishio, J.; Kodama, T.; Taniguchi, T.; Yanai, H. PGE2 induced in and released by dying cells functions as an inhibitory DAMP. *Proc. Natl. Acad. Sci. USA* **2016**, *113*, 3844–3849. [CrossRef] [PubMed]
24. Larsson, K.; Kock, A.; Idborg, H.; Arsenian Henriksson, M.; Martinsson, T.; Johnsen, J.I.; Korotkova, M.; Kogner, P.; Jakobsson, P.-J. COX/mPGES-1/PGE2 pathway depicts an inflammatory-dependent high-risk neuroblastoma subset. *Proc. Natl. Acad. Sci. USA* **2015**, *112*, 8070–8075. [CrossRef]
25. Xu, L.; Stevens, J.; Hilton, M.B.; Seaman, S.; Conrads, T.P.; Veenstra, T.D.; Logsdon, D.; Morris, H.; Swing, D.A.; Patel, N.L.; et al. COX-2 inhibition potentiates antiangiogenic cancer therapy and prevents metastasis in preclinical models. *Sci. Transl. Med.* **2014**, *6*, 242ra84. [CrossRef] [PubMed]
26. Xu, X.; Xie, K.; Li, B.; Xu, L.; Huang, L.; Feng, Y.; Pi, C.; Zhang, J.; Huang, T.; Jiang, M.; et al. Adaptive resistance in tumors to anti-PD-1 therapy through re-immunosuppression by upregulation of GPNMB expression. *Int. Immunopharmacol.* **2021**, *101*, 108199. [CrossRef]
27. Böttcher, J.P.; Bonavita, E.; Chakravarty, P.; Blees, H.; Cabeza-Cabrerizo, M.; Sammicheli, S.; Rogers, N.C.; Sahai, E.; Zelenay, S.; e Sousa, C.R. NK cells stimulate recruitment of cDC1 into the tumor microenvironment promoting cancer immune control. *Cell* **2018**, *172*, 1022–1037.e14. [CrossRef]
28. Narumiya, S.; Sugimoto, Y.; Ushikubi, F. Prostanoid receptors: Structures, properties, and functions. *Physiol. Rev.* **1999**, *79*, 1193–1226. [CrossRef]
29. Ma, X.; Holt, D.; Kundu, N.; Reader, J.; Goloubeva, O.; Take, Y.; Fulton, A.M. A prostaglandin E (PGE) receptor EP4 antagonist protects natural killer cells from PGE2-mediated immunosuppression and inhibits breast cancer metastasis. *Oncoimmunology* **2013**, *2*, e22647. [CrossRef]
30. Huang, H.; Aladelokun, O.; Ideta, T.; Giardina, C.; Ellis, L.M.; Rosenberg, D.W. Inhibition of PGE 2/EP4 receptor signaling enhances oxaliplatin efficacy in resistant colon cancer cells through modulation of oxidative stress. *Sci. Rep.* **2019**, *9*, 4954. [CrossRef]
31. Lin, X.; Li, S.; Zhou, C.; Li, R.; Wang, H.; Luo, W.; Huang, Y.-S.; Chen, L.-K.; Cai, J.-L.; Wang, T.-X.; et al. Cisplatin induces chemoresistance through the PTGS2-mediated anti-apoptosis in gastric cancer. *Int. J. Biochem. Cell B* **2019**, *116*, 105610. [CrossRef] [PubMed]
32. Bardhan, K.; Anagnostou, T.; Boussiotis, V.A. The PD1:PD-L1/2 pathway from discovery to clinical implementation. *Front Immunol.* **2016**, *7*, 550. [CrossRef] [PubMed]
33. Nguyen, L.T.; Ohashi, P.S. Clinical blockade of PD1 and LAG3–Potential mechanisms of action. *Nat. Rev. Immunol.* **2015**, *15*, 45–56. [CrossRef] [PubMed]
34. Ribas, A. Adaptive immune resistance: How cancer protects from immune attack. *Cancer Discov.* **2015**, *5*, 915–919. [CrossRef]
35. Kobayashi, K.; Kaira, K.; Kagamu, H. Recovery of the sensitivity to anti-PD-1 antibody by celecoxib in lung cancer. *Anticancer Res.* **2020**, *40*, 5309–5311. [CrossRef]
36. Fujita, M.; Kohanbash, G.; Fellows-Mayle, W.; Hamilton, R.L.; Komohara, Y.; Decker, S.A.; Ohlfest, J.R.; Okada, H. COX-2 blockade suppresses gliomagenesis by inhibiting myeloid-derived suppressor cells. *Cancer Res.* **2011**, *71*, 2664–2674. [CrossRef]
37. Mao, Y.; Sarhan, D.; Steven, A.; Seliger, B.; Kiessling, R.; Lundqvist, A. Inhibition of tumor-derived prostaglandin-E2 blocks the induction of myeloid-derived suppressor cells and recovers natural killer cell activity. *Clin. Cancer Res.* **2014**, *20*, 4096–4106. [CrossRef]

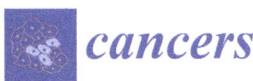

Article

Development of a Patient-Derived 3D Immuno-Oncology Platform to Potentiate Immunotherapy Responses in Ascites-Derived Circulating Tumor Cells

Thomas J. Gerton [1,†], Allen Green [1,†], Marco Campisi [2,†], Minyue Chen [2], Iliana Gjeci [3], Navin Mahadevan [2], Catherine A. A. Lee [4], Ranjan Mishra [5], Ha V. Vo [3], Koji Haratani [2], Ze-Hua Li [2], Kathleen T. Hasselblatt [6], Bryanna Testino [1], Trevor Connor [1], Christine G. Lian [4], Kevin M. Elias [6,7], Patrick Lizotte [3], Elena V. Ivanova [3], David A. Barbie [2,3,*] and Daniela M. Dinulescu [1,*]

[1] Division of Women's and Perinatal Pathology, Department of Pathology, Brigham and Women's Hospital, Harvard Medical School, Boston, MA 02115, USA
[2] Department of Medical Oncology, Dana-Farber Cancer Institute, Boston, MA 02215, USA
[3] Belfer Center for Applied Cancer Science, Dana-Farber Cancer Institute, Boston, MA 02215, USA
[4] Division of Dermatopathology, Department of Pathology, Brigham and Women's Hospital, Harvard Medical School, Boston, MA 02115, USA
[5] Whitehead Institute for Biomedical Research, Cambridge, MA 02142, USA
[6] Department of Obstetrics, Gynecology, and Reproductive Biology, Brigham and Women's Hospital, Harvard Medical School, Boston, MA 02115, USA
[7] Division of Gynecologic Oncology, Dana-Farber Cancer Institute, Boston, MA 02215, USA
* Correspondence: david_barbie@dfci.harvard.edu (D.A.B.); ddinulescu@bwh.harvard.edu (D.M.D.); Tel.: +1-617-632-6036 (D.A.B.); +1-617-732-5318 (D.M.D.)
† These authors contributed equally to this work.

Simple Summary: The clinical implementation of novel precision medicine strategies in high-grade serous ovarian cancer (HGSOC), the most common and aggressive ovarian cancer subtype, are urgently needed. Targeted immunotherapeutic combinations that maximize drug benefits are of particular interest. Unlike lung cancer and melanoma, immunotherapeutic responses using immune checkpoint blockade (ICB) in high-grade serous ovarian cancer have been lower than expected and longer-term remissions are uncommon. Evidence now demonstrates that global DNA hypermethylation plays a critical role in immune evasion. Consequently, epigenetic reprogramming strategies could be beneficial in potentiating immunotherapeutic responses by reversing tumor escape mechanisms and enhancing immune cell activation. The current study details the development of ex vivo 3D patient-derived platforms for rapid testing of immunotherapeutic combinations in high-grade serous ovarian tumor metastases and tumor ascites. It further proposes the implementation of epigenetic adjuvants to potentiate systemic ICB responses and eradicate circulating tumor cells responsible for wide, aggressive metastases in this poor prognostic disease.

Abstract: High-grade serous ovarian cancer (HGSOC) is responsible for the majority of gynecology cancer-related deaths. Patients in remission often relapse with more aggressive forms of disease within 2 years post-treatment. Alternative immuno-oncology (IO) strategies, such as immune checkpoint blockade (ICB) targeting the PD-(L)1 signaling axis, have proven inefficient so far. Our aim is to utilize epigenetic modulators to maximize the benefit of personalized IO combinations in ex vivo 3D patient-derived platforms and in vivo syngeneic models. Using patient-derived tumor ascites, we optimized an ex vivo 3D screening platform (PDOTS), which employs autologous immune cells and circulating ascites-derived tumor cells, to rapidly test personalized IO combinations. Most importantly, patient responses to platinum chemotherapy and poly-ADP ribose polymerase inhibitors in 3D platforms recapitulate clinical responses. Furthermore, similar to clinical trial results, responses to ICB in PDOTS tend to be low and positively correlated with the frequency of CD3+ immune cells and EPCAM+/PD-L1+ tumor cells. Thus, the greatest response observed with anti-PD-1/anti-PD-L1 immunotherapy alone is seen in patient-derived HGSOC ascites, which present with high levels of systemic CD3+ and PD-L1+ expression in immune and tumor cells, respectively. In addition, priming

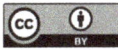

with epigenetic adjuvants greatly potentiates ICB in ex vivo 3D testing platforms and in vivo tumor models. We further find that epigenetic priming induces increased tumor secretion of several key cytokines known to augment T and NK cell activation and cytotoxicity, including IL-6, IP-10 (CXCL10), KC (CXCL1), and RANTES (CCL5). Moreover, epigenetic priming alone and in combination with ICB immunotherapy in patient-derived PDOTS induces rapid upregulation of CD69, a reliable early activation of immune markers in both CD4+ and CD8+ T cells. Consequently, this functional precision medicine approach could rapidly identify personalized therapeutic combinations able to potentiate ICB, which is a great advantage, especially given the current clinical difficulty of testing a high number of potential combinations in patients.

Keywords: PDOTS; ovarian cancer; ascites; epigenetic; methylation; ICB; PD-L1; PD-1

1. Introduction

High-grade serous ovarian cancer (HGSOC) represents more than 70% of all epithelial ovarian cancers and is responsible for the vast majority of gynecologic-related deaths [1–3]. Despite an initially robust clinical response to platinum-based chemotherapy, HGSOC has a high mortality rate, as patients often relapse within 2 years following diagnosis [4–7]. Patients with *BRCA*-mutated HGSOC receive additional treatment in the form of poly-ADP ribose polymerase inhibitors (PARPi), but regularly develop resistance to these therapies as well [8]. Unfortunately, there are no long-term viable therapeutic options for HGSOC patients with intrinsic or acquired platinum resistance, although some responses have recently been seen with a folate receptor alpha-targeted antibody-drug conjugate (ADC) [4–7,9]. Furthermore, despite impressive immuno-oncology (IO) advances in lung, head and neck cancers, and melanomas, several limitations remain. Multiple tumor subtypes, including HGSOC, are notoriously resistant to immunotherapy. Multiple clinical trials of ovarian cancer patients receiving immune checkpoint blockade alone (ICB) and in various combinations are currently being evaluated. To date, clinical trial response rates seen in HGSOC patients receiving immune checkpoint blockade have been limited (<15%) [10]. Current research in the field has shifted towards maximizing ICB efficacy through the use of combination treatments [11]. These combinations include PARPis, anti-angiogenic therapies, cytokine therapy, and chemotherapy [12,13]. Although these results are more promising compared to immunotherapy alone, there is still an urgent need to develop accurate testing platforms and ICB response biomarkers for use in clinical trials.

Several ICB inhibitors against cytotoxic T-lymphocyte-associated protein 4 (CTLA-4), programmed cell death protein 1 (PD-1), and/or programmed death-ligand 1 (PD-L1) have been approved by the FDA for the treatment of metastatic melanoma, advanced kidney cancer, metastatic non-small cell lung cancer, and unresectable or metastatic triple negative breast cancer [9,14,15]. These approved monoclonal antibodies (mAbs) for ICB therapy include ipilimumab (αCTLA-4), nivolumab (αPD-1), pembrolizumab (αPD-1), and atezolizumab (αPD-L1) [16,17]. A high tumor mutation burden and increased PD-L1 expression in cancer cells have often been associated with effective ICB responses and favorable prognosis in multiple tumor subtypes [18,19]. The presence of CD8+ T cells inside the tumor or at the tumor periphery, known as tumor-infiltrating lymphocytes (TILs), and increased PD-1 expression within T cells have also been associated with a more robust clinical response and outcome [18,19]. The current study further investigates the functionality of effector T cells in newly diagnosed HGSOC patients to better understand the low response to ICB in HGSOC clinical trials. To this end, we analyzed brisk (high) tumor-infiltrating lymphocytes (TILs) that infiltrate diffusely within the tumor and compared them to non-brisk (low) TILs that show only focal infiltration or absent TILs (no TILs or minimal TIL infiltration), respectively. We further sought to identify therapeutic strategies to potentiate immune activation and function.

Specifically, we employed epigenetic priming to reverse aberrant changes in DNA methylation, which is a key mechanism that enables tumor cells to evade the immune system, induce tolerance and develop resistance to ICB [20–38]. Specifically, DNA methylation is known to play a key role in modulating cytotoxic T cell function and exhaustion, while decreased tumor PD-L1 expression is associated with hypermethylation [20–38]. Consequently, epigenetic reprogramming strategies may be beneficial in cancer immunotherapy by modulating immune cell differentiation, proliferation and function while reversing escape mechanisms employed by cancer cells [20–39]. The discovery of the ten-eleven translocase (TET) family of 5-mC hydroxylases, including TET1, TET2 and TET3, which convert 5-methylcytosine (5-mC) to 5-hydroxymethylcytosine (5-hmC), has uncovered new layers of epigenetic modifications in cancer. Most importantly, global genome methylation levels and, specifically, changes in 5-hmC expression have been identified as a sensitive predictor for patient prognosis and therapeutic response in multiple solid tumors, including ovarian cancer [39]. Thus, global 5-hmC loss is associated with a decreased response to standard chemotherapy, shorter time to relapse and poor overall survival in patients newly diagnosed with HGSOC [39]. We have further identified a targetable pathway to reverse epigenetic 5-hmC loss, both genetically and pharmacologically [39]. Interestingly, epigenetic priming enables the rescue of 5-hmC loss, reduces the number of cancer stem cells, restores sensitivity to platinum chemotherapy, and increases overall survival in chemoresistant animal models [39]. Consequently, identifying prognostic epigenetic markers and altering therapeutic regimens to incorporate DNA methyl transferase inhibitors (DNMTi) in highly methylated tumors with poor prognosis could have important clinical implications for treatment in newly diagnosed HGSOC patients.

The current study shows that epigenetic priming potentiates ICB responses in tumor models and ex vivo 3D patient-derived platforms. Interestingly, epigenetic priming using 5-azacytidine (5-aza), a DNMTi, and givinostat, a histone deacetylase inhibitor (HDACi), prior to ICB delivery, enhances TIL infiltration and overall survival in the murine ID8 tumor model [40]. As outlined in the elegant study by Stone et al., the ID8-VEGF model is well suited and has been used extensively for ICB testing in ovarian cancer, as it is an immunocompetent model with an immunosuppressed tumor microenvironment (TME) [40]. However, it does not recapitulate HGSOC development since the ID8 parental cells are derived from the murine ovarian surface epithelium (OSE), while the vast majority of patient tumors originate in the distal fallopian tube rather than OSE [40]. More recently, novel syngeneic HGSC models, which have a fallopian tubal origin, key genetic alterations, and better recapitulate the clinical disease, have been described [41]. Consequently, additional research is needed to assess whether this potentially synergistic combination is effective in syngeneic models, which better recapitulate ICB responses [41], and in ex vivo testing platforms utilizing patient samples [42–44]. Our results indicate that epigenetic priming mediates the rapid secretion of key tumor-derived cytokines known to augment T and NK cell activation and cytotoxicity, including IL-6, IP-10 (CXCL10), KC (CXCL1), and RANTES (CCL5). It further upregulates the early activation of immune markers in both CD4+ and CD8+ T cells and potentiates ICB responses in ex vivo patient-derived platforms and in vivo syngeneic HGSOC models. The development of novel microfluidic devices embedded with patient-derived organotypic tumor spheroids (PDOTS) and autologous immune cells is key for the rapid IO testing of clinical samples. Here, we report the optimization of a 3D immuno-oncology PDOTS platform for ex vivo screening of HGSOC-derived ascites, which has broad implications for interrogating systemic immune and circulating tumor cell responses. The implementation of a predictive IO testing platform will allow for the rapid screening of a large number of personalized therapeutic combinations prior to their testing in patients.

2. Materials and Methods

2.1. Digital Spatial Profiling of the Tumor-Immune Microenvironment

Digital spatial profiling (DSP) of tumor samples was performed on the GeoMx platform (NanoString, Seattle, WA, USA) [45]. Regions of interest (ROIs) were selected by a board-certified pathologist. Immunofluorescence for pan-Cytokeratin (tumor marker), CD45 (immune marker), and SYTO 13 (DNA stain) (NanoString Technologies, GMX-PRO-MORPH-HST-12) guided the selection of ROIs. Samples were incubated with 77 oligonucleotide-conjugated and photocleavable antibodies (NanoString Technologies, GMX-PROCO-NCT-HICP-12, GMX-PROMOD-NCT-HICT-12, GMX-PROMOD-NCT-HIAS-12, and GMX-PROMOD-NCT-HIODT-12) as well as negative and positive controls. After incubation and imaging, the ROIs were segmented into pan-CK+ (tumor) and pan-CK− (stroma) areas. Oligo tags were released from the areas of illumination (AOIs) via targeted exposure to ultraviolet radiation, followed by hybridization and counting using the NanoString GeoMx nCounter system [45]. The GeoMx DSP Data Analysis Suite (v2.4.0.421) was used to evaluate the raw count data output from the nCounter platform. Initial QC was performed using the default parameters.

2.2. Tumor Cell Culture Assays

A2780Res and Kuramochi cells were cultured in RPMI base medium supplemented with 10% fetal bovine serum (FBS) and 1% penicillin-streptomycin. BPPNM, KPCA.A, KPCA.B, and KPCA.C cells were all cultured in a DMEM base medium supplemented with 10% FBS, 1% penicillin-streptomycin, 10 ng/mL epidermal growth factor (Sigma Aldrich, E4127-1MG), 5 mL of 100× insulin–transferrin–selenium (Fisher Scientific, 41400045, Waltham, MA, USA), and 100 ng/mL of cholera toxin (Sigma Aldrich, 227036-1MG, Burlington, MA, USA). Human ascites samples were cultured in a base medium of RPMI supplemented with 10% FBS and 1% penicillin-streptomycin.

Frozen peripheral blood mononuclear cells (PBMCs) purchased from STEMCELL (70025) were thawed and washed in 5 mL of RPMI with 10% human serum (Sigma-Aldrich, H5667), 1% penicillin-streptomycin, and 200 μM of L-Glutamine (Gibco, 25030149, Billings, MT, USA). The washed PBMCs were suspended in 1 mL of the complete medium at 37 °C for 45 min. Then, T cells were isolated using the EasySep™ Human T Cell Isolation Kit (STEMCELL, 17951, Tokyo, Japan), immediately followed by activation using the Human T Cell Activation/Expansion Kit (Miltenyi Biotec, 130-091-441, Bergisch Gladbach, Germany), according to the manufacturer's instructions. The activated T cells were cultured in the complete medium with 100 U/mL of human IL-2 (ThermoFisher, PHC0021, Waltham, MA, USA), and the medium and IL-2 were refreshed every three days. After 14 days of activation, the T cells were used for the downstream assay by day 35.

2.3. Assessment of Global Methylation (5-hmC) Levels in HGSOC

A2780Res, BPPNM, and KPCA.A cells were plated at 50,000 cells per well in a Falcon 8-well culture slide. After waiting 24 h for the cells to adhere, the medium was removed and replaced with 5-aza-treated medium. Aliquots of 5-aza (Sigma Aldrich, A2385-100MG) were thawed prior to each treatment and diluted to 1000× their final concentration in DMSO prior to a final 1:1000 dilution using the supplemented cell culture medium. Controls were treated with an equivalent volume of DMSO in supplemented cell culture medium. Treatment was readministered 48 h after initial cell plating; 72 h after initial cell plating, the cells were washed twice using 1× PBS and fixed for 30 min using 4% paraformaldehyde. After fixation, the cells were permeabilized for 15 min using 0.5% Triton X-100. Cell DNA was then denatured using 2N HCl for 30 min. The acid was then neutralized by adding 100 mM Tris-HCl (pH 8) for 10 min. All samples were then washed three times using 1× PBS supplemented with 0.6 μM EDTA. A blocking buffer consisting of 1× PBS supplemented with 5% goat serum and 0.3% Triton X-100 was then used to block the samples for 60 min. Then, 5-hmC (Active Motif, 39769, Carlsbad, CA, USA; 1:800) primary antibody dilutions consisting of 1× PBS with 1% BSA and 0.3% Triton X-100 were added to the respective samples and incubated overnight at 4 °C. The following day, the samples were washed three times with 0.1% PBS-T and incubated with an AF488 goat anti-rabbit secondary antibody (Invitrogen #A11008, 1:1000) for 60 min in the dark. After another three washes using 0.1% PBS-T, the samples were briefly dipped in deionized water to dissolve any excess salts from the PBS and DAPI was applied for nuclear staining. The samples were imaged on an EVOS FL Auto 2 microscope after adding coverslips. For quantification, three images were taken at 20× magnification and positive cells were counted using the ImageJ software (v1.53f).

2.4. Tumor-Derived Secreted Cytokine/Chemokine Profiling in Response to DNMTIs

KPCA.A, KPCA.B, and KPCA.C cell lines were seeded at 150,000 cells per well in a 6-well tissue culture plate and allowed to grow for 48 h. The cells were washed twice with 1× PBS and replenished with serum-free DMEM medium alone or containing 10 µM 5-aza. Azacytidine was replenished every 24 h. After 72 h, the cell culture supernatants were collected on ice, centrifuged to remove any cell debris, and then flash-frozen on dry ice. The secreted cytokines and chemokines were profiled using the Mouse Cytokine 44-Plex Discovery Assay from Eve Technologies (Calgary, AB, Canada).

2.5. Optimization of Patient-Derived Organotypic HGSOC Spheroids (PDOTS) in 3D Microfluidic Devices

Patient tissue studies reviewed and approved by the Institutional Review Board of Brigham and Women's Hospital (#2006P002438) and Dana Farber Cancer Institute (#02-051) were conducted in accordance with the Declaration of Helsinki. Patient-derived tumor ascites samples were collected using paracentesis and centrifuged into a cell pellet. The supernatant was aspirated, and the pellet was resuspended in ACK lysis buffer (Thermo Fisher, A1049201). After maximum hemolysis was observed, 1× PBS was added to the sample and centrifugation was repeated to ensure removal of red blood cells and hemolytic products. The final cell pellet was slightly agitated to promote the resuspension of the cells as spheroids. The resuspended sample was then filtered through 100 µm and 40 µm filters to generate three spheroid fractions: S1 (>100 µm), S2 (40–100 µm), and S3 (<40 µm). S2 fractions containing both tumor and immune cells within the tumor-immune microenvironment were used for ex vivo cultures of solid HGSOC tumor samples, as previously described [43,44]. S2 + S3 fractions containing circulating tumor spheroids and systemic immune cells were used for ex vivo cultures of HGSOC tumor ascites samples. On ice, a mixture of 3.00 µg/mL collagen, 1× phenol red, and distilled water was adjusted to a pH of 7.3–7.4 with 0.5 N NaOH. The S2 + S3 fraction of spheroids were pelleted again using centrifugation at 300× g for 3 min. This pellet was resuspended in the collagen mixture and 10 µL of this spheroid-collagen mixture was loaded into an IdenTx microfluidic device (AIM Biotech, DAX-1) as previously described [43,44]. The devices were incubated at 37 °C for 35–40 min to allow the collagen to polymerize and form a matrix. After polymerization, 300 µL of RPMI medium supplemented with 10% FBS, 1% penicillin-streptomycin, and 100 U/mL IL-2 (Miltenyi Biotec, 130097746) was divided equally between the four medium ports. For treatment conditions, various concentrations of 5-aza, HDACi, PARPi (Talazoparib, AbMole Biosciences, BMN637, Houston, TX, USA), αPD-1 (Fisher Scientific, 501360845), αPD-L1 (Fisher Scientific, 501360846), and cisplatin (Patterson Vet, 07-893-4099, Loveland, CO, USA) were administered. The medium was replenished on the third day of incubation for all conditions.

For tumor spheroid–T cell co-culture studies, Kuramochi tumor cells were cultured in a 6-well ULA plate (Corning, CLS3471-24EA, Corning, NY, USA) at 500,000 cells per well for 24 h. After spheroid formation occurred, the cells were filtered through a 100 µm filter and a subsequent 40 µm filter. The 40–100 nm spheroids isolated by filtration were collected and labeled as the S2 fraction. The S2 fraction was mixed with T cells isolated from PBMCs at a ratio of 1:3 in the collagen mixture listed previously. The co-culture was then loaded into the IdenTx microfluidic devices following the above procedure, with 40,000 cells loaded into each cell port. The medium used was composed of 5% human serum, 5% FBS, 1% penicillin-streptomycin, 100 µM L-glutamine, and 6000 U/mL IL-2. Media treatment conditions were 2 µM 5-aza and 2 µM HDACi; 200 µg/mL αPD-1 and αPD-L1; and 2 µM 5-aza, 2 µM HDACi, 200 µg/mL αPD-1 and αPD-L1. Devices were stained for live–dead analysis after 3 days of culture.

2.6. Immunofluorescent Imaging of PDOTS

After approximately 24 h in an untreated device, the medium was drained from the wells and replaced with a 1:100 dilution of FcR block (Miltenyi, 130-059-901, Tokyo, Japan) in 1× PBS. After a 15 min incubation, the blocking reagent was replaced with an antibody solution (Table S1) at 1:100 each with 1 µg/mL of Hoechst 33,342 in 1× PBS. Panel 1 was used for PDOTS derived from primary tumor samples, and panel 2 was used for PDOTS derived from ascites samples. After a 15 min incubation, the medium channels were washed twice with 1× PBS before imaging using an inverted Nikon Eclipse Ti microscope equipped with Nikon DS-Qi1Mc camera and NIS-Elements software. Live–dead analysis was performed on separate samples to determine cell viability in each treatment condition following 5–7 days of treatment. A 1:1 solution of AO/PI stain (Nexcelcom, CS2-0106, Lawrence, MA, USA) in 1× PBS was made and 20–30 µL of this solution was added to each device after the medium was drained. After a 5 min incubation with the stain, the devices were imaged using a Nikon Eclipse Ti microscope. Using this software, the number of live cells stained with acridine orange (AO) and dead cells stained with propidium iodide (PI) were quantified for analysis.

2.7. Identification of Early Markers of Immune Activation in CD4+ and CD8+ T Cells

Patient-derived solid tumor samples were collected surgically and cut into approximately 2 cm^3 pieces, avoiding any fatty or fibrotic material. 2 to 3 of these pieces were placed into a 15 mL centrifuge tube containing approximately 4 mL of warm digestion buffer composed of RPMI base medium supplemented with 10% FBS, 1% penicillin-streptomycin, 100 U/mL collagenase type IV (Gibco, 17104019), and 50 µg/mL Dnase I (Sigma-Aldrich, 04716728001). The tumor was minced with sterile scissors for approximately 2 min, after which the supernatant was transferred to a separate tube containing only RPMI with 10% FBS and 1% penicillin-streptomycin. The digestion medium was replaced, and this process was repeated about three times. The resulting cells were pelleted and resuspended in a 6-well ULA plate containing the RPMI medium supplemented with 10% FBS, 1% penicillin-streptomycin, and 100 U/mL IL-2. Separate wells were treated with the following conditions: control, 2 µM of 5-aza and 2 µM of HDACi, 200 µg/mL of αPD-1 and αPD-L1, and a combination of all therapies. The cells were left to incubate for 24 h.

2.8. Flow Cytometry of Immune Cells

In total, 1–2 mL of the S2 + S3 patient ascites fraction was centrifuged and trypsinized to dissociate tumor spheroids within the sample. After 5 min, the trypsin was quenched with medium, and the cells were pelleted. The cells were washed with 1× PBS and pelleted again. Afterwards, the samples were incubated in the dark with Zombie NIR viability dye (Biolegend, 423105, Tokyo, Japan) resuspended in 1× PBS for 15 min. The cells were then washed again with 1× PBS supplemented with 2% FBS (FACS Buffer) and pelleted. Blocking was done using a 1:100 FcR blocking reagent (Miltenyi, 130-059-901) in FACS buffer. After 15 min of blocking, the cells were stained with their respective antibodies (Table S2) and resuspended in FACS buffer for another 15 min. Panel 1 focused on T cells/PD-1 expression and consisted of antibodies for CD45, CD3, CD8, CD4, and PD-1. Panel 2 focused on PD-L1 expression and consisted of antibodies for CD45, EPCAM, and PD-L1. After staining, the cells were fixed with either 2% formaldehyde or 4% paraformaldehyde in the dark for 30 min, washed with 1.5 mL of FACS buffer, and pelleted. The cells were resuspended in 200 µL of the FACS buffer and analyzed using a BD LSR Fortessa. Data gating and analysis were done using the FlowJo 2 software. Gating descriptions can be found in Table S3. For the solid S1 patient sample, the above protocol was followed using the antibody panel listed in Table S4.

2.9. Assessment of Therapeutic Efficacy in Syngeneic HGSOC Models

The animal studies were reviewed and approved (#2016N000212) by the Institutional Animal Care and Use Committee (IACUC) of Brigham and Women's Hospital. Tumor engraftment was completed through intraperitoneal injection on 6-week-old immunocompetent C57BL/6J female mice (Jackson Laboratories, Strain #000664, Bar Harbor, ME, USA) with 3.7×10^6 KPCA.B cells resuspended in a 1:1 solution of $1\times$ PBS and Matrigel (Corning, 354234). The mice were treated with intraperitoneal injection of 5-aza resuspended in $1\times$ PBS at 4 mg/kg, HDACi resuspended in $1\times$ PBS at 2 mg/kg (Fisher Scientific, 0000001045), 50 µg of αPD-L1 (Bio X Cell, BE0101, Lebanon, NH, USA) diluted in a 6.5 pH dilution buffer (Bio X Cell, IP0065), and 50 µg of αCTLA-4 (Bio X Cell, BE0131) diluted in a 7.0 pH dilution buffer (Bio X Cell, IP0070). A total of four conditions were utilized: control, 5-aza and HDACi treatments four times a week on alternating weeks, αPD-L1 and αCTLA-4 treatments twice a week, and 5-aza and HDACi treatments four times a week on alternating weeks, with αPD-L1 and αCTLA-4 treatments twice every week. Tumor burden was quantified by isolating and measuring all tumors at necropsy. Tumor engraftment was considered successful if the final tumor mass was greater than 50 µg. Mice with unsuccessfully engrafted tumors (below threshold) were excluded in the study. Only mice that survived past day 30 had their tumor masses quantified.

2.10. Statistical Analysis

Statistical analysis was completed for immunofluorescent imaging, cytokine analysis, and live–dead imaging of patient-derived organoid tumor devices using the Prism 9 software. Paired two directional t-tests were used for cytokine analysis and a one-way ANOVA, with post hoc Tukey tests, was used for all other statistical analysis. The results were deemed significant if p values were equal to or less than 0.05 ($p \leq 0.05$). The results are shown as mean ± SD for in vitro studies and mean ± SEM for in vivo studies. The GeoMx DSP Data Analysis Suite (v2.4.0.421) was used to evaluate the raw count data output from the nCounter platform. As the counts for the three housekeeping control antibodies (Histone H3, GAPDH, and S6) were sufficiently high and concordant, we used the geometric mean of all three for normalization. For statistical testing, the negative controls (Ms IgG1, Ms IgG2a, and Rb IgG1) and the housekeeping genes (Histone H3 and GAPDH, S6) were removed, leaving 71 protein targets. Statistical significance was determined using t-tests with Benjamini–Hochberg correction for multiple testing.

3. Results

3.1. Digital Spatial Proteomic Profiling of Patient TILs in HGSOC

Unlike melanoma, immunotherapeutic responses in HGSOC have been lower than expected and longer-term cures have been hard to achieve with ICB, with clinical trial responses seen in 10–15% of patients [46]. Furthermore, the hypoxic and acidic TME seen in HGSOC can co-opt myeloid cells to promote a pro-tumorigenic and immune suppressive phenotype while blocking immune cell proliferation, activation, and infiltration [46,47]. Three formalin-fixed paraffin embedded (FFPE) primary ovarian cancer patient samples were selected for digital spatial proteomic (DSP) analysis by a board-certified pathologist. From these 3 slides, 24 tumor and 16 stroma segments were identified and evaluated for changes in immune-related protein expression. These segments were categorized according to their level of infiltration: absent TILs, low TILs, and high TILs (Figures 1 and S1).

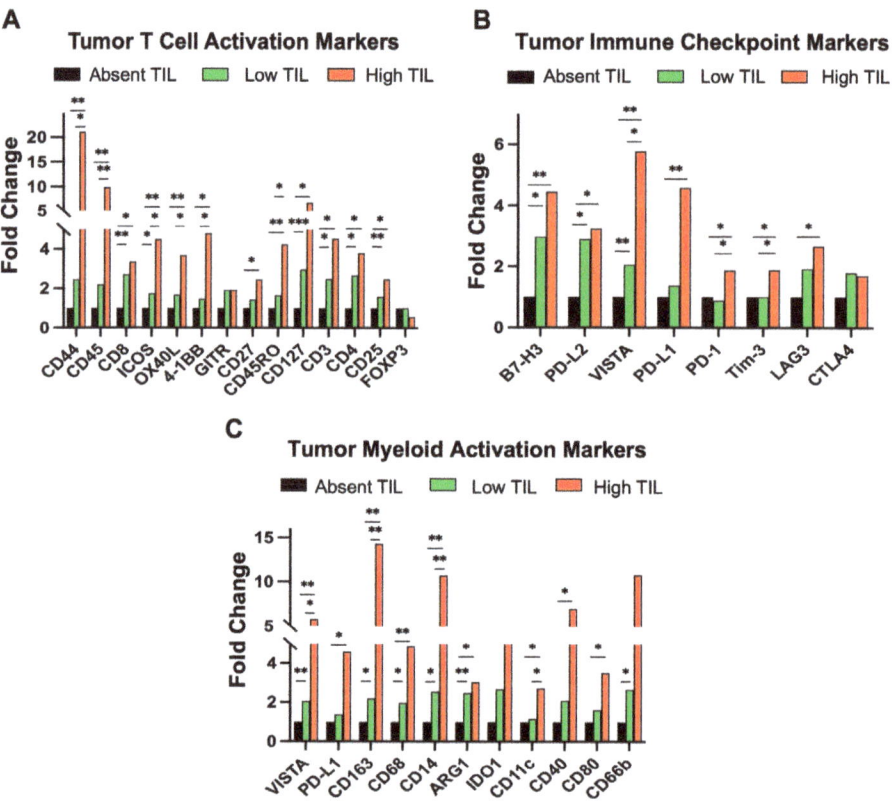

Figure 1. GeoMx digital spatial profiling. The signal from absent TIL was set as baseline. (**A**) GeoMx DSP proteomic analysis of tumor T cell activation markers; (**B**) tumor-immune checkpoint markers; (**C**) and tumor myeloid activation markers in patient samples with high TILs, low TILs, and minimal or absent TILs (* $p \leq 0.05$; ** $p \leq 0.01$; *** $p \leq 0.001$).

To investigate the functionality of effector T cells in heavily pretreated patients and better understand the low response to ICB in HGSOC clinical trials, we analyzed high (brisk) TILs that infiltrate diffusely within the tumor and compared them to low (non-brisk) TILs that show only focal infiltration and absent TILs. We used the Nanostring GeoMx platform, which allows spatial digital (microregional) single-cell proteomic profiling using 77 antibodies on a FFPE slide. Using this platform, we saw specific upregulation of tumor T cell activation, immune checkpoint, and myeloid activation markers. DSP analysis showed an increase by fold change (FC) in almost all T cell activation-associated markers in tumor regions with high TILs compared to low or absent TILs (Figure 1A). We found that immunostimulatory markers, such as CD25 ($p = 0.02$), CD127 ($p = 0.02$), and CD27 ($p = 0.01$), were all upregulated in high TILs. As expected, the total number of leukocytes in high TILs was higher than in absent TILs (CD45; $p = 0.002$). Additionally, high TILs showed higher levels of total T cells (CD3; $p = 0.02$), cytotoxic T cells (CD8; $p = 0.01$), T helper cells (CD4; $p = 0.01$), and memory T cells (CD45RO). CD44, a cell adhesion molecule involved in effector-memory T cell activation and cell migration [48], showed the largest fold change increase in high TILs ($p = 0.008$). The results were tumor-specific and stroma effects were relatively minor, although some markers followed similar trends (Supplementary Figure S1).

We also identified highly exhausted T cells with concurrent upregulation of multiple immune checkpoint markers in high TILs (Figure 1B). Upregulation of immune checkpoint markers characteristic of exhausted T cells was observed on high TILs, including PD-1, B7-H3, VISTA, Tim-3, and LAG3. B7-H3 inhibits tumor antigen-specific immune responses. Thus, brisk TILs showed increased expression of key immune checkpoint markers, such as VISTA ($p = 0.003$), PD-1 ($p = 0.03$), and B7-H3 ($p = 0.001$), which are associated with T cell exhaustion [49,50]. The functional severity of T cell exhaustion likely correlates with the number and magnitude of immune checkpoint protein expression, especially VISTA.

Myeloid cell activation-associated markers in high TILs followed the same trend as the T cell activation-associated markers (Figure 1C). Macrophage levels were found to be increased in high TILs (CD68; $p = 0.01$). These increases involved both M1-like macrophages (CD80; $p = 0.01$) and M2-like macrophages (CD163; $p = 0.003$). Interestingly, the largest increase involved immunosuppressive M2 macrophages (CD163). Upregulation of CD80, which has a crucial role in binding to CD28 and triggering activation of T cell immune function [51], was also noticed in high TILs. In addition, the upregulation of IDO1, which has immunosuppressive properties [52,53], was also present. Furthermore, neutrophils (CD66b) were elevated, and they have been correlated with worse progression-free survival and overall survival in other solid tumors [54,55]. Monocytes (CD14; $p = 0.001$), conventional dendritic cells (CD11c; $p = 0.04$), and antigen-presenting cells (CD40; $p = 0.01$) were all elevated in high TILs, with each being linked to either immunosuppression and/or tumor proliferation [56–58]. The low (non-brisk) TILs reflected these immune-associated differences, albeit to a lower extent, compared to non-TILs. Given the observed highly immunosuppressive tumor microenvironment and highly exhausted TILs, we sought to develop strategies that would enhance the potency of ICB immunotherapies, leading to the enhanced functionality, migration, and target engagement of T cells to tumor cells.

3.2. Epigenetic Priming Reverses Loss of 5-hmC and Mediates Upregulation of Key Tumor Cytokines

We previously reported that epigenetic priming increases sensitivity to standard chemotherapies [38]. Given the low responses seen in ICB clinical trials in HGSOC and the key role of DNA methylation in modulating responsiveness to ICB [20–37], we investigated whether epigenetic priming could potentiate immunotherapies in this tumor subtype. Similar to our previous results [38], we first confirmed that DNMTIs, such as 5-aza, can be used to reverse global 5-hmC loss in HGSOC. We quantified 5-hmC expression in response to 5-aza treatment in multiple tumor lines using immunofluorescence studies. The ovarian cancer cell lines included human chemoresistant A2780Res and several murine syngeneic HGSOC tumor lines with fallopian tubal origin and key genetic alterations found in patients: BPPNM ($Brca1^{-/-}$; $Trp53^{-/R172H}$; $Pten^{-/-}$; $Nf1^{-/-} Myc^{OE}$) and a series of KPCA ($Trp53^{-/R172H}$; $Ccne1^{OE}$; $Akt2^{OE}$; $KRAS^{G12V}$) tumor lines with varying degrees of immunotherapeutic resistance [39,41]. The KPCA cell line series consisted of a relatively responsive tumor line (KPCA.B), partially resistant (KPCA.A), and resistant (KPCA.C) tumor line to ICB therapy [59]. The percentage of 5-hmC positive cells showed a statistically significant increase in response to 10 µM 5-aza for all lines (Figures 2A–D and S2), indicating that 5-aza treatment leads to an increase in global demethylation in tumor cells similar to our previous findings [39]. Specifically, the A2780Res human chemoresistant cell line showed a significant increase in the percentage of 5-hmC positive cells at a concentration of 10 µM ($p \leq 0.05$) and the syngeneic murine HGSC BPPNM and KPCA.A lines exhibited similar trends at 10 µM with higher significance ($p \leq 0.001$, both) (Figure 2B–D).

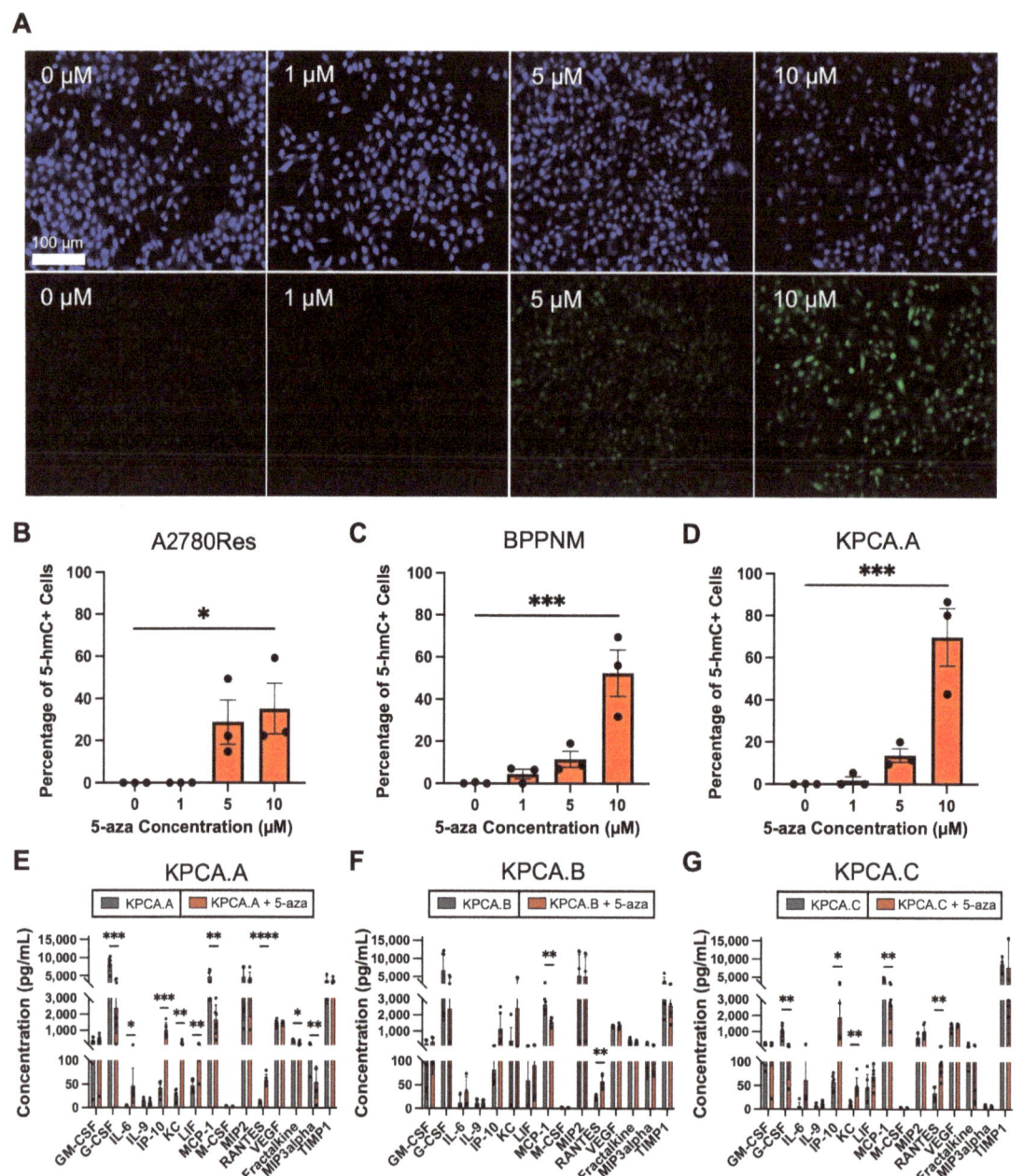

Figure 2. Effects of 5-azacytidine on tumor methylation and cytokine secretion. (**A**) Representative images of A2780Res human DAPI (**top**) and 5-hmC (**bottom**) immunofluorescent staining in response to increasing 5-aza concentrations. Scale bar, 100 μm; (**B**) Quantification of 5-hmC levels in response to 5-aza treatment for A2780Res; (**C**) BPPNM and (**D**) KPCA.A; (**E**) Quantification of cytokine expression with and without 5-aza treatment in KPCA.A; (**F**) KPCA.B and (**G**) KPCA.C ($n = 6$). (* $p \leq 0.05$; ** $p \leq 0.01$; *** $p \leq 0.001$; **** $p \leq 0.0001$).

Next, we sought to investigate a potential mechanism of action for DNMTis to prime and enhance the ICB response. We thus treated the three KPCA cell lines (KPCA.A, KPCA.B, KPCA.C) for 72 h with 5-aza and observed changes in tumor-derived cytokine secretion (Figure 2E–G). Conditioned tumor cell medium treated with 10 μM 5-aza showed upregulation of 4 key cytokines—IL-6, IP-10 (CXCL10), KC (CXCL1), and RANTES (CCL5)—which activate both adaptive and innate immune responses (Figure 2E–G). IL-6 is known to recruit neutrophils and promote the differentiation of T and B cells [59]. KC (CXCL1) can function as a neutrophil chemoattractant [60]. IP-10 (CXCL10) is a well-known chemoattractant that increases the expression of interferon genes and promotes effector CD8+ and NK tumor infiltration [61]. RANTES (CCL5) functions as a chemoattractant for monocytes, T effectors, and NK cells [62,63]. Statistically significant upregulation was observed for all four key markers as follows: IL-6 ($p \leq 0.05$, KPCA.A), IP-10 ($p \leq 0.001$, KPCA.A; $p \leq 0.05$, KPCA.C), KC ($p \leq 0.01$, KPCA.A and KPCA.C), and RANTES ($p \leq 0.0001$, KPCA.A; $p \leq 0.01$, KPCA.B and KPCA.C). Conversely, significant downregulation was observed for cytokines that confer a pro-tumor effect, such as G-CSF ($p \leq 0.001$, KPCA.A; $p \leq 0.01$, KPCA.C), MCP-1 ($p \leq 0.01$, all lines), and MIP3alpha ($p \leq 0.05$, KPCA.A) [64–66].

3.3. Optimization of Patient-Derived 3D Ex Vivo Platforms for Rapid Immunotherapeutic Testing of HGSOC Tumors and Ascites

Tumor spheroids, along with autologous immune cells, were isolated from patient ascites and processed via a standardized methodology (Figure 3A) to rapidly examine therapeutic combinations ex vivo. First, a primary tumor sample was loaded into the IdenTx device (Figure 3B) to demonstrate the standard morphology of a PDOTS sample. Subsequent immunofluorescent imaging (Figure 3C) showed that EpCAM-positive tumor cells were present in addition to regions of embedded CD45-positive immune cells. These findings were emulated with cells derived from patient ascites, as seen in images of the PDOTS in Figure 3D. This patient sample also demonstrated tumor spheroids, as seen by the EpCAM positivity and CD8 positive immune cells (Figure 3E). There also appear to be regions of PD-L1 positivity on the EpCAM tumor cells that are accessible to target with ICB immunotherapies (Figure 3E).

On selected patient ascites samples, we used standard-of-care therapies, such as platinum-based and PARPi therapy, to further validate our ex vivo platform. As seen in Figure 3F, when the devices were treated with 10 μM cisplatin, the only patient to show significant cell death compared to their control was patient 8, who was clinically diagnosed as platinum sensitive (Table S5). When the sample from patient 7 was first tested, the clinic informed our team that the patient was platinum sensitive. However, when cisplatin was tested on their sample, there was a reduced response. Upon following up with the clinic, we were told that the patient's chart was updated to indicate that the disease had become platinum resistant, which validates the sensitivity of our device. Patients with known *BRCA* mutations (Table S5) showed significant responses to PARPi (patients 2 and 8), while patient 5, with no known *BRCA* mutation, showed no significant response to PARPi (Figure 3G).

3.4. Epigenetic Priming Potentiates ICB in PDOTS and Upregulates Early Activation Immune T Cell Markers

A surgically resected primary HGSOC tumor was dissociated into PDOTS and treated for 24 h with 5-aza, HDACi and immunotherapies to observe the activation of immune cells. CD4+ and CD8+ T cells both had an observable downregulation of PD-1 (Figure 4A) in conditions treated with immunotherapies. We attribute the downregulation to the αPD-1 immunotherapy blocking the conjugated flow cytometry antibody from binding to the epitope, thus validating the treatment. Additionally, both CD4+ and CD8+ T cells treated with our 5-aza + HDACi treatment or the combination treatment had an upregulation of CD69 (Figure 4B), which is an early immune activation marker [67,68]. Another early immune activation marker, CD38 [69], was upregulated in CD4+ T cells when treated with the combination therapy (Figure 4C).

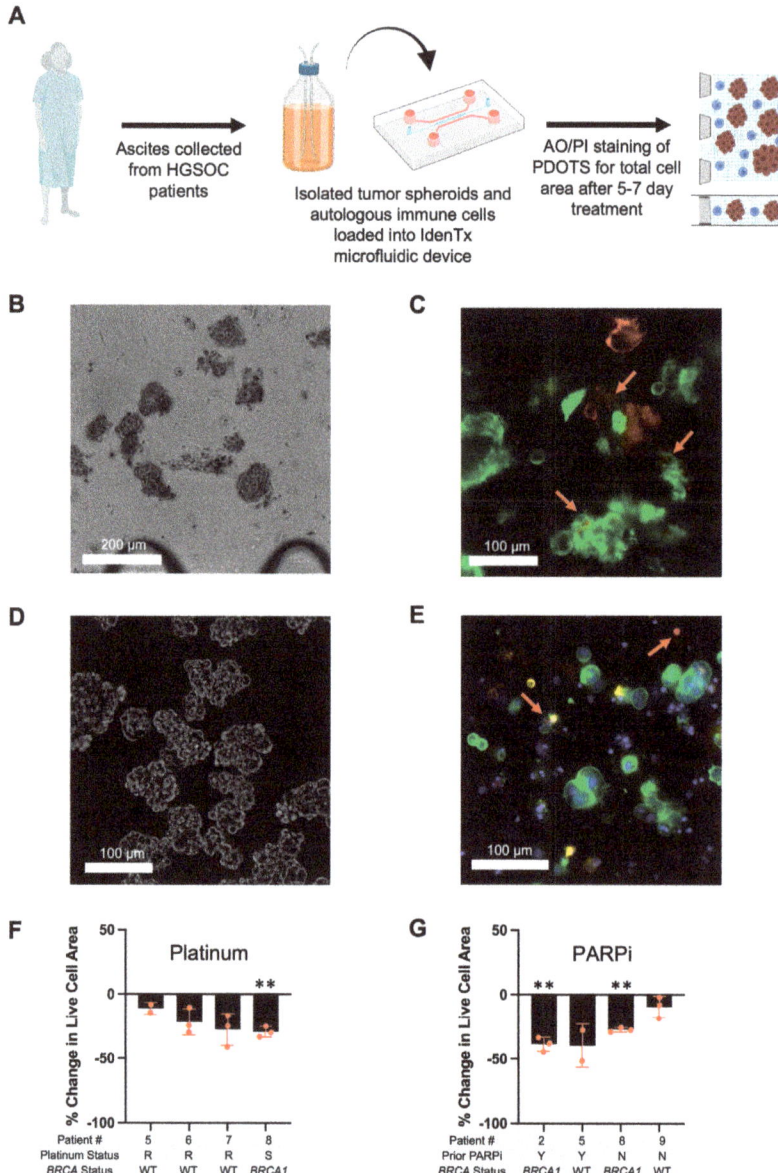

Figure 3. Scheme of PDOTS development, imaging of tumor spheroids, and clinically relevant treatments. (**A**) Scheme depicting how ascites samples were collected from ovarian cancer patients and processed to generate PDOTS; (**B**) Brightfield image of isolated primary tumor spheroids inside the IdenTx device. Scale bar, 200 µm; (**C**) Immunofluorescent image of PDOTS tumor spheroids from patient solid HGSC tumor stained with EpCAM (green) and CD45 (red). Red arrows indicate CD45+ immune cells. Scale bar, 100 µm; (**D**) Brightfield image of PDOTS tumor spheroids from patient ascites. Scale bar, 100 µm; (**E**) Immunofluorescent image of PDOTS tumor spheroids from patient HGSC tumor-derived ascites stained with Hoechst (blue), EpCAM (green), CD8 (red), and PD-L1 (gold). Red arrows indicate CD8+ immune cells. Scale bar, 100 µm; (**F**) Cumulative live–dead staining data of 10 µM of platinum treatment normalized to control of each patient; (**G**) Cumulative live–dead staining data of 1 µM of PARPi treatment normalized to control of each patient (** $p \leq 0.01$).

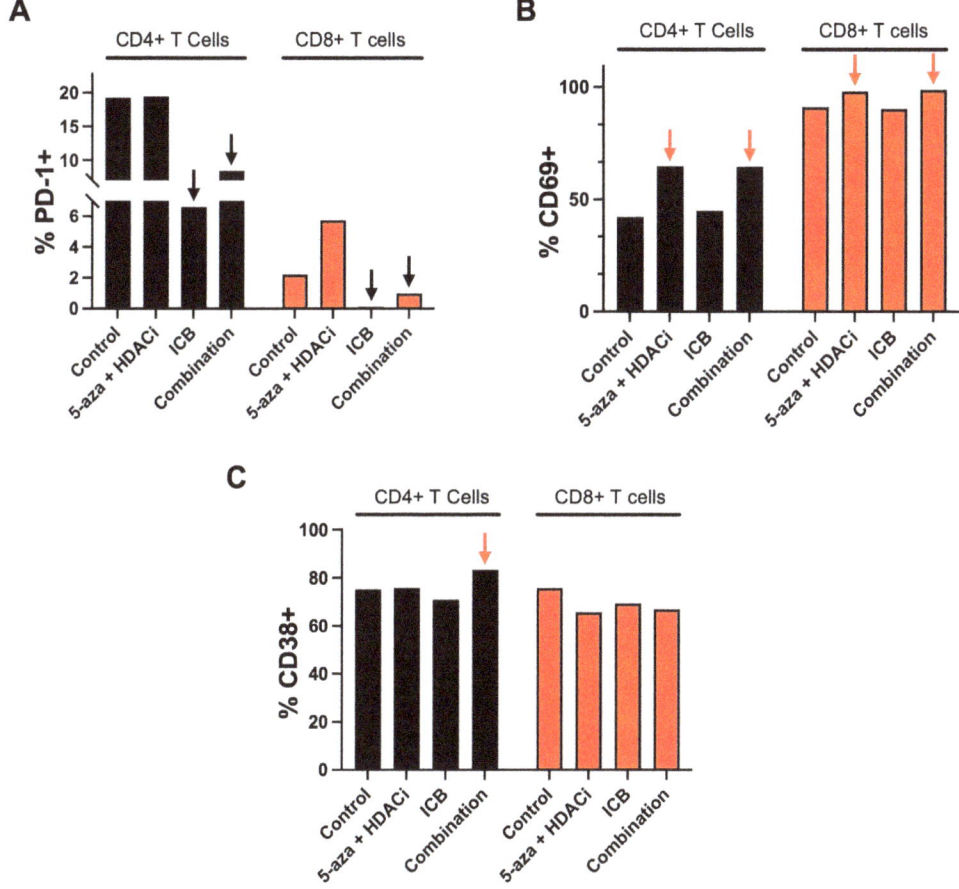

Figure 4. Immune profiling of solid HGSOC patient sample. After 24 h of treatment, markers for immune activation were quantified. Black arrows indicate downregulation and red arrows indicate upregulation. (**A**) Percentage of CD4+ and CD8+ T cells expressing PD-1; (**B**) Percentage of CD4+ and CD8+ T cells expressing CD69; (**C**) Percentage of CD4+ and CD8+ T cells expressing CD38.

Various combinations of 5-aza, HDACi, and immunotherapies were tested on ascites PDOTS to find a synergistic treatment that repeatedly gave significant results in the combination treatment. Response to treatments was measured by taking the area of live cells and dividing it by the total area of both live and dead cells (Figure S3A). Significance is determined by comparing it to the control. Of the seven tested patient ascites samples, 3/7 responded to treatment with epigenetic modulators, 1/7 responded to treatment with immunotherapies, and 4/7 responded to a combination of treatments (Figures 5A–C and S3B–E). The combination treatment indicates a trend whereby priming with epigenetic modulators can increase the effectiveness of immunotherapy treatments.

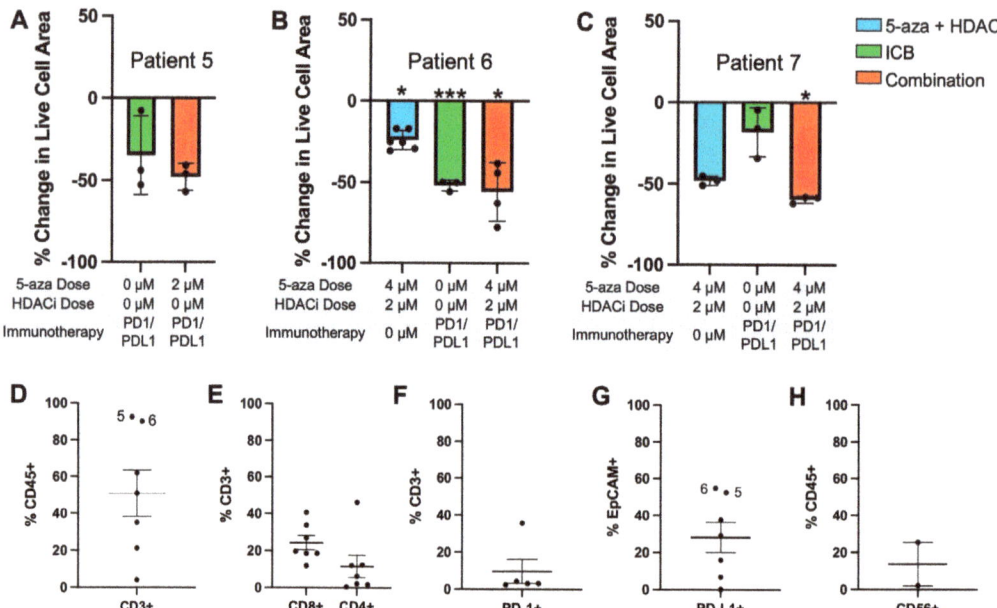

Figure 5. PDOTS utilizing circulating tumor from patient ascites and immune profiling. Cumulative live–dead staining data normalized to control. Significance is shown in comparison to each individual sample's control condition. (**A**) Patient 5; (**B**) Patient 6; (**C**) Patient 7; (**D**) CD3+ expression as a percentage of total CD45+ cells ($n = 7$). Patient sample 5 and 6 percentages indicated; (**E**) CD8+ and CD4+ expression as a percentage of total CD3+ cells ($n = 7$); (**F**) PD-1+ expression as a percentage of total CD3+ cells ($n = 5$); (**G**) PD-L1+ expression as a percentage of total EpCAM+ cells ($n = 7$); Patient sample 5 and 6 percentages indicated; (**H**) CD56+ expression as a percentage of total CD45+ cells ($n = 2$). (* $p \leq 0.05$; *** $p \leq 0.001$).

Of note, patient 5 (Figure 5A) did not show a significant response to αPD-1 and αPD-L1 immunotherapies alone, but the combination treatment did approach significance with a p-value of 0.06, showing a trend towards treatment synergism. Of the patient ascites samples, patient 6 (Figure 5B) was the only sample that showed significant cell death when treated with αPD-1 and αPD-L1 immunotherapies alone. Patient 7 (Figure 5C) was the only patient sample that responded to only the combination treatment and neither the epigenetic nor immunotherapy-alone conditions. Additionally, Kuramochi cells expressing the necessary HLA protein (Figure S4A) for non-autologous immune activation [70] also showed a significant response to the combination treatment when cocultured with T cells in the IdenTx devices (Figure S4B).

Flow cytometric analysis of the patient ascites samples (Figure 5D–H) showed large variability in fluid composition. CD3+ T cells made up about 50% of CD45+ immune cells (Figure 5D). Of these T cells, roughly 25% were CD8+ cytotoxic T cells and roughly 10% were CD4+ helper T cells (Figure 5E). Additionally, about 10% of CD3+ T cells were also PD-1+ (Figure 5F). EPCAM was utilized as a marker for circulating tumor cells, and roughly 30% of EPCAM+ cells were also PD-L1+ (Figure 5G). Notably, the only responders to the immunotherapy-alone condition (patient 5 and patient 6) correlated with an increased percentage of total CD3+ T cell populations (Figure 5D) and PD-L1 expression in EPCAM+ circulating tumor cells (Figure 5G).

3.5. Epigenetic Priming Increases Overall Survival by Potentiating ICB in Syngeneic HGSOC Models

In vivo experimentation was conducted with KPCA.B cells to identify a potential benefit in combining 5-aza, givinostat (HDACi), and ICB (PD-L1/CTLA-4) in syngeneic HGSOC tumor models that recapitulate the clinical disease and ICB responses [41]. The experimental design is outlined in Figure 6A. Overall, our results recapitulated previous tumor model studies [40], although we saw more subtle effects likely due to testing epigenetic priming in a tumor model relatively sensitive to ICB therapy. Most importantly, epigenetic priming increased overall survival, as all mice treated with combination therapy were alive at the end of the experiment (5/5) compared to immunotherapy-treated mice (4/6) and controls (5/10) (Figure 6B). The survival results of the control cohort were similar to those reported by Iyer et al. [41], who described the development of syngeneic HGSOC models. All remaining animals were sacrificed on day 35, when tumor burden endpoints were reached in the control cohort (Figure 6C). The tumor weights of all sacrificed mice are quantified in Figure 6C. The mice that were treated with 5-aza/HDACi/ICB combination had significantly smaller tumor masses than the control group ($p = 0.0001$) and the 5-aza/HDACi cohort ($p = 0.0381$) (Figure 6C). The control mice that were left untreated developed ascites consistent with previous animal models [40], while the other groups did not present ascites (Figure 6D). Overall, the combination-treated mice were a homogenous cohort in which all mice responded to ICB, had better overall survival, and had significantly lower tumor weights compared to the control and epigenetic therapy cohorts. The ICB-treated group was a more heterogenous group composed of both ICB responders and non-responders. Several mice that did not respond to ICB followed a survival pattern consistent with control mice and died before the 35-day mark. Mice that survived responded well and had low tumor weights comparable to those seen in combination-treated mice. These results, at least in this syngeneic tumor model, are more nuanced than the conclusions reached by previous ID8 studies [40] and appear to suggest that epigenetic priming likely confers additional benefit primarily to weak responders or non-responders to ICB therapy.

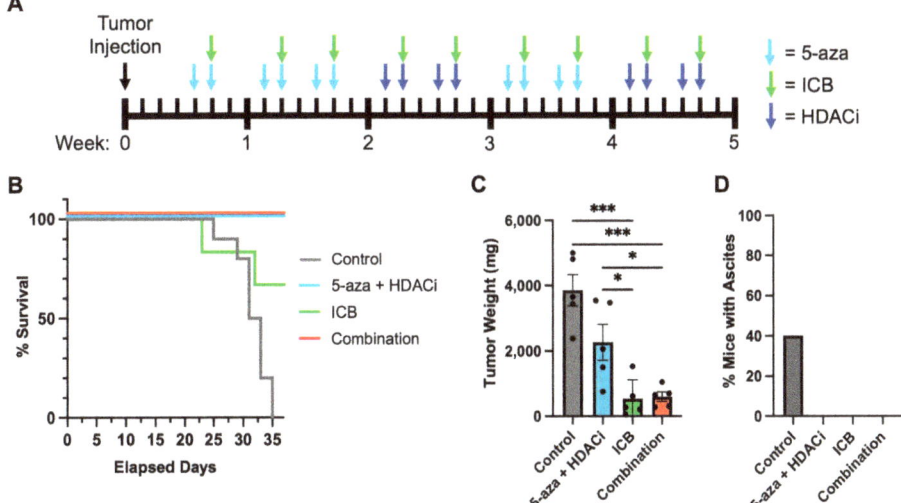

Figure 6. In vivo mouse model engrafted with KPCA.B cells. (**A**) Treatment schedule; (**B**) Survival curve of control ($n = 10$), 5-aza + HDACi ($n = 5$), ICB ($n = 6$), and combination ($n = 5$); (**C**) Quantification of tumor weights at sacrifice day (day 35) for the control cohort ($n = 5$), 5-aza/HDACi ($n = 5$), ICB ($n = 5$), and 5-aza/HDACi/ICB combination ($n = 5$); (**D**) Percent of mice that developed ascites in the controls at day 35 ($n = 5$), 5-aza + HDACi ($n = 5$), ICB ($n = 5$), and combination ($n = 5$) conditions. (* $p \leq 0.05$; *** $p \leq 0.001$).

4. Discussion

The main goal of our study is to develop 3D IO platforms to analyze patient responses and identify adjuvants, such as epigenetic drugs, that are able to potentiate systemic immunotherapy responses in tumor ascites. Towards this goal, we developed rapid, sensitive, and accurate functional systems based on ovarian patient-derived 3D PDOTS and expanded their use beyond solid tumors to study patient ascites. This allows us to study the complex and dynamic tumor-immune interactions in the systemic circulation and identify personalized profiles associated with the engagement of circulating tumor and immune cells that are primed for response to ICB immunotherapies. This patient-derived 3D platform fulfills a critical need for clinical tools that can accurately assess drug sensitivity and treatment responses in real time. While most investigations studying response to immunotherapies in ovarian cancer focus on characterizing biomarkers and immune cell infiltration in primary solid tumors, we instead concentrated on developing PDOTS containing both circulating ascites tumors and immune cells collected from the same patients in the setting of relapsed HGSC disease (either with pathogenic *BRCA1*, *BRCA2* mutations, or *BRCA* WT).

Most importantly, systemic responses are indicative of inefficient ICB responses seen in clinical trials. Moreover, we are showing that the 3D platform is predictive of clinical responses, as it accurately recapitulates responses to both platinum chemotherapy and PARPi responses in HGSC. Primary solid tumors are not relevant for ICB responses in ovarian cancer, since they are removed at diagnosis through surgical debulking. The main goal of ICB therapy in newly diagnosed HGSC patients following debulking or relapsed patients is to eliminate circulating tumor cells, which give rise to peritoneal metastases and contribute to disease progression. Consequently, this paper is novel and highly clinically relevant, as it allows the testing of readily accessible samples when solid tumors are not easily available or resectable. This includes liquid biopsies and tumor ascites through non-invasive methods of collection or as part of standard patient care.

A major aim of the current study was to identify biomarkers responsible for immune evasion in HGSOC, which could explain the low responses seen in ICB clinical trials for this tumor subtype. We employed digital spatial tumor profiling to investigate the functionality of effector T cells. Specifically, we analyzed TILs that infiltrate diffusively within the tumor and compared their functionality to non-brisk TILs that show only focal infiltration and also to non-TILs (no TILs or minimal TIL infiltration). Immunostimulatory markers, such as CD25 and CD27, were all upregulated in the brisk TIL sample. Additionally, the brisk TIL patient sample also showed significantly higher levels of total T cells (CD3), cytotoxic T cells (CD8), T helper cells (CD4), and memory T cells (CD45RO). CD44, a key activation marker for effector and memory T cells, showed the largest fold change increase between the brisk TIL sample and the absent TIL sample. CD45RO, which is expressed by memory T cells that have encountered antigens, was also upregulated in TILs. However, what we clearly saw was the presence of highly exhausted T cells and the upregulation of immune checkpoint markers. Upregulation of all immune checkpoint markers characteristic of highly exhausted T cells was seen on brisk TILs, including PD-1, B7-H3, VISTA, Tim-3, and LAG3. B7-H3 inhibits tumor antigen-specific immune responses. The functional severity of T cell exhaustion correlates with the number and magnitude of immune checkpoint protein expression. Most importantly, one of the biggest contributors to immune evasion is the presence of immunosuppressive M2-like macrophages, which show the highest elevation among myeloid immune cell markers. This suggests that therapies that trigger tumor-associated macrophage reprogramming from M2-like to M1-like phenotypes are likely to increase responsiveness to IO compounds. In addition, our results indicate that although TILs are present within the local immune microenvironment, they are highly exhausted and inefficient in detecting and destroying tumor cells located in their proximity. Consequently, epigenetic adjuvants, which induce demethylation of key sites, including PD1/PD-L1, could both reactivate and re-energize local and systemic immune responses. We thus suggest that combination treatments boosted by epigenetic priming could work synergistically to potentiate IO responses and more effectively target and eliminate tumor cells.

Immunofluorescence staining analysis for 5-hmC levels was performed to determine the extent of global methylation levels in response to 5-aza treatment. Similar to our previous studies [39], 5-hmC positive cells were observed to increase in response to 10 µM 5-aza; 5-aza-mediated global demethylation allows for the activation of genes targeted by immunotherapy, such as PD1/PD-L1. In turn, ICB can promote anti-tumor immunity [49]. As such, combining immunotherapy and 5-azacytadine administration can potentially have synergistic effects in the treatment of ovarian cancer. Epigenetic priming induces secretion of key cytokines that are involved in activation of innate and adaptive immunity. Thus, significant upregulation was observed for multiple key cytokines, specifically IL-6, IP-10, KC, and RANTES, in the KPCA HGSOC tumor lines in response to 5-aza. In addition, a significant downregulation was observed for G-CSF, MCP-1, and MIP3alpha cytokines following 5-aza treatment. Interestingly, the cytokines that were upregulated are those associated with increased immune activation [59–61,63], while those downregulated are associated with cell migration and metastatic phenotypes [64–66]. IL-6 is a proinflammatory cytokine and plays an important role in the immune response by recruiting neutrophils and promoting the growth and differentiation of T and B lymphocytes [59–61,63]. IP-10 functions as a chemoattractant for monocytes, macrophages, T cells, NK cells, and dendritic cells under physiological conditions. Several studies have suggested that IP-10 contributes to anti-tumor immunity. IP-10 promotes infiltration by CD8+ tumor-infiltrating lymphocytes as well as increasing the expression of interferon genes [59–61,63]. Several studies have shown increased expression of IP-10 in ovarian cancer cells following treatment with DNMTi, consistent with our results [59–61,63]. Stone et al. observed significant regulation of IP-10 by 5-aza both in vitro and in vivo in syngeneic ID8 tumor models as well [40]. Similarly, RANTES is involved in immune and inflammatory responses and it is a potent chemoattractant for monocytes, T effector, NK, and dendritic cells [59–61,63]. Interestingly, epigenetic priming has also been shown not only to activate effector T, helper T, and NK cells but also to decrease the percentage of immunosuppressive myeloid derived suppressor cells (MDSCs) and M2-like macrophages in the tumor microenvironment [40].

Consequently, we found that epigenetic priming potentiated ICB in patient-derived 3D ex vivo platforms and syngeneic tumor models, which recapitulated the HGSOC cell of origin and clinical disease [40]. The combination of epigenetic priming and IO yields the best overall responses and the highest overall survival in vivo. Of note, the tumor microenvironment of the HGSOC tumor models evaluated in the current study is heterogenous, similar to patients, which results in variable IO responses. The results of our in vivo study show that the IO non-responsive murine group derives the greatest benefit in response to epigenetic tumor priming. The ex vivo patient data are also in alignment with this conclusion. The analysis of patient samples indicates that epigenetic priming potentiates IO responses overall and especially in IO-resistant disease, which remains a critical priority clinically.

In addition, our studies indicate that ex vivo-based PDOTS platforms have the potential to bridge the gap between animal studies and clinical trials. When utilizing standard care treatments, such as platinum and PARPi, we found results consistent with those seen clinically in patients, which increases the validity and predictive ability of our platform. An increased response to anti-PD-1/anti-PD-L1 ICB alone correlated with a high frequency of CD3+ T cells and PD-L1+/EPCAM+ tumor cells and was seen in a small number of patients. A combination of epigenetic adjuvants and ICB drastically enhanced the potency of ICB therapeutics, with effective responses seen in the majority of patients. Interestingly, epigenetic priming alone and in combination with ICB immunotherapy in patient-derived PDOTS induced the rapid upregulation of CD69, a reliable early activation marker in both CD4+ and CD8+ T cells [67,68]. Furthermore, downregulation of anti-PD-1 was seen in both ICB alone and combination treatments, validating the target responses. Consequently, this functional precision medicine approach has the ability to rapidly identify specific combinations able to potentiate ICB, which is a great advantage, especially as we consider the current clinical difficulty of fast and accurate testing of a high number of potential combinations directly in patients. In addition, it could identify ineffective combinations and spare patients from deleterious toxic side effects. Recent findings by Huang et al. [38] synergize with our results by indicating that PD-L1 demethylation is key in potentiating the PD-1/PD-L1 interaction and enhancing tumor immunosurveillance. Conversely, PD-L1 hypermethylation, especially at the K162 site, critically inhibits the PD-L1/PD-1 interaction and is a negative predictive biomarker of ICB response in patients [38]. Furthermore, PD-L1 K162 methylation is abrogated in response to IL6 [38], which is the cytokine that we have shown to be upregulated in response to epigenetic priming of tumors. Therefore, it is highly likely that 5-aza promotes demethylation of PD-L1, including at the K162 site, enhances the PD-L1/PD-1 interaction, and potentiates ICB responses as a result.

Thus, by testing novel cancer immunotherapeutics in predictive ex vivo platforms using patient solid tumors or ascites, researchers can identify whether effective treatments transfer from murine models to human applications in a cost-effective and time-efficient manner. In recent years, the value of ascites for research has been recognized more and more [71,72]. The current findings are clinically relevant, as testing in PDOTS platforms could rapidly evaluate the most effective personalized immunotherapeutic options using solid tumors or circulating tumor cells in tumor-derived ascites. Identifying reliable response markers and assays, which could accurately predict response to immunotherapy and clinical outcome, is critical since functional ex vivo testing of individual patient samples will eliminate drugs to which the tumors are resistant, thus sparing patients unnecessary toxicity from ineffective treatment. In addition, it could allow the implementation of epigenetic reprogramming strategies capable of sensitizing immunoresistant tumors prior to or in conjunction with the delivery of ICB immunotherapies.

5. Conclusions

In this study, we sought to identify therapeutic strategies to potentiate immune activation and function. DSP analysis of patient tumor samples with varying levels of TILs showed an increased prevalence of immunostimulatory markers in high TIL samples. However, DSP also identified highly exhausted T cells with concurrent upregulation of multiple immune checkpoint markers in brisk TILs, including B7-H3, VISTA, Tim-3, LAG3, and PD-1, which could explain the low HGSOC responses seen in αPD-1 clinical trials. Additionally, we optimized a novel ascites-based ex vivo profiling assay using microfluidic devices that can be used to study liquid or circulating tumor cells in addition to solid tumors. Taken together, the results obtained in syngeneic HGSOC in vivo tumor studies and 3D PDOTS screening suggest that epigenetic adjuvants could potentiate the efficacy of ICB immunotherapies. The implementation of PDOTS platforms, in particular, will allow for a fast and effective method to screen drug combinations on solid tumors and ascites-derived patient samples with autologous immune cells. This functional precision medicine approach has the potential for wider research applications to interrogate local, systemic, and peripheral tumor immunity, since they all contribute to effective and durable IO responses. Furthermore, it will allow the identification of specific combinations that can reverse innate and acquired ICB resistance, which is a great advantage, especially as we consider the current difficulty of rapidly testing a high number of combinations in clinical trials.

Supplementary Materials: The following supporting information can be downloaded at: https://www.mdpi.com/article/10.3390/cancers15164128/s1, Table S1. Antibodies used for IF imaging of PDOTS. Table S2. Antibodies used for Flow Cytometry of Patient Ascites. Table S3. Gating used to Observe Cell Types or Protein Expression for Flow Cytometry of Patient Ascites. Table S4. Antibodies used for Flow Cytometry of Solid Patient Sample for Immune Activation. Table S5. Patient Data for Ascites Sample. Figure S1. GeoMx digital spatial profiling. Signal from absent TIL set as baseline. (A) GeoMx DSP proteomic analysis of stromal T cell activation markers, (B) stromal immune checkpoint markers, (C) and stromal myeloid activation markers. (*, $p \leq 0.05$; **, $p \leq 0.01$; ***, $p \leq 0.001$; ****, $p \leq 0.0001$). Figure S2. 5-hmC expression in tumor lines following 5-aza treatment. Representative images of human DAPI (top) and 5-hmC (bottom) immunofluorescent staining in response to increasing 5-aza concentrations in (A) BPPNM and (B) KPCA.A cell lines. Scale bar, 100 µm. Figure S3. Representative and cumulative live-dead results of patient ascites PDOTS and associated immune quantifications. (A) Images used from patient 1 to calculate live percent cell area. Live cells stained with acridine orange (green) and dead cells stained with propidium iodide (red). Cumulative live-dead staining data normalized to control with significance shown in comparison to each individual sample's control condition of (B) Patient 1, (C) Patient 2, (D) Patient 3, (E) and Patient 4. (F) Composition of CD45+ immune populations in patient derived ascites. (*, $p \leq 0.05$; **, $p \leq 0.01$). Figure S4. PDOTS utilizing co-culture of Kuramochi tumor line and T cells harvested from PBMCs. (A) HLA composition of Kuramochi tumor line. (B) Cumulative live-dead staining data normalized to control. Significance is shown in comparison to sample's control condition. (*, $p \leq 0.05$).

Author Contributions: Conceptualization, A.G., M.C. (Marco Campisi), D.A.B. and D.M.D.; methodology, T.J.G., A.G., M.C. (Marco Campisi), M.C. (Minyue Chen), N.M., C.A.A.L., H.V.V., K.H., Z.-H.L., C.G.L., E.V.I. and D.M.D.; validation, T.J.G., A.G., M.C. (Marco Campisi), and M.C. (Minyue Chen); formal analysis, T.J.G., A.G., I.G., C.A.A.L. and P.L.; investigation, T.J.G., A.G., M.C. (Marco Campisi), M.C. (Minyue Chen), I.G., R.M. and P.L.; resources, K.T.H., K.M.E., C.G.L., E.V.I., D.A.B. and D.M.D.; data curation, T.J.G., A.G., C.A.A.L., B.T. and R.M.; writing—original draft preparation, T.J.G. and A.G.; writing—review and editing, T.J.G., A.G., M.C. (Marco Campisi), N.M., T.C., D.A.B. and D.M.D.; visualization, T.J.G., A.G., M.C. (Marco Campisi), I.G. and P.L.; supervision, D.A.B. and D.M.D.; project administration, T.J.G. and A.G.; funding acquisition, D.A.B. and D.M.D. All authors have read and agreed to the published version of the manuscript.

Funding: This work was supported by DOD W81XWH-20-1-0342 (D.M.D.), DOD W81XWH-15-1-0089 (D.M.D.), NIH/NCI 1U01CA233360-01 (D.M.D.), NIH/NCI RO1CA142746 (D.M.D.), NIH/NCI R25CA174650 (D.M.D.), BWH Biomedical Research Institute Fund to Sustain Research Excellence Award (D.M.D.), and Canary Foundation (D.M.D.).

Institutional Review Board Statement: The study was conducted in accordance with the Declaration of Helsinki and approved by the Institutional Review Board of Dana-Farber Cancer Institute (#02-051) and Brigham and Women's Hospital (#2006P002438) for use of solid ovarian tumors and tumor-derived ascites. Animal studies were conducted following the guidelines provided by the Institutional Animal Care and Use Committee (IACUC) of Brigham and Women's Hospital under protocol 2016N000212.

Informed Consent Statement: Informed consent was obtained from all subjects involved in the study.

Data Availability Statement: Data can be accessed from corresponding author upon request.

Acknowledgments: The authors would like to acknowledge the Dana Farber Molecular Pathology Core for assistance with GeoMx data collection and the Dana Farber Cancer Institute GYN CRIS Team for coordinating the collection of patient ascites.

Conflicts of Interest: D.A.B. reports other support from Xsphera Biosciences and personal fees from Qiagen/N of One, Tango Biosciences, Exo Therapeutics; grants from Gilead Sciences, Novartis Oncology, BMS, Takeda, and Lilly/LOXO outside of the submitted work. There are no competing interests to declare by the other authors.

References

1. Zhang, L.-Y.; Han, C.-S.; Li, P.-L.; Zhang, X.-C. 5-Hydroxymethylcytosine Expression Is Associated with Poor Survival in Cervical Squamous Cell Carcinoma. *Jpn. J. Clin. Oncol.* **2016**, *46*, 427–434. [CrossRef] [PubMed]
2. Johnson, K.C.; Houseman, E.A.; King, J.E.; von Herrmann, K.M.; Fadul, C.E.; Christensen, B.C. 5-Hydroxymethylcytosine Localizes to Enhancer Elements and Is Associated with Survival in Glioblastoma Patients. *Nat. Commun.* **2016**, *7*, 13177. [CrossRef] [PubMed]
3. Yang, Q.; Wu, K.; Ji, M.; Jin, W.; He, N.; Shi, B.; Hou, P. Decreased 5-Hydroxymethylcytosine (5-HmC) Is an Independent Poor Prognostic Factor in Gastric Cancer Patients. *J. Biomed. Nanotechnol.* **2013**, *9*, 1607–1616. [CrossRef] [PubMed]
4. Kurman, R.J. Origin and Molecular Pathogenesis of Ovarian High-Grade Serous Carcinoma. *Ann. Oncol.* **2013**, *24*, x16–x21. [CrossRef] [PubMed]
5. Cho, K.R. Ovarian Cancer Update: Lessons From Morphology, Molecules, and Mice. *Arch. Pathol. Lab. Med.* **2009**, *133*, 1775–1781. [CrossRef]
6. Cho, K.R.; Shih, I.-M. Ovarian Cancer. *Annu. Rev. Pathol. Mech. Dis.* **2009**, *4*, 287–313. [CrossRef]
7. Patch, A.-M.; Christie, E.L.; Etemadmoghadam, D.; Garsed, D.W.; George, J.; Fereday, S.; Nones, K.; Cowin, P.; Alsop, K.; Bailey, P.J.; et al. Whole–Genome Characterization of Chemoresistant Ovarian Cancer. *Nature* **2015**, *521*, 489–494. [CrossRef]
8. Min, A.; Im, S.-A. PARP Inhibitors as Therapeutics: Beyond Modulation of PARylation. *Cancers* **2020**, *12*, 394. [CrossRef]
9. Hodi, F.S.; O'Day, S.J.; McDermott, D.F.; Weber, R.W.; Sosman, J.A.; Haanen, J.B.; Gonzalez, R.; Robert, C.; Schadendorf, D.; Hassel, J.C.; et al. Improved Survival with Ipilimumab in Patients with Metastatic Melanoma. *N. Engl. J. Med.* **2010**, *363*, 711–723. [CrossRef]
10. Hamanishi, J.; Mandai, M.; Ikeda, T.; Minami, M.; Kawaguchi, A.; Murayama, T.; Kanai, M.; Mori, Y.; Matsumoto, S.; Chikuma, S.; et al. Safety and Antitumor Activity of Anti–PD-1 Antibody, Nivolumab, in Patients with Platinum-Resistant Ovarian Cancer. *JCO* **2015**, *33*, 4015–4022. [CrossRef] [PubMed]
11. Palaia, I.; Tomao, F.; Sassu, C.M.; Musacchio, L.; Benedetti Panici, P. Immunotherapy For Ovarian Cancer: Recent Advances and Combination Therapeutic Approaches. *OTT* **2020**, *13*, 6109–6129. [CrossRef] [PubMed]
12. Chardin, L.; Leary, A. Immunotherapy in Ovarian Cancer: Thinking Beyond PD-1/PD-L1. *Front. Oncol.* **2021**, *11*, 795547. [CrossRef] [PubMed]
13. Kandalaft, L.E.; Odunsi, K.; Coukos, G. Immune Therapy Opportunities in Ovarian Cancer. *Am. Soc. Clin. Oncol. Educ. Book* **2020**, *40*, e228–e240. [CrossRef]
14. Hamid, O.; Robert, C.; Daud, A.; Hodi, F.S.; Hwu, W.-J.; Kefford, R.; Wolchok, J.D.; Hersey, P.; Joseph, R.W.; Weber, J.S.; et al. Safety and Tumor Responses with Lambrolizumab (Anti–PD-1) in Melanoma. *N. Engl. J. Med.* **2013**, *369*, 134–144. [CrossRef] [PubMed]
15. Pitt, J.M.; Vétizou, M.; Daillère, R.; Roberti, M.P.; Yamazaki, T.; Routy, B.; Lepage, P.; Boneca, I.G.; Chamaillard, M.; Kroemer, G.; et al. Resistance Mechanisms to Immune-Checkpoint Blockade in Cancer: Tumor-Intrinsic and -Extrinsic Factors. *Immunity* **2016**, *44*, 1255–1269. [CrossRef] [PubMed]
16. Alsaab, H.O.; Sau, S.; Alzhrani, R.; Tatiparti, K.; Bhise, K.; Kashaw, S.K.; Iyer, A.K. PD-1 and PD-L1 Checkpoint Signaling Inhibition for Cancer Immunotherapy: Mechanism, Combinations, and Clinical Outcome. *Front. Pharmacol.* **2017**, *8*, 561. [CrossRef]
17. Zou, W.; Wolchok, J.D.; Chen, L. PD-L1 (B7-H1) and PD-1 Pathway Blockade for Cancer Therapy: Mechanisms, Response Biomarkers, and Combinations. *Sci. Transl. Med.* **2016**, *8*, 328rv4. [CrossRef]
18. Gibney, G.T.; Weiner, L.M.; Atkins, M.B. Predictive Biomarkers for Checkpoint Inhibitor-Based Immunotherapy. *The Lancet Oncol.* **2016**, *17*, e542–e551. [CrossRef]
19. Seidel, J.A.; Otsuka, A.; Kabashima, K. Anti-PD-1 and Anti-CTLA-4 Therapies in Cancer: Mechanisms of Action, Efficacy, and Limitations. *Front. Oncol.* **2018**, *8*, 86. [CrossRef]
20. Wang, L.; Amoozgar, Z.; Huang, J.; Saleh, M.H.; Xing, D.; Orsulic, S.; Goldberg, M.S. Decitabine Enhances Lymphocyte Migration and Function and Synergizes with CTLA-4 Blockade in a Murine Ovarian Cancer Model. *Cancer Immunol. Res.* **2015**, *3*, 1030–1041. [CrossRef]
21. Wittenberger, T.; Sleigh, S.; Reisel, D.; Zikan, M.; Wahl, B.; Alunni-Fabbroni, M.; Jones, A.; Evans, I.; Koch, J.; Paprotka, T.; et al. DNA Methylation Markers for Early Detection of Women's Cancer: Promise and Challenges. *Epigenomics* **2014**, *6*, 311–327. [CrossRef] [PubMed]
22. Fu, S.; Wu, H.; Zhang, H.; Lian, C.G.; Lu, Q. DNA Methylation/Hydroxymethylation in Melanoma. *Oncotarget* **2017**, *8*, 78163–78173. [CrossRef]
23. Goode, E.L.; Block, M.S.; Kalli, K.R.; Vierkant, R.A.; Chen, W.; Fogarty, Z.C.; Gentry-Maharaj, A.; Toloczko, A.; Hein, A.; Bouligny, A.L.; et al. Dose-Response Association of CD8 + Tumor-Infiltrating Lymphocytes and Survival Time in High-Grade Serous Ovarian Cancer. *JAMA Oncol.* **2017**, *3*, e173290. [CrossRef] [PubMed]
24. Vilain, R.E.; Menzies, A.M.; Wilmott, J.S.; Kakavand, H.; Madore, J.; Guminski, A.; Liniker, E.; Kong, B.Y.; Cooper, A.J.; Howle, J.R.; et al. Dynamic Changes in PD-L1 Expression and Immune Infiltrates Early During Treatment Predict Response to PD-1 Blockade in Melanoma. *Clin. Cancer Res.* **2017**, *23*, 5024–5033. [CrossRef] [PubMed]
25. Gallagher, S.J.; Shklovskaya, E.; Hersey, P. Epigenetic Modulation in Cancer Immunotherapy. *Curr. Opin. Pharmacol.* **2017**, *35*, 48–56. [CrossRef]

26. Matei, D.; Fang, F.; Shen, C.; Schilder, J.; Arnold, A.; Zeng, Y.; Berry, W.A.; Huang, T.; Nephew, K.P. Epigenetic Resensitization to Platinum in Ovarian Cancer. *Cancer Res.* **2012**, *72*, 2197–2205. [CrossRef]
27. Wang, Y.; Cardenas, H.; Fang, F.; Condello, S.; Taverna, P.; Segar, M.; Liu, Y.; Nephew, K.P.; Matei, D. Epigenetic Targeting of Ovarian Cancer Stem Cells. *Cancer Res.* **2014**, *74*, 4922–4936. [CrossRef] [PubMed]
28. Dunn, J.; Rao, S. Epigenetics and Immunotherapy: The Current State of Play. *Mol. Immunol.* **2017**, *87*, 227–239. [CrossRef]
29. Peixoto, P.; Renaude, E.; Boyer-Guittaut, M.; Hervouet, E. Epigenetics, a Key Player of Immunotherapy Resistance. *CDR* **2018**, *1*, 219–229. [CrossRef]
30. Kim, K.; Skora, A.D.; Li, Z.; Liu, Q.; Tam, A.J.; Blosser, R.L.; Diaz, L.A.; Papadopoulos, N.; Kinzler, K.W.; Vogelstein, B.; et al. Eradication of Metastatic Mouse Cancers Resistant to Immune Checkpoint Blockade by Suppression of Myeloid-Derived Cells. *Proc. Natl. Acad. Sci. USA* **2014**, *111*, 11774–11779. [CrossRef]
31. Oda, K.; Hamanishi, J.; Matsuo, K.; Hasegawa, K. Genomics to Immunotherapy of Ovarian Clear Cell Carcinoma: Unique Opportunities for Management. *Gynecol. Oncol.* **2018**, *151*, 381–389. [CrossRef] [PubMed]
32. Saleh, M.H.; Wang, L.; Goldberg, M.S. Improving Cancer Immunotherapy with DNA Methyltransferase Inhibitors. *Cancer Immunol. Immunother.* **2016**, *65*, 787–796. [CrossRef] [PubMed]
33. Sato, E.; Olson, S.H.; Ahn, J.; Bundy, B.; Nishikawa, H.; Qian, F.; Jungbluth, A.A.; Frosina, D.; Gnjatic, S.; Ambrosone, C.; et al. Intraepithelial $CD8^+$ Tumor-Infiltrating Lymphocytes and a High $CD8^+$/Regulatory T Cell Ratio Are Associated with Favorable Prognosis in Ovarian Cancer. *Proc. Natl. Acad. Sci. USA* **2005**, *102*, 18538–18543. [CrossRef]
34. Zhang, L.; Conejo-Garcia, J.R.; Katsaros, D.; Gimotty, P.A.; Massobrio, M.; Regnani, G.; Makrigiannakis, A.; Gray, H.; Schlienger, K.; Liebman, M.N.; et al. Intratumoral T Cells, Recurrence, and Survival in Epithelial Ovarian Cancer. *N. Engl. J. Med.* **2003**, *348*, 203–213. [CrossRef]
35. Zhao, P.; Li, L.; Jiang, X.; Li, Q. Mismatch Repair Deficiency/Microsatellite Instability-High as a Predictor for Anti-PD-1/PD-L1 Immunotherapy Efficacy. *J. Hematol. Oncol.* **2019**, *12*, 54. [CrossRef]
36. Asgarova, A.; Asgarov, K.; Godet, Y.; Peixoto, P.; Nadaradjane, A.; Boyer-Guittaut, M.; Galaine, J.; Guenat, D.; Mougey, V.; Perrard, J.; et al. PD-L1 Expression Is Regulated by Both DNA Methylation and NF-KB during EMT Signaling in Non-Small Cell Lung Carcinoma. *OncoImmunology* **2018**, *7*, e1423170. [CrossRef]
37. Emran, A.A.; Chatterjee, A.; Rodger, E.J.; Tiffen, J.C.; Gallagher, S.J.; Eccles, M.R.; Hersey, P. Targeting DNA Methylation and EZH2 Activity to Overcome Melanoma Resistance to Immunotherapy. *Trends Immunol.* **2019**, *40*, 328–344. [CrossRef] [PubMed]
38. Huang, C.; Ren, S.; Chen, Y.; Liu, A.; Wu, Q.; Jiang, T.; Lv, P.; Song, D.; Hu, F.; Lan, J.; et al. PD-L1 Methylation Restricts PD-L1/PD-1 Interactions to Control Cancer Immune Surveillance. *Sci. Adv.* **2023**, *9*, eade4186. [CrossRef]
39. Tucker, D.W.; Getchell, C.R.; McCarthy, E.T.; Ohman, A.W.; Sasamoto, N.; Xu, S.; Ko, J.Y.; Gupta, M.; Shafrir, A.; Medina, J.E.; et al. Epigenetic Reprogramming Strategies to Reverse Global Loss of 5-Hydroxymethylcytosine, a Prognostic Factor for Poor Survival in High-Grade Serous Ovarian Cancer. *Clin. Cancer Res.* **2018**, *24*, 1389–1401. [CrossRef]
40. Stone, M.L.; Chiappinelli, K.B.; Li, H.; Murphy, L.M.; Travers, M.E.; Topper, M.J.; Mathios, D.; Lim, M.; Shih, I.-M.; Wang, T.-L.; et al. Epigenetic Therapy Activates Type I Interferon Signaling in Murine Ovarian Cancer to Reduce Immunosuppression and Tumor Burden. *Proc. Natl. Acad. Sci. USA* **2017**, *114*, E10981–E10990. [CrossRef]
41. Iyer, S.; Zhang, S.; Yucel, S.; Horn, H.; Smith, S.G.; Reinhardt, F.; Hoefsmit, E.; Assatova, B.; Casado, J.; Meinsohn, M.-C.; et al. Genetically Defined Syngeneic Mouse Models of Ovarian Cancer as Tools for the Discovery of Combination Immunotherapy. *Cancer Discov.* **2021**, *11*, 384–407. [CrossRef] [PubMed]
42. Campisi, M.; Shelton, S.E.; Chen, M.; Kamm, R.D.; Barbie, D.A.; Knelson, E.H. Engineered Microphysiological Systems for Testing Effectiveness of Cell-Based Cancer Immunotherapies. *Cancers* **2022**, *14*, 3561. [CrossRef] [PubMed]
43. Aref, A.R.; Campisi, M.; Ivanova, E.; Portell, A.; Larios, D.; Piel, B.P.; Mathur, N.; Zhou, C.; Coakley, R.V.; Bartels, A.; et al. 3D Microfluidic Ex Vivo Culture of Organotypic Tumor Spheroids to Model Immune Checkpoint Blockade. *Lab Chip* **2018**, *18*, 3129–3143. [CrossRef]
44. Knelson, E.H.; Ivanova, E.V.; Tarannum, M.; Campisi, M.; Lizotte, P.H.; Booker, M.A.; Ozgenc, I.; Noureddine, M.; Meisenheimer, B.; Chen, M.; et al. Activation of Tumor-Cell STING Primes NK-Cell Therapy. *Cancer Immunol. Res.* **2022**, *10*, 947–961. [CrossRef]
45. Merritt, C.R.; Ong, G.T.; Church, S.E.; Barker, K.; Danaher, P.; Geiss, G.; Hoang, M.; Jung, J.; Liang, Y.; McKay-Fleisch, J.; et al. Multiplex Digital Spatial Profiling of Proteins and RNA in Fixed Tissue. *Nat. Biotechnol.* **2020**, *38*, 586–599. [CrossRef] [PubMed]
46. Peng, H.; He, X.; Wang, Q. Immune Checkpoint Blockades in Gynecological Cancers: A Review of Clinical Trials. *Acta Obstet. Gynecol. Scand.* **2022**, *101*, 941–951. [CrossRef]
47. Leary, A.; Tan, D.; Ledermann, J. Immune Checkpoint Inhibitors in Ovarian Cancer: Where Do We Stand? *Ther. Adv. Med. Oncol.* **2021**, *13*, 175883592110398. [CrossRef]
48. Senbanjo, L.T.; Chellaiah, M.A. CD44: A Multifunctional Cell Surface Adhesion Receptor Is a Regulator of Progression and Metastasis of Cancer Cells. *Front. Cell Dev. Biol.* **2017**, *5*, 18. [CrossRef]
49. Castellanos, J.R.; Purvis, I.J.; Labak, C.M.; Guda, M.R.; Tsung, A.J.; Velpula, K.K.; Asuthkar, S. B7-H3 Role in the Immune Landscape of Cancer. *Am. J. Clin. Exp. Immunol.* **2017**, *6*, 66–75.
50. Catakovic, K.; Klieser, E.; Neureiter, D.; Geisberger, R. T Cell Exhaustion: From Pathophysiological Basics to Tumor Immunotherapy. *Cell Commun. Signal.* **2017**, *15*, 1. [CrossRef]

51. Horn, L.A.; Long, T.M.; Atkinson, R.; Clements, V.; Ostrand-Rosenberg, S. Soluble CD80 Protein Delays Tumor Growth and Promotes Tumor-Infiltrating Lymphocytes. *Cancer Immunol. Res.* **2018**, *6*, 59–68. [CrossRef] [PubMed]
52. Amobi-McCloud, A.; Muthuswamy, R.; Battaglia, S.; Yu, H.; Liu, T.; Wang, J.; Putluri, V.; Singh, P.K.; Qian, F.; Huang, R.-Y.; et al. IDO1 Expression in Ovarian Cancer Induces PD-1 in T Cells via Aryl Hydrocarbon Receptor Activation. *Front. Immunol.* **2021**, *12*, 678999. [CrossRef] [PubMed]
53. Liu, M.; Wang, X.; Wang, L.; Ma, X.; Gong, Z.; Zhang, S.; Li, Y. Targeting the IDO1 Pathway in Cancer: From Bench to Bedside. *J. Hematol. Oncol.* **2018**, *11*, 100. [CrossRef] [PubMed]
54. Wu, L.; Saxena, S.; Singh, R.K. Neutrophils in the Tumor Microenvironment. In *Tumor Microenvironment*; Birbrair, A., Ed.; Advances in Experimental Medicine and Biology; Springer International Publishing: Cham, Switzerland, 2020; Volume 1224, pp. 1–20, ISBN 978-3-030-35722-1.
55. Templeton, A.J.; McNamara, M.G.; Šeruga, B.; Vera-Badillo, F.E.; Aneja, P.; Ocaña, A.; Leibowitz-Amit, R.; Sonpavde, G.; Knox, J.J.; Tran, B.; et al. Prognostic Role of Neutrophil-to-Lymphocyte Ratio in Solid Tumors: A Systematic Review and Meta-Analysis. *JNCI J. Natl. Cancer Inst.* **2014**, *106*, dju124. [CrossRef] [PubMed]
56. Kwiecień, I.; Rutkowska, E.; Raniszewska, A.; Rzepecki, P.; Domagała-Kulawik, J. Modulation of the Immune Response by Heterogeneous Monocytes and Dendritic Cells in Lung Cancer. *WJCO* **2021**, *12*, 966–982. [CrossRef]
57. Osugi, Y.; Vuckovic, S.; Hart, D.N.J. Myeloid Blood CD11c+ Dendritic Cells and Monocyte-Derived Dendritic Cells Differ in Their Ability to Stimulate T Lymphocytes. *Blood* **2002**, *100*, 2858–2866. [CrossRef]
58. Kim, C.W.; Kim, K.-D.; Lee, H.K. The Role of Dendritic Cells in Tumor Microenvironments and Their Uses as Therapeutic Targets. *BMB Rep.* **2021**, *54*, 31–43. [CrossRef]
59. Tanaka, T.; Narazaki, M.; Kishimoto, T. IL-6 in Inflammation, Immunity, and Disease. *Cold Spring Harb. Perspect. Biol.* **2014**, *6*, a016295. [CrossRef]
60. Son, D.-S.; Parl, A.K.; Montgomery Rice, V.; Khabele, D. Keratinocyte Chemoattractant (KC)/Human Growth-Regulated Oncogene (GRO) Chemokines and pro-Inflammatory Chemokine Networks in Mouse and Human Ovarian Epithelial Cancer Cells. *Cancer Biol. Ther.* **2007**, *6*, 1308–1318. [CrossRef]
61. Lunardi, S.; Lim, S.Y.; Muschel, R.J.; Brunner, T.B. IP-10/CXCL10 Attracts Regulatory T Cells: Implication for Pancreatic Cancer. *OncoImmunology* **2015**, *4*, e1027473. [CrossRef]
62. Aldinucci, D.; Borghese, C.; Casagrande, N. The CCL5/CCR5 Axis in Cancer Progression. *Cancers* **2020**, *12*, 1765. [CrossRef]
63. Crawford, A.; Angelosanto, J.M.; Nadwodny, K.L.; Blackburn, S.D.; Wherry, E.J. A Role for the Chemokine RANTES in Regulating CD8 T Cell Responses during Chronic Viral Infection. *PLoS Pathog.* **2011**, *7*, e1002098. [CrossRef]
64. Kumar, J.; Fraser, F.W.; Riley, C.; Ahmed, N.; McCulloch, D.R.; Ward, A.C. Granulocyte Colony-Stimulating Factor Receptor Signalling via Janus Kinase 2/Signal Transducer and Activator of Transcription 3 in Ovarian Cancer. *Br. J. Cancer* **2014**, *110*, 133–145. [CrossRef] [PubMed]
65. Alvero, A.B.; Montagna, M.K.; Craveiro, V.; Liu, L.; Mor, G. Distinct Subpopulations of Epithelial Ovarian Cancer Cells Can Differentially Induce Macrophages and T Regulatory Cells Toward a Pro-Tumor Phenotype: IMMUNE REGULATION BY OVARIAN CANCER CELLS. *Am. J. Reprod. Immunol.* **2012**, *67*, 256–265. [CrossRef]
66. Singh, S.; Anshita, D.; Ravichandiran, V. MCP-1: Function, Regulation, and Involvement in Disease. *Int. Immunopharmacol.* **2021**, *101*, 107598. [CrossRef] [PubMed]
67. Yu, L.; Yang, F.; Zhang, F.; Guo, D.; Li, L.; Wang, X.; Liang, T.; Wang, J.; Cai, Z.; Jin, H. CD69 Enhances Immunosuppressive Function of Regulatory T-Cells and Attenuates Colitis by Prompting IL-10 Production. *Cell Death Dis.* **2018**, *9*, 905. [CrossRef]
68. Cibrián, D.; Sánchez-Madrid, F. CD69: From Activation Marker to Metabolic Gatekeeper. *Eur. J. Immunol.* **2017**, *47*, 946–953. [CrossRef] [PubMed]
69. Sandoval-Montes, C.; Santos-Argumedo, L. CD38 Is Expressed Selectively during the Activation of a Subset of Mature T Cells with Reduced Proliferation but Improved Potential to Produce Cytokines. *J. Leukoc. Biol.* **2004**, *77*, 513–521. [CrossRef] [PubMed]
70. Wang, C.; Xiong, C.; Hsu, Y.-C.; Wang, X.; Chen, L. Human Leukocyte Antigen (HLA) and Cancer Immunotherapy: HLA-Dependent and -Independent Adoptive Immunotherapies. *Ann. Blood* **2020**, *5*, 14. [CrossRef]
71. Ford, C.E.; Werner, B.; Hacker, N.F.; Warton, K. The Untapped Potential of Ascites in Ovarian Cancer Research and Treatment. *Br. J. Cancer* **2020**, *123*, 9–16. [CrossRef]
72. Rickard, B.P.; Conrad, C.; Sorrin, A.J.; Ruhi, M.K.; Reader, J.C.; Huang, S.A.; Franco, W.; Scarcelli, G.; Polacheck, W.J.; Roque, D.M.; et al. Malignant Ascites in Ovarian Cancer: Cellular, Acellular, and Biophysical Determinants of Molecular Characteristics and Therapy Response. *Cancers* **2021**, *13*, 4318. [CrossRef] [PubMed]

Disclaimer/Publisher's Note: The statements, opinions and data contained in all publications are solely those of the individual author(s) and contributor(s) and not of MDPI and/or the editor(s). MDPI and/or the editor(s) disclaim responsibility for any injury to people or property resulting from any ideas, methods, instructions or products referred to in the content.

MDPI
St. Alban-Anlage 66
4052 Basel
Switzerland
www.mdpi.com

Cancers Editorial Office
E-mail: cancers@mdpi.com
www.mdpi.com/journal/cancers

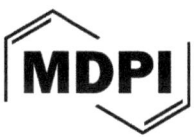

Disclaimer/Publisher's Note: The statements, opinions and data contained in all publications are solely those of the individual author(s) and contributor(s) and not of MDPI and/or the editor(s). MDPI and/or the editor(s) disclaim responsibility for any injury to people or property resulting from any ideas, methods, instructions or products referred to in the content.

www.ingramcontent.com/pod-product-compliance
Lightning Source LLC
LaVergne TN
LVHW070436100526
838202LV00014B/1610